ORTHOPEDIC MEDICINE
A New Approach to Vertebral Manipulations

Orthopedic Medicine

A New Approach to Vertebral Manipulations

By

ROBERT MAIGNE, M.D.

Head, Physical Medicine and Rehabilitation Center
Hotel Dieu Hospital
Lecturer, Faculty of Medicine
University of Paris
Paris, France
President, International Federation of Manual Medicine

Translated and Edited by

W. T. LIBERSON, M.D., Ph.D.

Professor, Physical Medicine and Rehabilitation
Abraham Lincoln Medical School, University of Illinois
Chicago, Illinois
Visiting Professor, Pharmacology
Stritch School of Medicine, Loyola University
Hines, Illinois
Physician in Residence
Veterans Administration Hospitals
Washington, D.C.
Senior Attending Physician, Little Company of Mary Hospital
Evergreen Park, Illinois
Consultant in Neurology, MacNeal Memorial Hospital
Berwyn, Illinois
Vice-President, North American Academy of Manipulative Medicine

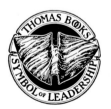

CHARLES C THOMAS · PUBLISHER
Springfield · Illinois · U.S.A.

Published and Distributed Throughout the World by

CHARLES C THOMAS • PUBLISHER

BANNERSTONE HOUSE

301-327 East Lawrence Avenue, Springfield, Illinois, U.S.A.

NATCHEZ PLANTATION HOUSE

735 North Atlantic Boulevard, Fort Lauderdale, Florida, U.S.A.

With THOMAS BOOKS *careful attention is given to all details of
manufacturing and design. It is the Publisher's desire to present books
that are satisfactory as to their physical qualities and artistic possibilities and appropriate for their particular use.* THOMAS BOOKS *will
be true to those laws of quality that assure a good name and good will.*

This translation of the 1968 French edition
has been revised by author and editor.

Printed in the United States of America

N-1

Editor's Introduction

DOCTOR MAIGNE WAS BORN in 1923 in one of the central regions of France. He graduated from the Faculty of Medicine, Sorbonne, Paris. At the very beginning of his medical career, he specialized in rheumatology and was interested in physical treatments of patients with arthritis, as well as in their rehabilitation. He was particularly intrigued by the problems offered by minor derangements of the spine, as he was the physician for a team practicing judo (of which he is an expert.) It was in 1947 that he started to develop his therapeutic system. He went to England (1950-1951) and studied relevant techniques there, including those of osteopaths. This is how he progressively arrived at developing the strictly medical methodology that is presented in this book.

Doctor Maigne is one of the founders of the French National Society of Physical Medicine and Rehabilitation (1952). He has been secretary of this organization for a number of years. He also is one of the founders of the French Society of Manual Medicine and served as its President from 1964 to 1966. He is now President of the International Federation of Manual Medicine. He is a physician of the Hotel Dieu Hospital affiliated with the University of Paris School of Medicine, where he directs a Physical Medicine and Rehabilitation Service and, assisted by a team of specialized physicians, contributes to the training of students and physicians interested in physical medicine in general, manual medicine in particular.

Doctor Maigne has also contributed to training physicians on this side of the Atlantic. During several lecture tours, he has given a great number of demonstrations of his methodology in Canada and in the United States. His courses in this country are always fully attended.

I first met Doctor Maigne in 1962 when he was invited to give some lectures and demonstrations at Hines. I was at once won

over by the precision and elegance of his handling of patients and
by the logic of the presentation of his system of manual therapy.
This impression grew during multiple contacts which I had with
him on the occasions of several international meetings and mutual visits. So naturally, I was pleased to translate and edit his first
monograph for presentation to the English-speaking physician.

As it turned out, I had just finished the translation of his first
book when I learned that Doctor Maigne was preparing to publish a second, much enlarged monograph on the same subject. We
felt that it would be disappointing to the English readers to be
offered an English edition of Doctor Maigne's first book while his
second book was appearing in French. Therefore, we decided to
combine the two.

For about two years we tried to extract from the second book
additional information to complete the first one, only to realize
that it would be unfair to the English readers to omit practically
anything from the second book. As a result, the English edition
which we are now presenting contains all of the material which
was included in the second monograph with the exception of
a few sections related to specific problems such as the delivery of
health services in France.

The book has already been translated into several languages.
The English edition, however, is completely different from the
French one insofar as the order of presentation of subject matters
is concerned. In reorganizing the content of this book, I was
guided by the following considerations:

The monograph of Doctor Maigne is much more than a presentation of his system of manipulation. He has written very helpful chapters concerning functional anatomy and pathophysiology
of the spine. The monograph describes in detail techniques of
other forms of manual therapy, such as maneuvers of relaxation
and mobilization. It also presents an extremely vivid and systematic description of clinical conditions frequently faced by
physiatrists, rheumatologists, and orthopedic surgeons. The mem-
bers of these medical specialties may, therefore, derive considerable benefit from studying it even if they do not intend to practice
manipulations.

For the above reasons, I suggested to Doctor Maigne that we place the chapters on techniques of manual therapy at the end of the book. In the French edition, this part of the book occupies the middle core of the monograph and the clinical indications are presented at the end. The same considerations caused us to extract from the part of the book devoted to techniques, the sections related to regional anatomy and pathophysiology, as well as those devoted to the examination of patients with painful spine and/or the upper and lower extremities and to present them in the first part of this book.

The reader of this monograph will see that this reshuffling of the subject matter for the English edition does not in any way decrease the importance of the discussion of manipulative techniques from either general or specific points of view. The introduction of the *"rule of no pain and free movement"* to this field is obviously a most welcome innovation in this therapeutic methodology, and Doctor Maigne's presentation of "star diagrams" makes the technique well standardized. His masterful step-by-step description of techniques of maneuvers of relaxation, mobilization, and manipulation, illustrated by superb photographs and didactic diagrams, makes this book a most refreshing addition to the literature, useful to the experienced practitioner and novice alike.

Recently, interest in manipulation has increased among physiatrists, with the North American Academy of Manipulative Medicine now leading the way. It is time that research in this field be encouraged as it has been lagging far behind practical achievements. It is the opinion of this editor that the explanation for the efficacy of these maneuvers will be found to be much less mysterious than it may seem at the present time. If the "minor vertebral derangements" are due to local muscle spasms, any procedure which may bring about a sudden inhibition of these spasms may have great therapeutic success. This is true of cooling sprays applied to the skin, whether at the trigger points or not; certain intranasal reflex procedures; or needling of the involved fasciculi. We recently showed with Paillard that simple rubbing of the plantar region of the foot may bring about a profound segmental spinal cord inhibition. By pulling vertebral structures in certain directions, one may exert such segmental inhibition. The success of the "rule of no pain and free movement" suggests that the structure which is pulled may be only reflexly related to the involved tissues inducing in certain cases "reciprocal inhibition."

One may wonder whether such an explanation will be accepted, inasmuch as reflex inhibition usually lasts a very short time, much shorter than the after-effects of a therapeutic act. One should, however, keep in mind the fact that a contracted muscle interferes with the circulation of blood and lymph, thus contributing to an accumulation of pain-inducing metabolites. By sudden inhibition of the contracted muscle, circulation may be re-established at once, and the pain-producing "vicious cycle" broken for a much longer time than the duration of the inhibition proper. In addition, when considering the mode of action of manipulation, one should keep in mind the more prolonged autonomic nervous system reflex actions discussed in this book by Doctor Maigne.

The recognition of the importance of manipulative therapeutic maneuvers does not mean that other physiatric methods applied to the same kind of patients should be abandoned, even if they may require more time for full therapeutic effects. As Doctor Maigne states, "Not every one is able to practice manipulation, or spend the necessary long time for self training, or finding an adequate teacher, just as not every one is able to play billiards, or musical instruments." For these physicians, the book remains of great value because of the material which is not necessarily related to manipulations. Thus, the universality of the contribution which this book makes to the general field of manual and physical medicine cannot be overestimated.

We trust that this monograph will convince the most recalcitrant readers that, when logically and skillfully applied by a specialized physician, manipulations have "equal rights" among other medical procedures. Although they were introduced in the dark ages of medical practice under false pretenses and have been indiscriminantly applied by nonphysicians, one should not be prejudiced by such beginnings, since under favorable conditions, manipulations can bring quick relief to the patient. After all, contemporary surgery also had dark beginnings in the hands of barbers before the time of anesthesia.

The title of this English edition of Doctor Maigne's book has also been changed. The first French edition was called *Vertebral Manipulations*. The second, more extensive book has the title, *Pain of Vertebral Origin and Treatments by Manipulations*. In view of the revision of this book and the reorganization of the material, as it now stands in the English edition, it appeared to us that a more general title was appropriate. It was Cyriax's idea that that part of physical medicine with which the physiatrist deals in his everyday practice and which covers complaints related to the neck, back, shoulders, elbows, etc., belongs in fact to the field of orthopedic medicine, to be differentiated from orthopedic surgery. Manual medicine, including manipulations, is certainly a part of it.

It is for these reasons that we adopted the new title for this monograph, *Orthopedic Medicine—A New Approach to Vertebral Manipulations*.

W.T.L.

Preface to French Edition

Our first monograph on vertebral manifestations, which appeared in 1960, was devoted to manipulative techniques and their clinical applications, their indication, contraindications, and limitations. We aimed at reintegrating this therapeutic method into medical practice and eliminating some erroneous concepts and peculiar jargon used in connection with its exercise. We proposed terminology permitting a clear definition of each maneuver and formulated new rules governing their application; in particular, the "rule of no pain and free movement." Favorable acceptance of this book in France and abroad expressed new interest in this method which the medical profession thus manifested. Three French editions were published in rapid succession by French Scientific Expansion; and a German edition is now out of print. We gratefully acknowledge the elogious preface which Professor de Sèze wrote at that time. We also thank Professor Junghanns, well known by his work related to spine, who introduced the German translation by Mrs. Junghanns. Finally, Professor Liberson of Chicago honored us by proposing to edit an English translation to be published by Charles C Thomas. We are grateful to him for this task.

In the present book, we continue to study manipulative and other manual treatments applicable to the spine. We analyze the maneuvers in use in order to better understand the need for their precision. Recent studies of anatomophysiology and anatomopathology allow one to better understand "minor vertebral derangements." They permit us to formulate hypotheses in order to imagine the processes which elicit a painful vertebral syndrome during an awkward spontaneous movement and to understand how a manipulation may relieve the patient.

A large part of this book is devoted to methods of examining the patient and to therapeutic rationale. We are aware of the difficulty in learning manipulations in a manual. Prolonged training under guidance is indispensable; moreover, not everyone will be able to manipulate, just as not every one is able to play billiards or golf. Vertebral manipulations in fact have been strongly criticized. The grievances are many: "brutal and blind treatment" some say; "occasional good results do not compensate for the accidents which may be produced"; "it is a dangerous form of psychological treatment."

Although these criticisms most often are spelled out by those who have never attended a session of well-conducted manipulation, it should be recognized they are not without foundation and it is regrettable that therapy as valuable as this attracted the interest of so many disputable practitioners and did not generate serious research by physicians.

During the reign of Napoleon, Doctor Corvisart, the Physician-in-Chief of the Emperor and Queen, used to visit the royal couple twice a week. Only occasionally did he need to dispense his professional services. His treatments were simple and benign, since the Emperor enjoyed excellent health. It is said, however, that once he was called to see Napoleon who was suffering from violent lumbago. After asking everyone to leave the room, he asked the Emperor to disrobe and lie across a table. He then administered a slap on the buttocks which was violent and well aimed. The Emperor turned in fury but during the sudden twisting of his body, the painful contracture of the lumbar muscles miraculously subsided and the insolence of the celebrated physician was immediately pardoned. This is how the first famous successful manipulation was transmitted through history. The difficulty in finding the exact point of application of force in this maneuver causes us to avoid it in our practice. We propose in this book other maneuvers for the treatment of lumbagos and other conditions. We regret that they are less spectacular but pleased that they are more reliable. However, we have asked ourselves the following question: How, despite such a prestigious example, have manipulations been so little appreciated for such a long time?

R.M.

Contents

PART III

Clinical Applications

PART IV

Techniques

Contents xv

ORTHOPEDIC MEDICINE
A New Approach to Vertebral Manipulations

PART I

ANATOMY, PHYSIOLOGY, AND MECHANICAL DISTURBANCES OF THE INTERVERTEBRAL MOBILE SEGMENT

Introduction

A FORCED PASSIVE MOBILIZATION, which is a definition of a manipulation, can, obviously, act only upon the mobile structures of the spine: the disc, the posterior joints, the ligaments and the muscles, the elements of articulation and those of motor control. We are indebted to Junghanns for having considered these elements as forming the "mobile segment" (Fig. 1). The study of this functional unit must then precede the study of the mobilization techniques. We shall first study anatomo-physiology, then physiopathology, and finally different pain-producing lesions which may be found within the "mobile segment."

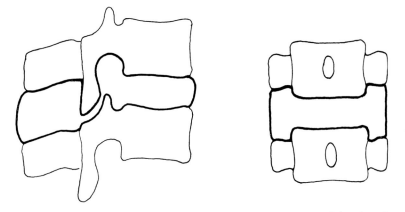

Figure 1. Mobile segment of Junghanns. *Left,* lateral view; *Right,* AP view.

The vertebral column comprises 23 "mobile segments," each representing one mobile unit of the spine. An intimate relationship which exists between the elements of the mobile segment and those of the intervertebral foramen must be noted at the very onset of this discussion.

This concept leads to a more functional than anatomical approach to pathology. The intervertebral joint forms a unit as a whole. Every mechanical perturbation of one of the elements obviously affects the other. The disc permits intervertebral movements, while the posterior articulations control their amplitude and direction.

One should mention that there are no discs between the atlas and the occiput and the atlas and the axis.

Chapter 1

Anatomical Review

W E SHALL STUDY BRIEFLY the following constituents of the intervertebral joints: (1) disc, (2) posterior joints, (3) connecting ligament system, (4) muscles, (5) intervertebral foramen, and (6) nerves.

THE INTERVERTEBRAL DISC

The intervertebral disc is composed of two parts: (1) the peripheral or annulus fibrosus and (2) the central, or nucleus pulposus.

The annulus fibrosus is formed of concentric fibrocartilaginous layers. The fibers of each layer are oblique and of reverse obliquity from one layer to the other. This type of successive orientation of fibers permits better resistance to the *torsional movements.* The annulus inserts itself on the vertebral body. The marginal insertional fibers (fibers of Sharpey) are particularly tough. The weakest point is located posteriorly. It can be stretched elastically, and it absorbs the pressures which are transmitted to it by the central core while maintaining the vertebrae together (Fig. 2).

The nucleus pulposus is a gelatinous substance which is located more posteriorly than anteriorly, at a union of two-thirds anterior and one-third posterior of the disc. This core may be deformed but is incompressible. It behaves like a pocket of water, preserving the same total volume. It functions like a joint for the intervertebral movements and transmits, without any loss, the pressure which it receives to the annulus fibrosus. It presents, moreover, an internal tension, which, as well as its elasticity, is directly related to its water content. Very rich in water at birth (88%), the nucleus pulposus dehydrates progressively with age: 80% at 14 years, 70% at 70 years. The annulus fibrosus dehydrates relatively little with age: 79% at birth, 70% at old age (Keyes and Compere, 1932).

The disc is not vascularized in the adult. Its nutrition is as-

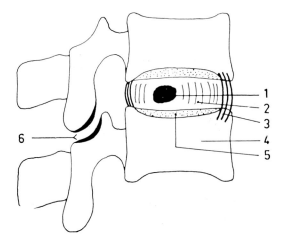

Figure 2. Cross section of the disc. (1) nucleus pulposus; (2) annulus fibrosus with (3) Sharpey fibers which are firmly inserted over the edges of the vertebrae; (4) vertebral body; (5) cartilagenous plate which for Schmorl and Junghanns is an integral part of the disc; and (6) posterior articulations.

sured by its osmotic properties through the cartilaginous layer of the vertebral body. Thus, the "correct distension of the discs" depends on the permeability of the cartilaginous layer and the osmotic property of the nucleus pulposus. An alteration of these properties of imbibition can, according to Mitchell *et al.* (1961), perturb the vertebral stability.

The innervation of the disc is not very well known. It seems, however, according to most investigators, that the sinu-vertebral nerve which innervates the posterior longitudinal ligament, also innervates the peripheral fibers of the annulus, at least its posterior portion. The nucleus pulposus has no nerve supply.

Cloward (1960), who directly stimulated the anterior part of the cervical disc, was able to provoke pain in the scapula, demonstrating the innervation of the annulus even in its anterior part by the sinu-vertebral nerve, and its importance in the vertebral pain syndrome.

THE POSTERIOR JOINTS

From a strict anatomical viewpoint the posterior joints are the only true joints of the spine, having an articular capsule with a synovial membrane. Their form and their orientation vary according to the different segments of the vertebral column. They determine the amplitude and the direction of the movements within each intervertebral segment (Figs. 3 and 4).

Each joint is maintained by a dense articular capsule which is quite elastic and which covers it like a hat. According to some in-

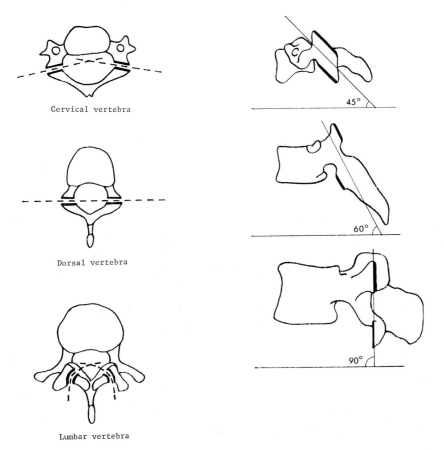

Figure 3. Posterior articular surfaces. *Left,* Orientation of the facets (after Olivier). *Right,* Angle with the horizontal line.

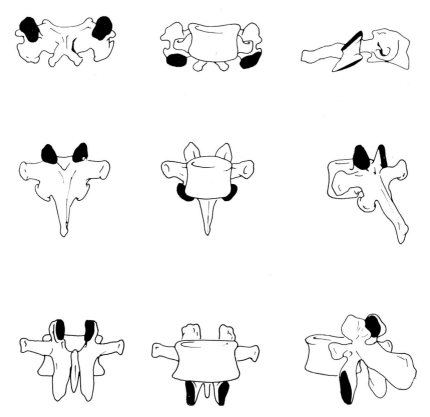

Figure 4. Posterior articular facets. *Top,* cervical vertebra; *Center,* dorsal vertebra; *Bottom,* lumbar vertebra. *Left,* posterior view; *Center,* anterior view; *Right,* lateral view (¾ for the dorsal and lumbar vertebrae).

vestigators, there are small semilunar "menisci" which originate from this capsule, penetrating intra-articular space, filled with small adipose cushions (Schmincke and Santo, 1932; Töndury, 1953). These investigators believe that the lesions of these small menisci play an extremely important role in the minor traumatic pathology of the spine. They are not the true menisci but rather synovial fringes, comprising: 1) a capsular attachment made of conjunctive tissue; 2) a central area, richly vascularized and innervated and 3) a very thin free border made of chondroid tissue devoid of blood vessels. The articulations are the most richly innervated structures of the entire vertebral column (Töndury, 1932). This rich innervation responds, without doubt, to the need to permit the proximal and distal structures of body support to adapt themselves to the continuous variations of tension to which the articular capsule is exposed. This explains why the minor derangements of these joints can have an extremely painful effect (Taillard, 1957).

Posterior articulations and disc form the mobile elements of the intervertebral joint. The ligaments and the muscles form a system which tie them together (see also Tiry, 1957).

THE LIGAMENTS (Fig. 5)

The anterior longitudinal ligament forms a long, fibrous network running from the anterior tubercle of the atlas to the sacrum. It forms a bridge over the anterior edge of the disc without being inserted on it. It has a high resistance to traction and is generally preserved in vertebral compression.

The posterior longitudinal ligament, contrary to the anterior ligament, is inserted on the disc itself. At this level it is widened, while it narrows at the level of the vertebral body. Thus, it reinforces the disc posteriorly.

The ligamentum flavum, which interconnects the lamina, is elastic and thick. Its color is due to the "elastine" which it contains. It checks the movements of the interapophysary articulations.

The interspinous ligaments which connect the vertebral spines are very important for the stability of the spinal column. They are reinforced, especially at the level of the dorsal and lumbar spine, by the supraspinous ligament.

In addition, there are intertransverse ligaments.

THE MUSCLES

The motor elements of the mobile segment comprise short and long paraspinal muscles. The former exert their action directly, while the latter act indirectly, affecting distal segments.

Their description, even a brief one, is too complex for this monograph. These muscles are innervated by the posterior

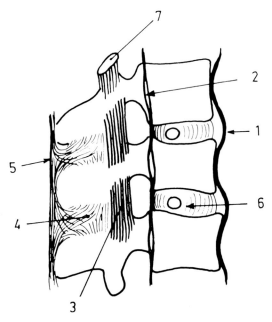

Figure 5. Vertebral ligaments. (1) common anterior longitudinal ligament; (2) common posterior longitudinal ligament; (3) ligamentum flavum; (4) interspinous ligament; (5) supraspinous ligament; (6) disc with its annulus fibrosus and its nucleus pulposus; (7) posterior and superior articular facet. (Note: The common anterior ligament adheres to the vertebral body, but makes a bridge from the edge of one vertebra to the edge of the other without adhering to the disc. The posterior ligament adheres to the disc.)

branches of the spinal nerves which thus play a very important part in the vertebral mechanical pathology.

The proper functioning of the mobile segment demands a perfect synergy of the different muscles. A movement which is not anticipated, or poorly estimated, can bring about a harmful distribution of forces upon the intervertebral joint. Certain elements of this joint, acting as levers, may be submitted to traction or compression beyond their capacity for resistance. One should try to achieve through therapeutic reeducation of the spine, a correct synchronization of these muscles rather than an increase of the strength of different muscle groups. The spasm of these muscles undoubtedly constitutes a major factor in the genesis of painful spine susceptible to treatment by manipulation.

INTERVERTEBRAL FORAMEN

The intervertebral foramen is more of a short canal than orifice (Fig. 6) ; it is formed by the superposition of two neighboring pedicles, formed posteriorly by the posterior articular apophyses and anteriorly by the posterolateral part of the disc as well as by the vertebral body. "It has an elipsoid form, but in view of the great mobility of intervertebral joints the slightest change of the interrelation of the articular facets modifies the intervertebral foramen. While the vertebral foramina of the dorsal and lumbar vertebrae are opened laterally and are directed straight to the left and right, the intervertebral foramen of the cervical spine is oriented slightly forward forming an angle of about 15 degrees with the axes of the dorsal and lumbar foramina" (Dechame *et al.*, 1961).

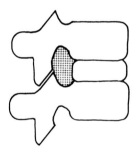

Figure 6. Intervertebral foramen.

The canal is covered by fibrous structure connected to the annulus fibrosus and the articular capsule of the posterior joints. Macroscopically, the ventral root (motor) and the dorsal root (sensitive) are fused in the canal, but microscopically, they are still separated at the outlet of the intervertebral foramen. The dorsal root contains the spinal ganglion.

The sinu-vertebral nerve, which is called "nerve of Luschka", after the anatomist who discovered it in 1850, (Ramus meningus nervi spinalis) is formed by the junction of two roots, one spinal and the other sympathetic. It originates from these roots outside of the canal of conjugation, then penetrates it again by a recurrent path. The vascular pocket is made of a voluminous veinous plexus and a small radial artery.

The irritation or compression of these elements of the canal by different disturbances of the intervertebral joint is responsible for numerous painful disorders of spinal origin.

THE INNERVATION OF THE MOBILE SEGMENT

The "mobile segment" is innervated by (1) the posterior branch of the segmental nerve and (2) the sinu-vertebral nerve.

The Posterior Branch of the Segmental Nerve

Paravertebral articulations and muscles are innervated by the posterior branches of the segmental nerves. The posterior branches of the two first segmental nerves are many times larger than the anterior branches. This is the reverse of all the other segmental nerves. These nerves are both motor and sensory.

The joint between the atlas and the occipital bone and between the atlas and the axis are innervated by the anterior branch of the first two cervical nerves, while the posterior branch of the second cervical nerve innervates the joint between C2 and C3 (Lazorthes, 1955, 1966; Lazorthes *et al.,* 1965).

All the other intervertebral joints are innervated by the posterior branches of the segmental nerves with many rami incorporated into the articular structures, especially at the level of the cervical spine (Lazorthes). This explains the vulnerability of the nerves to arthritic or traumatic lesions of these joints. At the edge of the intervertebral foramen the nerve divides into two or three branches which run towards the anterior part of the articular facet. (Lazorthes, 1966). The paravertebral muscles and the skin are also innervated by the posterior branches of the segmental nerves. They take a descending course while innervating deep short segmental muscles.

The Sinu-vertebral Nerves

The sinu-vertebral nerves (Fig. 7) are the size of a large thread (Hovelacque, 1927). They are formed by the union of a spinal and a sympathetic root whose relations vary according to the level of the spine. The distribution of these terminal branches has been described by Lazorthes *et al.* (1965). This distribution is purely segmental. They ascend toward the vertebral bodies, the pedicles and the adjacent disc by numerous rami. The disc located below the corresponding vertebra is supplied by the only branches that have a descending course. They also supply posterior longitudinal ligament, the epidural tissues as well as the dura itself (Lazorthes, 1962; Lazorthes and Poulhes, 1947), the anterior longitudinal ligament, and the annulus fibrosus. According to Töndury (1937), the ascending and descending rami form anastomoses between themselves as well as with the neighboring nerve fibers and also interconnect through horizontal branches (see also Jung and Brunschwig, 1932).

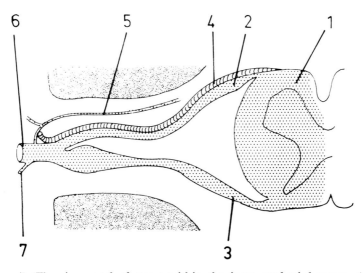

Figure 7. The sinu-vertebral nerve within the intervertebral foramen (after Testut). (1) Spinal cord; (2) ventral root; (3) dorsal root; (4) anterior branch of the radicular artery; (5) nerve sinu-vertebral; (6) anterior branch of the spinal nerve; (7) posterior branch of the spinal nerve.

Chapter 2

Physiological Review

T HE DISC PLAYS the role of a joint for intervertebral movements while the posterior articulations limit and direct the movement (Fig. 8) .

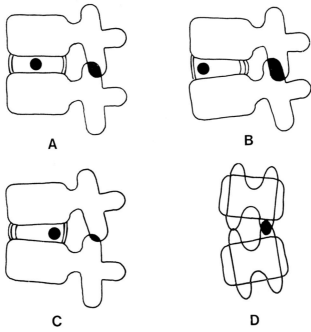

Figure 8. Movement of the intervertebral joint. *A,* normal position; *B,* in extension; *C,* in flexion; *D,* in left lateral bending (anterior view) .

In the movement of flexion, there is (1) a slight gliding movement backwards of the nucleus pulposus; (2) a separation or, better, a divergence of the articular facets.

In the movement of extension, there is (1) a gliding movement forwards of the nucleus pulposus; (2) a convergence of the articular facets.

In the movement of *lateroflexion,* to the left, for example, there is (1) a gliding of the nucleus to the right; (2) a divergence of the right articular facets; (3) convergence of the left articular facets.

It is, in effect, impossible to consider intervertebral mobility while taking into account the disc by itself. The combined structure of posterior joints and of the discs must be studied instead. In effect, if we block the two posterior joints with a pin or screw, there will no longer be any movement in the mobile segment. If we block only one posterior joint (Brugger, 1961), the dynamics of the joint are greatly modified.

In reality, the intervertebral movement is far from being as simple as we have described it above. For example, we said that in the movement of forward flexion there is a dorsal gapping of the posterior disc and a divergence of the facets. We have recently taken a large number of slow motion cineradiographic films of normal and pathological cervical columns and have been able to observe that there exists only a very small ventral pinching of the disc at the time of the forward flexion. The upper vetebra acts like a hood, rolling over the disc located immediately underneath it, as if it were a ball-joint, while the facets also glide one over the other without losing their contact. We have found a marked ventral pinching only when there has been discal deterioration. We conclude from the study that this pinching is the first radiological sign of deterioration of a cervical disc (Fig. 9).

By contrast, during extension (backward flexion), there is ventral gapping and dorsal pinching between the vertebrae as well as an analogous mechanism of dorsal rolling over the discal "ball."

At each segment of the column, the physiodynamics of the intervertebral joint change. There is a great difference between the movement of a "mobile segment" at the level of the cervical spine and at the level of the lumbar spine. The vertical dimensions of the disc in relation to that of the vertebral body, the width of the disc in relation to its height, as well as the form and the orientation of the articular facets govern the movement in each mobile segment and, in a large measure, predetermine the tech-

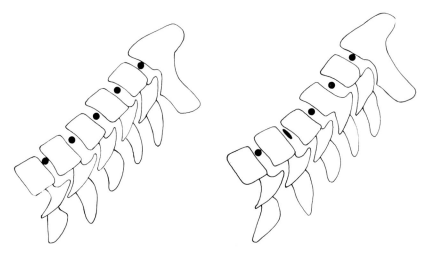

Figure 9. Movements of anterior flexion. *Left,* normal spine; *Right,* degeneration of the C5-C6 disc; it shows a ventral pinching in the movement of flexion at this level.

nique of manipulations carried out. We will return to this point when we study these techniques.

STRESSES ACTING UPON THE INTERVERTEBRAL JOINT

The intervertebral joint is subjected to considerable compression (Fig. 10). Certain authors, in particular, Herbert (1953), in France, have calculated approximately, the forces of pressure

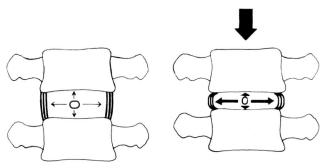

Figure 10. Stresses upon a normal disc. *Left,* erect position. *Right,* in a subject carrying a heavy load on his shoulder.

exerted upon the intervertebral joint and the traction to which it is submitted in different body positions, without load and with lifting a load. The reader is referred for details to the publication of Herbert. We shall simply give some examples (Fig. 11) :

1. In a subject standing without a load (Fig. 11a) the lumbar disc is subjected to

    a) a pressure of 15 kg/cm² of the nucleus; the pressure is transmitted to the annulus stretching it.

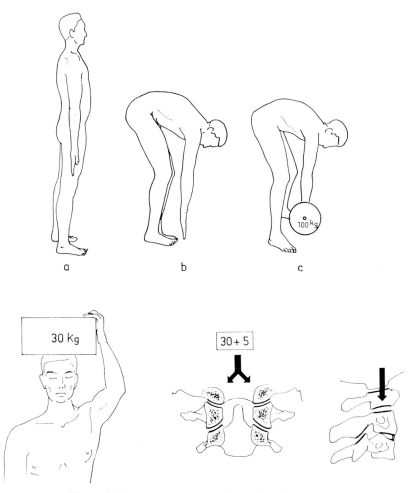

Figure 11. Stresses upon a cervico-occipital junction.

    b) a shearing force of 13 kg in the corresponding articular facets.

    2. In a subject bending forward (Fig. 11b), the lumbar disc is subjected to

    a.) a pressure of 58 kg/cm^2 at the nucleus and a corresponding stretching of the annulus.

    b) a shearing force of 47 kg in a perpendicular plane to the axis of the spine, absorbed by compressed facets.

    3. In a subject in complete forward flexion, lifting a weight of 100 kg (Fig 11c),

    a) the disc undergoes a compression of 144 kg/cm^2 at the nucleus and corresponding stretching of the annulus.

    b) a shearing force of 126 kg acts upon compressed facets.

In this case the total pressure on the nucleus is on the order of 1000 kg. In other words, the intervertebral segments are submitted to enormous stress. It is true that a certain amount of correction must be made with regard to these figures, as one must also account for intra-abdominal pressure. In fact, the compressive force of 1000 kg would be exerted only if there were no contraction of abdominal muscles. But, as is known, some lumbar effort is supported by the abdominal contraction. The intra-abdominal structures absorb a part of the force: 30 percent for Morris *et al.* (1961). The contraction of the abdominal muscles can be replaced or aided by the resistance given by a corset or a girdle (the girdle of weight lifters). In this case the intra-abdominal pressure is increased because of an effort in the same manner, but there is no contraction or there is less contraction of the abdominal muscles. In other words, it is important to have strong abdominal muscles in order to protect the lumbosacral spine (see also Bartelink, 1957).

The lumbar spine, however, is not the only one subjected to such stress. In order to be convinced of the importance of the stress elsewhere in the spine, it is sufficient to examine the cervico-occipital joint. Despite the smallness of the diameter of the corresponding bony structures and the articular facets, they support that large ball of approximately twelve pounds that is a man's head and assure its mobility. The head is balanced over two articular facets small as nails, and yet it may be mobilized in all directions. Some individuals may carry on their heads a load of more than 120 pounds, entirely supported by the joints of the two upper cervical vertebrae, as there is no other structure at that level which may share such a load with them (Fig. 11, bottom).

Chapter 3

Effects of Aging on the Intervertebral Joint

W<small>ITH</small> <small>AGE</small> <small>OR</small> as a result of various pathological processes, the constituents of the "mobile segment" lose some of their essential qualities. This affects their mobility and resistance. This fact is due essentially to the deterioration of the disc (Fig. 12). Discal deterioration and its prevention have been well studied in Germany by Schmorl and Junghanns (1956) and in France by de Sèze and his school (1939).

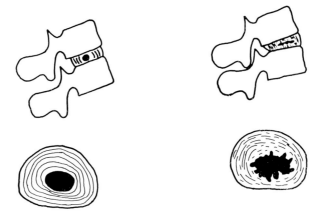

Figure 12. Degeneration of the disc. *Left,* normal disc; *Right,* degenerated disc.

The nucleus is dehydrated, becomes flat, and fragments. As a result of these changes, the pressure transmitted to the spine is distributed unevenly against the annulus fibrosus, which splits. Normally, this commonly observed process occurs without clinical manifestation. "During the same time as the disc ages, the ligaments also harden and progressively limit the movements of the spine. Moreover, the man to whom they belong ages likewise and progressively reduces his physical activity. Thus an equilibrium can most often be established between a fragile disc and reduced discal mobility" (de Sèze, 1953).

However, the disc can, for various reasons (traumatisms, for example), age sooner than the man to whom it belongs. The disc can be old at 35 and thus becomes vulnerable. It is, in general, the posterior part of the annulus fibrosus (the weakest) which receives the most pressure and which gives up if it is either compressed and displaced or fragmented prior to its posterior herniation. In other cases, under some specific influence, combined or not with age, the deterioration of the nucleus pulposus occurs gradually, while the annulus fibrosus becomes progressively compressed and displaced not posteriorly but towards the periphery, where the discal material will meet the ligamentary formations of the spine and where an ossifying process will contribute to the formation of an osteophytic collar around the disc (de Sèze, 1953).

The osteophytes originate from the vertebral body in the space found between the annulus fibrosus and the anterior ligament. The latter, as we recall, is inserted on the vertebral body and not on the disc. They mold themselves on that ligament which, because of the discal collapse, bulges out more and more.

This explains the horizontal orientation of the osteophytes, since the deteriorated disc is very flat. X-ray pictures of the profiles of these osteophytic flanges resemble beaks; thus, the reason for the name "Parrot's beaks" given by French radiologists and "spurs" from the English literature (Fig. 13).

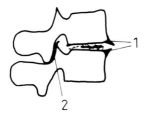
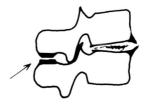

Figure 13. Effects of deterioration of the disc. (1) Formation of osteophytes; (2) disturbance and arthrose of the posterior joints.

Figure 14. Interspinal arthrose: Baastrup syndrome.

This flattening of the disc, especially if the ligamentary system is not hardened, creates an instability of the intervertebral joint and in certain cases a hypermobility of the joint (Junghanns, 1958). The flattening of the disc will necessarily affect the other elements of the "mobile segment": posterior joints and the interspinal ligaments. In the latter case if there is a hyperlordotic spine, two neighboring spinal processes may enter into contact ("kissing spines"). Sometimes a true arthrosis may be formed (syndrome of Baastrup, 1933) (Fig. 14). All these consequences of discal wear are seen with the greatest predominance in the case which de Sèze (1959) has described under the name of "trophostatic syndrome of postmenopausal women" (Fig. 15).

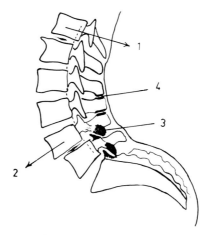

Figure 15. Post-menopausal "trophostatic" syndrome (de Sèze). (1) Retrolisthesis of D12 over L1 by flattening of D12 over L1 resulting from a pull of articular joints and their capsule and from the pull of the supraspinous ligament; (2) interspinal arthrose L2, L3, L4; (3) forward gliding of L4 following the flattening of the disc L4-L5 with deterioration and arthrosis of the posterior joints while the supraspinous ligament is stretched (4).

The overweight and the slackening of the abdomen, associated with postural collapse and with the relative compression of the vertebral column, leads to the following deformations: hyperlordosis which together with the discal deterioration increases the pressure over the posterior joints at the level of the lower lumbar vertebrae. This results in arthrosis of the posterior joints and a tendency toward a ventral vertebral gliding. At the same time, the vertebrae of the upper lumbar region are, for the same reason (relative collapse of the disc), in a receding position in relation to the vertebrae immediately underneath, with the tendency to a shearing of the posterior articulations. It is in these lumbar vertebrae that one sees the emergence of an interspinal arthrosis as the spinal processes approach each other. Aging also directly affects the supraspinal ligament. The degenerative lesions of this very strong dorsal structure contributing to the maintenance of the posture (a truly "posterior disc"), are often noted at the level of the lumbar column. In a study carried out on thirty autopsy examinations of subjects between 30 and 70 years of age, Rissanen (1964) was able to show that there was an impressive parallelism between degeneration of the disc and that of the supraspinal ligament (equal percentage). These lesions can be brought into evidence radiologically by injecting a contrasting substance on each side of the ligament. A normal ligament gives the picture of a homogenous spindle of fusiform shape different from that of an injured one which is penetrated by an opaque fluid.

The intervertebral foramen is also subject to the modifications of aging which results in its shrinking due to discal collapse and the osteophytic proliferation. This is particularly noticeable at the level of the cervical spine because of the existence of uncinate processes and the formation of disco-osteophytic nodules. Also arthrosis of the posterior joints may be often observed in such cases. The disco-osteophytic nodules shrink the foramen in front and the arthrosis of the posterior joints shrink it posteriorly. This is especially noticeable in the upper part of the intervertebral "canal," its lower part being involved only in the advanced stages of the arthrosis. These formations have repercussion at the level of the cervical spine not only on the elements contained in the intervertebral foramen but also on the vertebral artery which climbs through the foramen of the transverse processes. This is clearly evidenced by arteriographies, although one cannot state whether or not these deformities as well as the arthrosis itself play a direct pathological role, since one may see arterial deformities in the absence of any symptomatology (see also Barcelo and Vilaseca, 1956; Bradford and Spurling, 1945).

Chapter 4

Minor Mechanical Disturbances
of the Intervertebral Joint or
"Minor Intervertebral Derangements"

INTRODUCTION

T HE LESIONS of the spinal column due to aging are generally quite well tolerated and are not directly responsible for pain or other complaints. They often bring about simple stiffness, perceived by the patient as "rustiness," or they may even remain completely silent. Nevertheless these deteriorations facilitate transitory or prolonged pain (which may be light or severe) that is provoked by stress, false movements, or various traumatisms. It is this minor mechanical pathology which interests us when we study vertebral manipulations. It is certainly better known insofar as their clinical manifestations are concerned than in its innermost mechanisms. Improved knowledge of anatomopathology, however, permits a more interesting approach. We shall look at the different possible lesions of each of the elements of the intervertebral joint; then we will consider the pain that is elicited experimentally from each of these elements. Then we will have occasion to compare the experimentally produced pain to that which we encounter daily in our clinical practice.

It goes without saying that we are only interested here in minor mechanical derangements. This excludes fractures, dislocations, and the entire inflammatory pathology, as well as the tumors. Certain minor mechanical derangements that can be present in the different elements of the intervertebral joint: (disc, posterior joints, ligamento-muscular system) are well known in their clinical manifestations and their anatomopathology. The others remain unknown and the role of certain anatomical structures in vertebral pathology, although very probable, is still quite hypothetical.

In order to designate these small lesions of traumatic or static origin, we found it convenient to use the term "minor intervertebral derangements." This term has the merit of prejudging neither the injured element or the nature of the lesion, nor the mechanism responsible for the pain. When the manipulation was effective, we can say that it was a remedy for a reversible intervertebral derangement; the latter could have been anatomical or functional. This does not hinder any analysis from being made in order to discover the real causes of the observed clinical facts or to add any complementary information which may increase the precision of the observable phenomenon.

PATHOGENESIS AND CLINICAL MANIFESTATIONS

Discal Lesions

We have seen the physiological alterations of the constituents of the intervertebral disc due to aging. We know that its central portion dehydrates progressively and that it is gradually replaced around the age of 60 years by an amorphus mass, sometimes with calcifications. At the same time some lacerations may occur in the annulus fibrosus, which becomes thinner. But all this is not a sufficient explanation of discal hernias, since we know that sciatica, for example, is a disease of the thirties, and that it can be seen in adolescents. The more frequent stresses at middle age are without doubt the favoring factors.

Classically, the disc can be subject to a variety of mechanical lesions. The occurrence of least severity is exemplified by the "intradiscal blockage," the most severe being represented by the discal hernia.

Intradiscal Blockage

The most benign discal derangement is due entirely to the fact that in the course of a movement, especially in the course of an effort to flex the trunk, a fragment of this nucleus can catch itself in a posterior fissure of the annulus (Fig. 16) .

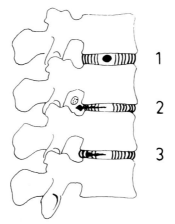

Figure 16. Lesions of the disc. (1) Normal disc; (2) posterior herniation; (3) posterior intradiscal block by a fragment of the nucleus.

The bulging out of the posterior part of the disc and of the posterior ligament, which this accident occasions, and perhaps a pressure against the dura mater, is painful because these elements are very richly innervated. It is commonly admitted that this intradiscal blockage is the cause of acute lumbago (de Sèze).

It is probable that other intradiscal blocks exist that do not elicit any direct disturbance, but produce involvement of another element of the mobile segment, thus causing minor intervertebral derangements amenable to manipulations (see Mode of action of manipulations p. 173).

Discal Hernia

The more severe disturbance is represented by the hernia of the disc (Fig. 16). The gelatinous nucleus makes an eruption through the annulus fibrosus and therefore breaks it. It then compresses the nerve root. This discal hernia is accompanied by a strong congestive local reaction which is responsible in part for the symptoms. We know that hernia of the disc L5-S1, compresses the root S1, while that of the disc L4-L5 compresses the root L5. But, a massive hernia at the lumbar level can compress both roots or even the roots of the cauda epuina.

Most of these cases are amenable to medical treatment, although in some, surgery is the only solution. The numerous surgical verifications have permitted some very valuable comparisons in order to establish in a precise manner the semeiology of these discal hernias. There are, nevertheless, cases where we must have recourse to myelographies in order to affirm the presence of discal herniation and its level.

The lumbar column does not possess exclusive rights to discal herniation. It is, however, at this level that we encounter them with maximum frequency. In a statistical study of 294 public aid cases by the University Clinic of Neurosurgery of Zurich, the following levels were found:

Discal Hernias	Location
1,098	L5-S1
1,667	L4-L5
135	L3-L4
14	L2-L3
7	lower dorsal spine
20	two lower cervical segments.

Lesions of the Posterior Joint

A number of authors have fixed their attention on the role of these articulations in the pathology of low back pain (Putti, 1927; Brocher, 1948; Taillard, 1957; Lazorthes, 1966). According to the German author Junghanns (1939, 1958, 1959, and 1966), a blockage of one of these articulations can be produced by the jamming of articular villosities or of the small interapophysary menisci which can be subject to folds or tears. This implies an acute pain originating in these small articulations, especially if the other elements of the intervertebral joint conserve their mobility; each movement painfully affects the torn joint structures inasmuch as the capsule of these articulations is the most innervated structure of the spine (Tondury, 1937; Lazorthes, 1949, 1955; Lazorthes *et al.*, 1965). It is not contrary to common sense to think that this is one logical explanation of these numerous complaints of vertebral pain provoked by false movements and in which the role of the disc cannot be involved without some reservation. It is the considered opinion of Lazorthes (1966) that "vertebral and paravertebral pain generally originate from the conflict between the discal or arthro-radicular structures. But certain clinical evidence and certain therapeutic results demonstrate that this hypothesis cannot explain all the cases of vertebral radicular pain."

Lazorthes showed that the posterior branch of the spinal nerves is a part of the posterior vertebral arch. It is distributed in the interapophysary articulations, in the vertebral laminae, and in the muscles of the back, from the vertex to the coccyx. "The richness of the vertebral apophysary innervation makes us presume that the pain most often originates at the level of the posterior joints."

"Edema, the involvement of the capsuloligamental structures, peri-articular hematoma constitute many factors of irritation of the posterior branch of the spinal nerve which finds itself laying against this articulation."

Can we find in the anatomy of the posterior joints other reasons for derangement? We suggested a subject for a thesis related to this discussion to Freudenberg (1967). His work was done in the anatomical laboratory of the Faculty of Medicine of the University of Paris under the direction of C. Gillot. Some very interesting information emerged from this investigation. First, the extreme variability of size and shape of the posterior articulated lumbosacral apophyses. Fifty-four out of 100 were normal. Among the others, a significant number had a bony surface which showed irregularities, forming transverse ridges which the cartilage covered uniformly, although their presence remained very visible. Some ridges even had true facets. We know that the form of the posterior articulations is peculiar to the lumbar region where they have the shape of a segment of a cylinder. This shape facilitates the movement of flexion and extension and prevents rotational movement, except if there is a flexion and associated lateral inclination. Freudenberg (1967) has been able to show on an anatomical specimen that when an articular facet shows the above-described small ridges, a combined anterior and lateral flexion imposed on the 5th lumbar vertebra is followed at the time of return in the direction of extension by a manifest blocking of the movement or at least a temporary arrest, with a secondary rebound. A sudden separation of the articular apophyses produced in this way is clearly visible on the anatomic specimen but is certainly too small to be uncovered by contemporary radiography. Therefore, this sharp rebound may produce a disturbance in the smooth course of the movement which will effect the ligamentary and muscular systems. It is perhaps in this kind of disturbance that one will find an explanation of certain low back pain, and more specifically, of those cases where the patients are subject in the course of their lives to numerous lumbagos without at any time presenting a full-blown picture of discal sciatica.

Lesions of the Supraspinous Ligament

In all "derangements" of the mobile intervertebral segment, there is also more or less marked involvement of the supraspinous ligament, which is pulled or pinched. We can thus reach the conclusion that the deterioration of the supraspinous ligament can disturb the proper functioning of the mobile segment and produce an instability in the latter. A lesion of this ligament, degenerative or traumatic, no longer assures its satisfactory maintenance, which favors the mechanical derangements of the disc or of the posterior joints. Moreover, the slightest and yet unusual pull on the injured ligament risks provoking pain which would not happen with normal ligament. Hackett (1956) attributes to the "slackening" of this ligament certain aches which he treats by (sclerotic) injections. But it appears that he attributes all abnormal ligamentary sensibility to a "slackening" of this structure which is very debatable. Good results which this therapeutic method can elicit do not justify this interpretation.

Interaction of the Lesion in the Intervertebral Joint

It must be remembered that the intervertebral joint is a total functional unit and that the lesion of one of the constituents affects all the others: thus, the intervertebral blockage caused by discal herniation affects the posterior intervertebral articulations as well as the interspinal ligaments. The herniated disc acts as a wedge between the vertebral bodies, therefore modifying the reciprocal relationships of the posterior articulations and their functionings so that either (1) they assume the position which they occupy in a hyperflexion movement, or that is to say, in the position of maximum divergence (if the hernia is posterior and central), or (2) they assume an asymmetric position, which they occupy in a movement of lateroflexion (if the hernia is postero-lateral). In such case one finds one joint in maximum convergence, the other in maximum divergence.

Moreover, the herniated nucleus modifies the dynamics of the joint mainly in moving back the axis of the intervertebral movement. When the vertebral segment corresponding to the site of the lesion participates in a global movement of the spine, the posterior articulations, already brought to the extreme limit of their joint action, become quite painful. Posterior joint disorders are an important cause of pain in the case of discal herniations (Copeman, 1953; Taillard, 1957) (Fig. 17). Yet one must remember that interspinal ligaments can in certain cases constitute the source of the troublesome sequellae of a discogenic disease.

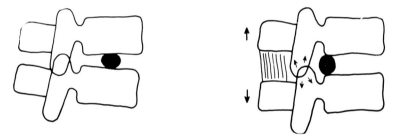

Figure 17. Effect of posterior discal herniation upon posterior joints. Posterior discal herniation elicits a separation of the posterior joints and a painful pull of the capsule as well as of the supraspinous ligament.

The Role of the Muscle Spasm in the Persistence of These Derangements (a Functional Derangement)

The common consequence of all these minor intervertebral "derangements" is the partial loss of the mobility of the affected segment. It is a vicious circle in which the muscular contracture plays a role which may be all the more dominant when the structural derangement is least pronounced. A voluntary vertebral movement is in effect a global movement. It brings into play an important number of muscle fascicles inserting each in a different fashion and which must function in most perfect synergy. The harmonious development of the successive contractions of these fascicles determines the proper execution of the movement. If it is disturbed by whatever incident (false movement, poorly estimated movement, etc.) an isolated involuntary contraction of a fascicle may be elicited, which occurs at a wrong phase of the total movement and therefore may lead to a deep painful vertebral cramp.

When a similar incident is produced at the level of an extremity, it may be easily remedied by a spontaneous corrective movement (Terrier, 1959). For example, we can relieve a cramp of the calf by stretching the sore muscles, that is to say by forced dorsiflexion of the foot. But at the level of the spine the effective voluntary movement is impossible and every local attempt of this sort may only increase the local contracture. If there is no mechanical or static defect present at that level of the spine, the contracture yields spontaneously. But, if there is a weak structure point and if it produces a mechanical derangement, the muscle spasm provokes a more or less persistent functional block which may often even outlast the cause of the disorder. This then produces a *functional derangement* of the intervertebral joint, that is to say a dysfunctioning by persistent muscular contraction, after the mechanical original cause has disappeared. This neuromuscular element may be the main point in this pathology of vertebral pain and consequently is important to consider for the act of manipulation. We will discuss below what we call "partial durable contractions" which involve only some muscle fascicles but which may maintain a painful low back or facilitate its relapse.

"Spasmophilic Constitution"

It is possible that neuromuscular hyperexcitability, such as that encountered in various cases favors the appearance or persistence of such contractures. We have, in effect, noted the great frequency with which we find during electromyographical examinations the signs of marked neuromuscular instability in patients showing chronic or repeated vertebral pain.

Pain and Disturbances Elicited in Each Element of the Intervertebral Joint

It is interesting to consider pain which can be experimentally provoked at the level of the different elements of the intervertebral joint and compare these experimental findings with cases encountered in clinical practice. We will consider successively (1) the pain that can originate from the disc itself; (2) the pain originating in the posterior intervertebral joints; (3) the pain originating from the interspinal ligaments and from the paravertebral muscles.

Pain Elicited from the Disc Itself

After probing the sensitivity of the different anatomic vertebral structures at both lumbar and cervical levels, in conscious patients under local anaesthetic, Wiberg (1949) came to the following conclusion insofar as the lumbar spine was concerned.

1. The pressure on the ligamentum flavum is not painful.

2. The pressure on the posterior surface of the disc and on the posterior ligament always elicits a lumbosacral pain. It is a deep pain lateralized to the side of the stimulation.

3. Direct pressure on the nerve root provokes a sharp pain in the territory of the corresponding dermatome.

4. If the root is anesthetized, it is still always possible to elicit pain by pressure on the disc.

Cloward (1960) repeated the experiment of Wiberg and came to the same conclusions. By stimulating the superficial fibers of the hemilumbar disc, one elicits pain, radiating to the sacro-iliac region, the hip, and the buttocks on the same side. It is concluded that this pain is due to the irritation of the sinu-vertebral nerve which innervates the peripheral fibers of the disc and the ligaments which surround it.

Cloward differentiates this "discal" pain from "neural" pain related to the irritation of the spinal root. During cervical discography, with injection of an opaque fluid into the disc, no pain is elicited if the disc is normal and the quantity of the injected fluid does not exceed 0.2 to 0.3 cc. However, if the fibers of the annulus are torn, so that the injected opaque solution under pressure reaches the periphery of the disc, pain is elicited. Its localization, character, and intensity will depend on the localization and the extent of the tear in the disc (Cloward, 1960).

This opinion has, however, been disputed. In practically all 148 discograms obtained on fifty young volunteers free from any vertebral or root pain, Earl P. Holt (1964) has shown that intradiscal injection of contrasting substance was regularly painful, and therefore no consistent relationship of this pain to a tear of the annulus could be established. It remains true that all the authorities agree that the puncture of the peripheral layer of this disc by the needle during discography, or any other mechanical or electrical stimulation, provokes regional pain. It is interesting to note that at the level of the cervical spine where experimentation is easiest, it has been stated that the pain is different for the anterolateral part of the annulus and for its posterior part (Cloward, 1960).

1. Pressure on the superficial part of the disc in its posterior and posterolateral part produces a pain, even when the corresponding root is anesthetized. This pain is lateralized to the stimulated side and is regionally projected (shoulder, upper arm) (Falconer *et al.,* 1948; Cloward, 1960).

2. On the contrary, the pressure on the anterolateral part of the cervical disc provokes an interscapulary muscular pain (analogous to that obtained while irritating the motor root) (Cloward, 1960; Frykholm, 1951) (see also Inman and Saunders, 1947).

Pain Originating from the Posterior Joints

Taillard (1957) has been able to provoke radiating pain with a pseudoradicular topography when he stimulated the capsule of the posterior joints in subjects under local anesthesia. He states,

It is interesting to consider again the observations made in the course of surgery conducted under local anesthesia. It is easy to make a good infiltration of novocaine of the subcutaneous tissues, the lumbar aponeurosis, the paravertebral muscles and the periosteum of the lamina. This anesthesia is not generally sufficient to insensitize the capsules of the small joints. We could almost always, while pinching the capsule at the involved level, reproduce exactly the pain which patients habitually endure according to their reports. We elicited in this way, not only the lumbago, but the radiating sciatic pain in the thigh, the calf and sometimes even the foot.

These radiations of pain are elicited by a needle placed at the level of the posterior joints. Like other authors, we have seen such radiating pain vanish after an injection of Novocain® or hydrocortizone at the level of posterior joints. The radiation is frequently lumbogluteal for the middle lumbar spine and towards the iliac crest and the posterior aspect of the buttocks and of the thigh in the case of the posterior joints of the lower lumbar spine.

Pain Originating from the Interspinous Ligaments

Kellgren (1939), while injecting some hypertonic saline solution in the interspinous ligaments in patients after anesthesia of the skin, has been able to elicit both local and deep pain. The topography of this pain is nearly identical to that of the corresponding spinal roots; however, there are some differences at the level of the extremities. The infiltration of the ligament at the L1 level, for example, provokes a pain in the region of the root L1. But, this pain bears a resemblance to that of an attack of kidney stones and is accompanied by a retraction of the testicle and a painful contraction of the inferior part of the abdominal wall.

The supraspinous ligament is not the only ligament whose irritation can provoke deep pain. For example, irritation of the iliolumbar ligament by a needle provokes a pain in the external aspect of the buttocks and especially in the groin. It is certainly the cause of the pain in the groin which we encountered so frequently in typical radicular sciatica, almost always L5 and which we can temporarily relieve by injecting the ligament. Lewis and Kellgren (1939) state that the pain is independent of the technique of stimulation. Therefore, it is entirely logical to think that an intervertebral ligament submitted to a mechanical irritation can cause local or distant pain, according to a radicular topography without direct involvement of the root.

If the interspinal pain is due to an "intervertebral derangement" which manipulation can control, it can also relieve the pain originating from this ligament by normalizing the articular function. We frequently find in clinical practice, pain originating from the supraspinal ligament. The temporary relief (without correcting the casual derangement) which we can obtain by anesthetizing (Novocain) this ligament demonstrates quite well its responsibility in the origin of the pain.

Pain Which Originates in the Muscle Itself

When one injects into the gluteal intramuscular mass a small amount of irritative substance one often elicits a pseudosciatic pain, propagating along the entire thigh, although the injection is made in a point of the lateral iliac fossa, far from the course of the sciatic nerve. Kellgren and Lewis have studied the projection of pain obtained by injecting an irritating solution in different muscles and tendons after anesthesia of the skin. Whereas the pain provoked by the injection of the tendons remains a local pain, the one elicited by the intramuscular injection is projected at a distance. For example, an injection in the lower part of the triceps gives rise to a pain which extends to the medial aspect of the forearm and travels to the 5th finger. An injection in the trapezius gives rise to a pain irradiating to the occipital region. Kellgren (1939) has established some precise localizations of these projections, and numerous experiments have permitted him to conclude the following:

1. The distribution of the pain for a given muscle is the same for all individuals, although the projection is more or less distal according to the part of the muscle injected. There can, however, be variations from one individual to another, some having a dorsal predominance, others a ventral one.

2. The projections obtained depend upon the nerve root which innervates the muscle concerned in such a way that the muscles which are innervated by this same root have a common locus of projection.

3. The topography of the projection coincides with that of the corresponding spinal root (see Fig. 18) .

4. The pain is independent of the mode of stimulation. The pain can be experimentally elicited by the injection of hypertonic solution, by electrical stimulation, in the course of certain surgical

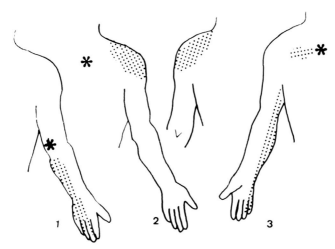

Figure 18. An irritant, hypertonic saline, is injected in the muscles. It elicits radiating pain (Kellgren). Example: (1) Brachial triceps; (2) rhomboid; (3) first intercostal. The injected point is indicated by a star.

operations, or finally by Lewis' maneuver in which a garrot is placed at the root of the extremities and repeat contractions of the distal muscles provoke an insupportable muscular pain, necessitating the cessation of the movement.

Such is the information derived from experimentation. We can correlate this information with certain clinical evidence to which we have drawn attention (see p. 305) : if we palpate with care the mass of gluteal muscles, in the course of certain types of sciatica, we discover that there exist areas particularly sensitive to pressure. They are most often located at the level of the gluteus medium or minimus. We thus reproduce or exaggerate the spontaneous pain of the lower extremity by pushing a "bell button" as it were.

The local anesthesia of a myalgic point (Novocain) can bring complete relief of the sciatic pain, generally temporary, but sometimes quite lasting. A careful palpation of these tender muscular zones shows a consistency different from that of a normal muscle: there are muscular bundles which appear hard and tight, and even sometimes like cords. We can find analogous consistency at the level of the quadriceps in femoral neuralgias or in the muscles of the upper extremity in certain cervicobrachial neuralgias. The treatment directed strictly to these muscles by stretching them or by appropriate massage and local injections remarkably relieves these patients.

We find similar phenomena at the level of the paravertebral muscles. Their careful palpation permits us to recognize at the involved level a modification of their consistency: the impression of hardness and the presence of very tender small cordlike formations. A local injection of an irritating substance exaggerates the complaints and reproduces spontaneous pain of the patient, which sometimes is perceived at a great distance. Certain relaxing maneuvers affecting only the muscles, without any mobilization of the vertebral segment, sometimes suffice to relieve immediately and lastingly a radiated or projected regional pain. Without doubt this explains the success of infiltration of various other techniques achieving the same result: either acting on the cause which elicits the muscle changes, or affecting the muscle itself so as to break self-sustained circular mechanism. We shall return to these "partial and lasting indurations of the muscles" in the following chapter, since we see them so often in cases of a root involvement provided that the muscle is supplied by the same root.

We can conclude from these experiments that the capsule of the posterior joints or the supraspinal ligament, or the paravertebral muscles, originate not only a local pain but also a radiating pain in the region approximately the same as that of the corresponding root. One may recall that all these elements are innervated by the posterior branches of the spinal nerves.

Pain Provoked by the Irritation of the Elements of the Intervertebral Foramen

After having considered the pain which can be originated from the disc, the posterior joints, and the supraspinal ligament, it is necessary to consider the consequences of an irritation or compression of the spinal or sympathetic nerves which pass through the intervertebral foramen (Figs. 19 and 20). The pain induced by the involvement of the dorsal and of the ventral roots

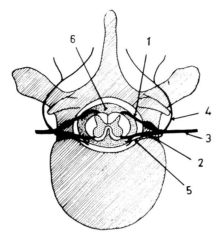

Figure 19. Diagrammatic representation of the formation of the spinal nerve (after Rouviere). (1) Dorsal root; (2) ventral root; (3) anterior branch; (4) posterior branch; (5) sinu-vertebral nerve; (6) subarachnoid space.

are well known (sciatica, cervicobrachial neuralgia, etc.). Usually one considers the posterior branch of the spinal nerve to a much lesser degree than the spinal root. Yet this branch plays a very important role in vertebral pain (Lazorthes, 1966).

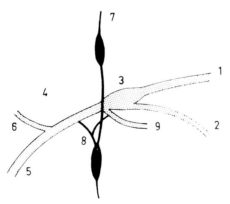

Figure 20. Division of the spinal nerve into two terminal branches (after Testut). (1) Dorsal root; (2) ventral root; (3) spinal ganglion; (4) spinal nerve proper; (5) its anterior branch; (6) its posterior branch; (7) sympathetic chain; (8) ramus communicans; (9) sinuvertebral nerve.

We wish to stress the findings which seem to us of interest, although they have escaped general attention. We have in view not only some tender cordlike muscle fascicles which are supplied by the involved root but also a tender infiltration of the skin belonging to the same segmental dermatome. Although the explanation of these findings is not easy, one should not underestimate their importance from the therapeutic viewpoint.

PAINFUL DORSAL ROOT. The compression or irritation of the dorsal root elicits a sharp pain in the dermatome corresponding to this root. In clinical practice, this is the case of sciatica or of cervicobrachial neuralgia involving the neck, the shoulder, or the upper extremity. The involved dermatome makes it possible to localize the corresponding root. For example, the L5 pain propagates to the posterior aspect of the thigh, to the lateral aspect of the lower leg, and to the dorsal aspect of the foot, traveling toward the big toe. The involvement of S1 will be manifested by pain radiating to the posterior aspect of the thigh and of the lower leg, traveling under the heel to the lateral aspect of the foot. However, the pain may involve only a part of this dermatome, or be replaced by paresthesias which have the same localizing value. There are, for example, cases of radicular pain of cervical origin localized to the fingers (so-called "painful cervical finger" of Arlet, 1952, 1954) without any painful manifestation at the arm or forearm. There are cases when just the opposite is observed. In most cases pain constitutes the total clinical picture, although when the involvement of sensory fibers is more complete, there is additional objective evidence of defects of sensory perception: hypoesthesia, hyperesthesia, sometimes involving the touch or the perception of a prick of a pin, particularly in the distal part of the dermatome.

It may be a change of tendon reflexes, the ankle jerk for S1 root, the bicipital reflex for C6, or tricipital for C7. In fact, the pain is not elicited solely by pressure; mechanical irritation of the root induces its symptomatic inflammation. It is this inflammation which is responsible for the pain. For Granit, Leksell, and Skoglund (1944), the immediate cause of the sciatica is an intrinsic alteration of the nerve leading to a formation of an artificial synapse. Thus the nerve impulses generated by excitation of a motor fiber will be transmitted to a damaged sensory fiber passing alongside by "induction."

For Burke (1964), irritation or compression of a sensory fiber does not generate the usual pain of radicular neuralgias. According to him, irritation or compression of the root elicits a momentary sharp pain like an electric discharge which does not persist despite continuous compression, the patient having in such cases only a perception of numbness. Frykholm assumes that the compression of a root in the case of a fibrous herniated disc, at the cervical level, is tolerated for a long time without any pain and is generated only when dura mater becomes involved or when another mechanical derangement, even a minimal one, is suddenly added.

INVOLVEMENT OF THE VENTRAL ROOT. If the fibers of the ventral root are involved, motor deficiences as well as muscle atrophy are seen. Their distribution, obviously different from that of sensory disturbances, corresponds to the involved segment. Thus the plantar flexors are involved in S1 root disturbance and the dorsiflexors in the L5 segmental involvement. Motor deficiencies are rare in the cervical involvement.

Fasciculations are often seen in cases of segmental pain. These are limited contractions, due to a sudden involuntary activation of one or many muscle fascicles. They undoubtedly constitute a manifestation of the irritation of the ventral root. We should not forget, however, that such fasciculations may be due to other causes: muscle fatigue resulting from static contractions or amyotrophic lateral sclerosis. In the latter case they appear as a most consistent clinical manifestation.

Muscle cramps may be present in cases of segmental pain. They are characterized by a painful, involuntary and transitory contraction of a muscular group or of only a few muscle fibers. They are mostly observed as sequellae of sciatica or femoral neuralgia. They occur most often when the muscle is completely relaxed. In addition to these classical findings, it is appropriate to cite the work of Cloward (1960) and that of Frykholm (1947, 1951), who showed that direct stimulation of a ventral root is pain-inducing. However, this pain is different from that elicited by the stimulation of the dorsal root. The stimulation of the motor root elicits a sharp interscapulary pain located at a different level according to the segment corresponding to the stimulated root. The same pain is obtained by stimulating the anterolateral portion of the annulus of lower cervical discs. Frykholm considered two types of radicular pain:

1. A myalgia consisting of deep exasperating pain which can be reproduced by stimulation of the ventral root.

2. A neuralgia (like an electric current) which can be reproduced by stimulation of the dorsal root.

SYNDROME OF THE POSTERIOR BRANCH OF THE SPINAL NERVES. It is necessary to consider not only the anterior branch of the spinal nerve, but also its posterior branch, which can be injured near the intervertebral foramen. Lazorthes has given the particular symptomatology of such an injury the name of "syndrome of the posterior branch of a spinal nerve." Lazorthes *et al.* state the following:

> The posterior branches of the spinal nerves innervate all the formations dependent on the posterior vertebral arch.
>
> Their motor distribution is in the muscles acting on the axial skeletal structures.
>
> Their segmental sensory distribution covers a large skin area extended without interruption from the vertex to the coccyx and spreading out at certain levels: the posterior regions of the scalp, scapulary regions, and gluteal regions.
>
> Their role in the rich innervation of the posterior joints is now well known.
>
> These nerve branches closely adhere to the articular bony structures being fixated by fibrous formations. The nature, the shape, and the importance of these structures certainly varies from one level of the spine to another. Their constant coexistence implies an inexorable intimacy of the relationships between the posterior spinal nerves and the articular vertebral column.
>
> The intimate relationships which unite at each level, the posterior branch of the spinal nerve and the articulations of the vertebral arches, should be taken into consideration in the interpretation of some types of back pain, more from the pathological than from the clinical point of view.
>
> The posterior branches of the spinal nerves must be affected by

the derangement of the system of posterior joint whether they are acute or chronic.

Involvement may be acute and brutal, being secondary to a non-physiological movement of great amplitude. The nerve is then involved either directly, by traction (in particular at the lumbar level), or indirectly by edema, periarticular hematoma, or the ligamentocapsular tears. During chronic derangements, a pericapsular fibrosis of the posterior articular structures, and the marginal osteophytosis, just as other conditions susceptible to damaging the nerves, may be contributing factors. We have often noted these changes while dissecting cases with arthrosis of the spine.

. . . .

The posterior spinal nerve is a mixed nerve. The manifestations of its distress are always both sensitive and motor. The pain is limited to the juxavertebral region relatively localized. It is very often spontaneous, but can be relieved by deep paravertebral pressure near the spinal process capable of affecting the periarticular zone through the muscle masses. Finally the same pain may often be elicited by those movements of the spine which involve mostly the posterior joints, that is to say, essentially the movements of rotation. Contracture is another muscular consequence of the irritation of the nerve: it results from a true regional reflex elicited in response to the irritation of the sensitive proprioceptive fibers of articular origin. This contracture, often very pronounced, is followed by various complications and deformities such as torticollis, scoliosis, etc.

SYMPATHETIC NERVE INVOLVEMENT. It can also be irritated in the intervertebral foramen. Recalling the ideas of Leriche (1930) concerning sprains in general, we can agree with Dechaume *et al.,* (1959, 1961) that vertebral sprains can, by a reflex mechanism involving vasomotor components, generate a chain reaction. Guilleminet and Stagnara (1952) write: "if we imagine that the same reaction of pseudoinflammatory edema which commonly occurs in a case of a sprained ankle or knee, can exist at the level of vertebral articulations, we must admit that the nerve root must suffer being in their immediate vicinity."

Dechaume *et al.* state:

Apophysary or unco-vertebral sprain compresses the other elements of the intervertebral foramen at the same time as the root: the sinu-vertebral nerve as well as the artery, veins, and the sympathetic nerve; hence, new vasomotor reactions affecting the nerve formations may ensue. Thus, one should not exclude from the intricate mechanical, circulatory, and nervous factors which intervene in the course of traumatisms the participation of the sympathetic nerve either directly or through a reflex mechanism.

Moreover, one should recall that for Frykholm (1951), sympathetic fibers travel in the ventral root, which may explain the pain of a sympathetic type associated with vasomotor and trophic disorders which accompany the radicular compression.

OTHER SYMPTOMS ASSOCIATED WITH RADICULAR NEURALGIA. It might be of interest to stress certain manifestations which are not discussed classically but which are frequently associated with radicular neuralgia. At the end of this chapter we will discuss in detail certain partial intramuscular indurations which seem to us to have particular interest. We will first mention, however, tender tendinous insertions and tender periosteum, the occurrence of which has been already stressed by Lacapère (1950). We should also mention certain cellular infiltration of particular interest to manual physicians and rheumatologists, who can thus explain persistence of an intractable pain in these patients.

Painful Cutaneous Infiltrations in Root Involvements

It is common to note areas of infiltration of the skin in radicular neuralgia. The cutaneous and subcutaneous tissue appears to be infiltrated so that skin-rolling maneuver gives the impression of the skin being thicker on one side than that on the other side. In addition, this maneuver elicits a rough sensation and sometimes reveals the presence of small nodules which are extremely tender.

The "cellulalgia" has a distribution in strips with preferential localized zones: supraspinal fossa of the scapular region, the lateral aspect of the shoulder, at the level of the deltoid insertion, the lateral aspect of the lower part of the arm, the sacral region, the buttocks, the lateral aspect of the thigh; the external aspect of the lower leg, the medial aspect of the knee, etc. These areas of "cellulalgia" which appear with neuralgia can also disappear when the neuralgia disappears. But sometimes they outlast the disappearance of the neuralgia, causing a persistent pain whose authenticity is doubtful up to the day when it will vanish under the influence of a few sessions of massage (see Fig. 112).

These zones of cellular infiltration should be looked for during the very first examination; however, they should be treated only if they persist after the acute phase is over. Comparative examination of the non painful side is evidently of crucial significance. In particular, one should not confuse these areas of "cellulalgia" with the gross pockets of cellulitis found in obese women. The infiltrations considered in this chapter are strictly unilateral, corresponding to an affected vertebra which is either manifest or to be revealed by further examination.

It is necessary to think of these "cellulalgic" infiltrations since they can lead to locally projected pain which often is misleading and is the source of diagnostic errors, especially if they are found in the precordial, abdominal or epigastric regions and also if they are located near an articulation (knee or elbow for example). One should not conclude that local tenderness is related to an articular lesion without first trying to make it disappear by appropriate massage of the cutaneous tissue using the skin-rolling technique. Such massage may be associated with local anesthesic infiltrations which may be helpful if the correction of the responsible derangement is not sufficient.

In effect, before making a local treatment, it is necessary to be absolutely sure by careful examination of the corresponding vertebral segment that there is no longer any sign of intervertebral derangement. If it persists and if an appropriate manipulation may correct it, the tenderness of the skin subsides very quickly, sometimes instantaneously. If it remains uncorrected, the local treatment may only irritate the tissue.

Tender Tendinous Insertions and Periosteum in Root Involvement

It is quite often found, in the course of certain radicular neuralgias, that the patient complains of tenderness of various bony structures. When the examiner strokes this area lightly with his finger he exacerbates the pain. The localization is that encountered most often in association with a typical radicular pain: epicondyle and radial styloid, for example, in the course of some cervicobrachial neuralgias of C6 origin; the trochlea in the C8 cervicobrachial neuralgia; the trochanter in certain cases of sciatica, etc. The pain can accompany these radicular syndromes or it can succeed them or outlast them. It also can be a unique manifestation of this syndrome although its vertebral origin can be ascertained later on. An epicondylitis is one of the examples. It goes without saying that it can have an entirely different origin and that one must not refer systematically to the spine all epicondylites or "trochanterites." But this possibility must not be overlooked because of the therapeutic option which it offers.

Intramuscular Partial Indurations

We should like to direct attention once more to the observations which we made concerning certain muscles supplied by a compressed or irritated root at the level of the spine. A careful palpation may reveal hardened fascicles in these muscles which appear to be stretched and tender. They seem to us to be associated with the genesis of radicular neuralgia and to be capable of contributing to their persistence. Despite their frequent occurrence, surprisingly, they have not been considered or investigated from this point of view in the literature. The mechanism of their genesis is not too clear and their presence is quite difficult to understand as a manifestation of a purely neurogenic etiology. It is, however, necessary to be able to reveal them in order to consider their true nature.

The muscles supplied by the affected root may be hypotonic or even atrophied. This fosters a soft consistency of the muscle. However, what we consider here are small segments of the muscle with a consistency of a hardened cord, contrasting with that of the surrounding hypotonic muscle where they are found. They are tender; their size varies from that of a thin cord to that of a thick pencil of 2 to 10 cm in length; sometimes it is a mass which occupies a large part of the muscle. If one palpates these formations, barely exercising any pressure between two fingers which can grasp them through the muscle tissue, a sharp pain, quite localized, resembling a cramp, may be elicited, which the patient often identifies with the spontaneous pain that he experiences during an acute attack. The femoral biceps, the soleus, sometimes the gluteus maximus, may contain these indurations in a case of sciatica of S1 origin; it is the gluteus medius which may contain them in a patient with sciatica at L5 origin, or the quadriceps in the case of femoral neuralgia.

When it is difficult to identify the muscle which contains these indurated fascicles, one should ask the patient to contract isometrically the muscle under examination against the resistance offered by one hand of the operator, while the other is free to palpate the muscle so that a precise analysis of the findings may be completed.

For a given muscle, the location of such indurated fascicles is quite consistent. Thus, for example, in the femoral biceps they are almost always found in its lower part, near the tendon. The direction of these "cords" or "pencils" is the same as that of the muscle fibers. Their responsibility in perseveration of pain (even when the root compression has been removed) is easy to determine, since it may be sufficient to inject novocaine into the most tender point of the muscle in order to obtain total relief. This improvement, either transitory or persistent, not only of the local tenderness, but also of the radiating segmental pain, is all the more impressive, since the same injection localized one to four inches from this point will remain without any therapeutic effect upon the painful syndrome.

These indurated fascicles may be the origin of some cramps, particularly if the muscle is somewhat compressed as happens when the patient is in a sitting position or when the muscle remains completely relaxed for some time (or with a flexed knee, in this example) or when the muscle suddenly contracts maximally against resistance. One is, therefore, led to consider these indurated and tender muscle fascicles, as in a state of true "chronic cramp," particularly so since stretching of the muscle is the best maneuver for their relaxation. The EMG recordings which have been done in many cases have been quite inconclusive, as they usually do not show any particular pattern. These results should be considered with great caution as it is very difficult to sample these formations with an EMG needle. We have asked Aullas to resume these investigations. In the recent cases which he reported, using common procedures of facilitation he found in most of these patients repetitive activity characteristic of "spasmophilia." A "spasmophilic constitution" may therefore be contributory to this phenomenon.

We shall abstain from formulating hypotheses concerning the nature and pathogenic mechanisms of these partial indurations of the muscle, so surprising to find in a root involvement. However, we should recall the occurrence of cramps as a part of the clinical radicular syndrome and the fact that some authors stress the presence of myalgias as a component of radicular pain elicited by irritation of a root (Frykholm, 1947, 1951). These indurations or "partial contractures" may, therefore, well be another manifestation of such myalgia.

TREATMENT OF MYALGIA. The aim of the treatment is above all the suppression of vertebral mechanical conflict. It is astonishing to see in certain cases, and especially when the gluteal muscles are involved, that the tenderness of these indurated bundles suddenly subsides after an appropriate and properly conducted manipulation on the spine. Often, this is not sufficient and one should proceed with a local treatment, the best appearing to be stretching the muscle. The latter may be obtained by making the patient assume forced positions, variable according to the muscle reaction. Novocain injections or even those of saline solution may bring about a favorable therapeutic effect, in case of small size of the indurations and particularly in those cases where a localized pressure elicits a sharp momentary pain. Different forms of massage may be effective: petrissage, local vibration, or pressure. Then with the tips of the fingers, going from the surface of the skin towards the deep tissues, one should explore the muscles.

We have been trying to find analogous phenomena in paravertebral muscles. They are much more difficult to reveal at that level. The patient should be placed in a favorable position (supine for the neck, prone for the lumbar region, or in sitting position for the back). Slow and deep maneuvers will relax the regional muscles at the levels of the spine. With some practice one will generally perceive at the affected level (often somewhat below) and only on one side, one or two small hard cords, tense and extremely tender if the pressure upon them is sufficiently precise. They generally disappear after a successful manipulation. A question remains: Does manipulation suppress the conflict responsible for the genesis of these cords, or is the therapeutic effect due to the stretching of the muscle? What is remarkable is that when by local massage or stretching of the muscles, without manipulation, we succeed in reducing the muscular tension of these fascicles, the patient is at once relieved of all distress and feels free not only from local pain (lumbar, dorsal, or cervical) but often of the radiating pain. An injection of Novocain, often difficult to accurately localize, can give the same result.

These particular muscular states can be compared with those described under the name of "myogelose" or "tenoperiostose." These terms refer to painful, functional muscle disturbances (acute or chronic) without any known humeral or anatomo-pathological cause that one can encounter in any muscle, although they usually occur with certain regional predisposition.

They are attributed to the physical strain of one or several muscles generated by unaccustomed work which is either too prolonged or repeated. This physical strain can also be the cause of static disorders or an involvement of a joint (coxarthrose, gonarthrose) disturbing the normal functioning of the muscles and bringing about abnormal fatigue in some of them. The frequency of the hip muscles pain has been mentioned as a sequel of discal sciatica. It was attributed, however, to the involvement of the posterior joints and was treated by infiltration of these joints. Travell (1955) has studied in great detail particular examples of muscle pain which are held responsible for projected pain. She considers them as very common phenomena and treats them in infiltrating the most tender points (trigger points, the irritation of which is responsible for the projected pain) (see also Kohlrausch, 1961).

PHYSICAL DIAGNOSIS OF THE MINOR
INTERVERTEBRAL DERANGEMENTS

In the acute painful syndromes such as lumbago, sciatica, torticollis, etc., the spinal involvement manifests itself by a marked contracture, an antalgic attitude, a stiffness, and a definite limitation of the movement in certain directions. It is on these elements, as well be seen later, that is based the system we propose for the choice of various manipulative techniques to be used.

However, in many cases of vertebral pain that are essentially chronic, such as lumbago, dorsalgia, and cervico-occipital pain, the specific spinal symptomatology is much less marked and sometimes appears as nonexistent during an examination of the spine, if conducted according to the classical technique. Yet, in chronic cases, just as in a case of acute disturbance with a marked muscular contracture, there is generally only one vertebral level which is responsible for the distress of the patient. Hence the importance of being able to reveal and determine, as precisely as possible, the origin of this distress in order to conduct treatment by manipulation.

The localization of the level which is involved in such chronic cases has not been of principal interest in order to apply classical treatments. It is only in the case of pain related to a discal hernia, when surgery is contemplated, that such precision becomes indispensable. Even then, it is not so much the examination of the spine itself, with the exception of the search of the pain elicited by local pressure radiating from there, that determines the segmental diagnosis, but rather the neurological signs: topography of the pain, reflex changes, muscle weakness, or the results of an EMG examination, as well as radiological signs of de Sèze *et al.* (1951). But in the final analysis, it is the myelography which will demonstrate, in doubtful cases, the presence of discal herniation.

Thus, the physician is more dependent upon the signs of radicular character than on the signs provided by local examination of the spine itself for the diagnosis. And yet, it is in cases of discal herniation that the signs of intervertebral derangement should be most marked.

But how do we make a diagnosis when these radicular signs are absent? What is the local expression of these minor derangements currently observed in clinical practice?

It is certainly the absence of a clear and indisputable semiology that accounts for the opinion so often held that these derangements are only imaginary. It appears, however, quite difficult to deny their existence after having discussed their nature. It is indeed fortunate that here anatomopathology comes to the rescue of common sense in showing that their somatic reality is not unreasonable to assume.

The purpose of this chapter is to make a rapid, critical review of the signs that we can reveal in such cases. We do not mean to imply that they permit us to affirm the existence of a mechanical derangement or the necessity of manipulative treatment. They are simply the expression of local distress and do not prejudice their cause. They have nothing specific and even the most evocative manifestation, resulting from a lateral pressure in the opposite direction of two successive spines, one below the other, brings only a presumptive evidence. It is on the basis of the medical history, the clinical examination, the radiological evidence, and the complementary tests that the diagnosis of a minor mechanical derangement at a particular vertebral level can be made.

The local examination will simply allow us to recognize its existence, to localize its level, and to delineate its characters as precisely as possible. This last point is of threefold interest:

1. To reveal the necessary criteria for the therapeutic decision and, if manipulative therapy is indicated, to choose a specific maneuver.

2. To determine the effect, beneficial or not, of the treatment by the changes of these objective signs, in addition to the subjective reports of the patients.

3. To evaluate more specifically the degree to which the problem is truly resolved (disappearance of the local signs) or, only partially improved (partial persistence of the signs) when the patient is relieved of pain or discomfort.

In the last case a complementary treatment (the nature of which is to be determined) should be presented or a permanent fragility of the segment under consideration ascertained. One must not expect to find very marked signs but one must know how to analyze them with precision. They can be validated only if compared with the findings at neighboring levels or on the opposite side. These are essentially discrete signs, revealed by palpation (conducted with a particular technique) and by applying local pressure. Such pressure should be quite light and easily graded. A sudden persistent pressure, exerted by an unrestricted finger, will be painful for anyone and anywhere. It must be done lightly and firmly, never forcefully.

We shall first take a look at examinations using *pressure,* then we shall see what can be achieved by palpation.

Pressure Maneuvers

Axial Pressure on the Spine (Fig. 21)

A moderate axial pressure on the spine, which should be painless at the uninvolved segments, is a well-known maneuver very often used during the examination of vertebral pain. It reveals only whether or not there is something abnormal at one particular

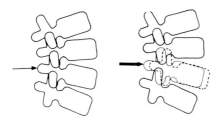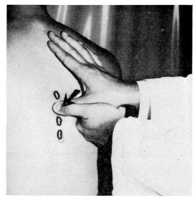

Figure 21. Axial pressure over a spinal process. *Left* and *Center* show different degrees of pressure. *Right* shows the way maneuver is carried out. Slight pressure or even simple rubbing elicits an acute superficial tenderness in case of a simple "apophysitis" *(Left)*. A more vigorous pressure exerted with the thumb, preferably with the other thumb being interposed between the patient and the pressing thumb *(Center* and *Right)* mobilizes the vertebra and may elicit discal pain or tenderness in the posterior joints.

level. In case of induced pain, one may deal as well with a mechanical derangement as with a tumor or infection. In certain cases of discal hernias, it arouses a radiating pain.

A cause of error should be avoided, namely the presence of an apophysitis (Tavernier, 1949), characterized by a particular sensitivity of the apex of the spine, a common disturbance which is benign and often due to repeated rubbing (e.g. on a chair back) or a superficial tramatism. But in the case of apophysitis, the pressure arousing tenderness may be relieved by a very superficial injection of Novocain. It is quite different from the deep pain aroused by slow and steady pressure, which one may exert through the interposed thumb of the other hand. This maneuver indicates the presence of a local disturbance. The latter can painfully affect the vertebrae itself or the intervertebral joints located immediately above and below it.

We will extend the analysis a little further with the following maneuver:

Lateral Pressure in the Opposite Direction Upon the Spinous Processes of the Two Adjacent Vertebrae (Figs. 22 and 23)

We have tried to determine a maneuver which facilitates a search of painful movements at a precise level of the spine. The one which we describe here is essentially a maneuver of forced rotation.

The patient is in the most comfortable position (seated for an examination of the dorsal region or lying prone across a table for an examination of the lumbar region), in such a way that his spinous processes stick out clearly. We exert pressure, with the thumb, toward the left side on all the spinous processes of the region; then we press toward the right side. This pressure must be quite delicate, tangential to the surface of the skin. In a case of local derangement, this maneuver will not be painful at the level of all the vertebrae except one. And, generally, it will only be painful in one direction (toward the right or left side). It is, as a rule, the same vertebra, which is painful during the axial pressure of the spinous process.

Next, while maintaining lateral pressure on the spinous pro-

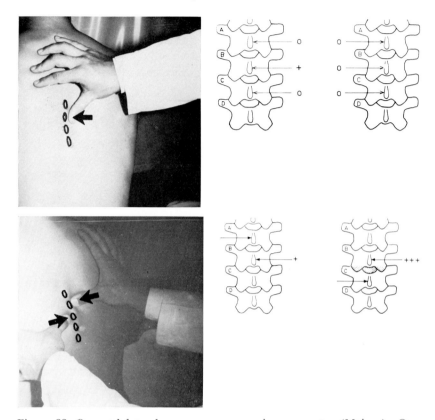

Figure 22. Opposed lateral pressure over a spinous process (Maigne). One exerts a lateral pressure (from right to left, and from left to right) over the spines if they are accessible *(Top left)*. Let us consider an example where the pressure over the spine of *B* vertebra is painful from right to left *(Top center)* and not painful from left to right *(Top right)*. In order to localize the involved segment, one exerts simultaneously with a painful pressure a counter pressure over the spine *A* located just above *(Bottom left and center)*, then over the spine *C* of the vertebra located just below *(Bottom right)*; the pain is exaggerated when the corresponding segment is involved *(Bottom right)* and is not changed in the other case *(Bottom middle.)*

cess in the painful direction, we will exert pressure in the *opposite direction* on the adjacent spinous process above, then on the adjacent spinous process below. One of these maneuvers will clearly

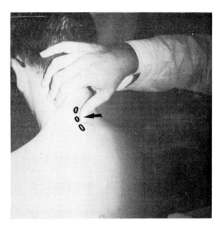

Figure 23.
Lateral pressure over the spinal process of a lower cervical vertebra.

increase the provoked pain, the other will not. This clearly reveals the pain while twisting a vertebral segment in one direction and not in the other. It is quite analogous to what one finds in the discal sciaticas during a global maneuver of the spine: free rotation in one direction, painful and blocked rotation in the other. This finding is quite evocative of mechanical derangement, since in the tumoral affections or in infections, the pain is generally elicited in both directions. Moreover, this examination is the only one which brings indispensable information as to the application of direct manipulation according to the system which we propose ("rule of no pain and free movement"). Let us insist again on the fact that it is an excellent means by which one can determine with precision the level of a discal hernia. This maneuver obviously cannot be used for the middle and lower cervical spine.

Pressure on the Supraspinous Ligament

This is done with the ring of a key that is held lightly between two adjacent spinous processes (Fig. 24). Such pressure on the normal ligament is painless. If we look for it, we will find with a certain frequency, this ligamentary pain. It is a constant sign of an intervertebral microderangement, or it may constitute a sequel of partial derangements, or it can be encountered under other circumstances. It is not rare to see this ligamentary tenderness being a residual of a discal herniation, causing by itself a pro-

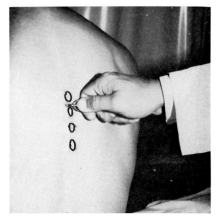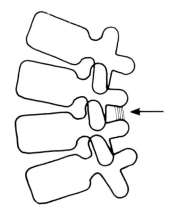

Figure 24. Pressure over the supraspinous ligament. This pressure is preferably exerted with a key ring.

tracted low back pain which only appropriate treatment will relieve. It may also be the case of cervical post-traumatic derangements, where abnormal sensitivity of the supraspinal ligament can maintain an intractable pain. In the case which interests us, it is the association with other signs which makes this finding so important, and above all the fact that it localizes precisely the painful level.

The Paramedian Posterior Point of the Painful Posterior Joint

We are concerned here with a tender point which is practically always found in minor vertebral derangements (Fig. 25). It is localized one finger's width from the midline. It is very precise and always present in this position. According to the radiological controls which we have conducted, it corresponds to the posterior joint with an adjacent posterior branch of the spinal nerve. It is unilateral, so that identification of this tender point is made by comparison with the opposite side and with the adjacent levels. The finger pressure should be moderate. We are aware of limitations of the diagnostic value that may be accorded to a "tender point." The one which is described here does not escape this prudent rule. Nevertheless, the fact of arousing sharp tenderness

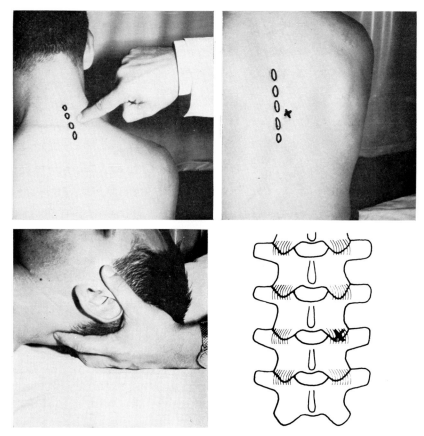

Figure 25. The paramedian posterior articular tender point. It is located one fingerwidth from the midline and is practically always found in the minor intervertebral derangements. It seems to correspond to the bony structures of the posterior joint (diagram). In the case of the cervical spine, the patient preferably should be in a lying position; in case of the dorsal spine, he should preferably be in a sitting position. This tender point is very precise so that even a moderate pressure elicits acute pain, while pressure over the symmetrical point is painless.

at a particular level on only one side in the case of dorsal or cervical pain, draws attention to this segment and calls for a more detailed analysis.

A more meticulous examination will show that this point

corresponds to a modification of the local tissue, an observation to which we will return when we will consider information furnished by palpation. Besides, it may be much more relevant and interesting to proceed in the reverse order, that is to say, not looking first for the tender pressure point but proceeding at the beginning of the examination with a careful superficial palpation of the paravertebral groove, using the tips of the fingers only, with the technique described in the following section.

Information Furnished by Soft Tissue Palpation

If for us palpation is only one of the elements of diagnosis, it constitutes for osteopaths an essential element of vertebral examination. The information that they look for is threefold:

1. A modification of the paravertebral tissue.

2. A modification of the relative position of the spinous and the transverse processes.

3. Especially, a modification of the interspinal mobility.

Let us add that we are referring to an extremely light palpation in which the fingers of the operator do not exert any pressure. We will come back to the osteopathic examination because of its historical interest. But, let us say from the outset, that we cannot consider as valid the apparent modification of the relative position of the spinous or of the transverse processes which plays such an important role in the osteopathic examination. Anatomy teaches us that the spinous processes never are aligned and that the interspinal spaces that we are able to palpate are as much a function of the form of the processes as of the distance between them. As for the transverse processes, the muscular and cutaneous tissues that cover them make illusory all attempts to estimate the difference of few millimeters which differentiates the normal from the pathological. Nor will we consider any further the evaluation of the minimal differences between the comparative movements in flexion or extension of the spinous processes which signify to the osteopath the existence of a "lesion." On the other hand, we consider important the information furnished by a careful palpation of the paravertebral tissues. It is always surprising for a patient, as well as for the observer, to see the trained doctor locate, with the help of palpation, the painful level of the spine, and to find that the pressure exerted at the level of a small zone characterized by modification of the local tissue is susceptible to arouse the usual pain of the patient, with its usual radiation. This area, which is only one or two square centimeters wide always corresponds to the paramedian tender point at a finger's width from the midline.

The Technique of This Examination

The patient must be in a relaxed position, lying supine for the neck, seated for the dorsal region, and prone for the lumbar region. The operator uses the tip of the index or the middle finger. He runs his finger, without pressing, along a line parallel to the line of spinous processes, about a finger's width from it. It is on this line that the modifications are best perceived.

In a case of minor vertebral derangement, we may find a small zone at only one vertebral level and on only one side from the midline where the consistency of the superficial tissue is different, giving the impression of a light local edema, while, in depth, some muscular fascicles seem to be stretched, contracted, sometimes even giving the impression of a veritable small cord. This zone is very small, one or two square centimeters, with maximal signs in its center. It is at this point, as mentioned above, that the slightest pressure gives rise to an acute tenderness that one does not find at the adjacent level or on the opposite side. Such symptomatology, admittedly quite discreet, is found in all cases of intervertebral derangements. This finding is very difficult to evaluate in the lumbar region, or when there is a marked contracture, but this symptomatology is quite obvious for those who have the skill to look for it, at the level of the neck, or dorsal region, in both subacute or chronic involvements. It is clearly not pathognomonic of a mechanical disorder, but it gives some interesting information for the doctor. He will appreciate the efficacy of his treatment as much by the attenuation of the patient's complaints as that of this local sign. The response of these tissues to different modalities of brisk or slow maneuvers, pressing or stroking, repeated or not, will be a valuable guide for their choice.

These trophic modifications and muscular contractions are due either to a particular reaction around the posterior joints or to an irritation of the posterior branch of the spinal nerve. They should be considered in the framework of the syndrome of the posterior branch of the spinal nerve (Lazorthes *et al.,* 1965). They constitute a constant component of the minor reversible intervertebral derangements, generating pain and discomfort and responding best to manipulative therapy.

The following chapter offers a more systematic description of the examining procedures in relation to a review of functional anatomy applied to manual medicine of the spine.

Chapter 5

Review of Regional Functional Anatomy Applied to Manual Medicine

THE CERVICAL SPINE

Anatomy

T HE CERVICAL SPINE is composed of seven vertebrae and offers a curvature with a forward convexity (cervical lordosis). The apex of this curvature corresponds to C4 and its arc continues down to D2 (Figs. 26 and 27).

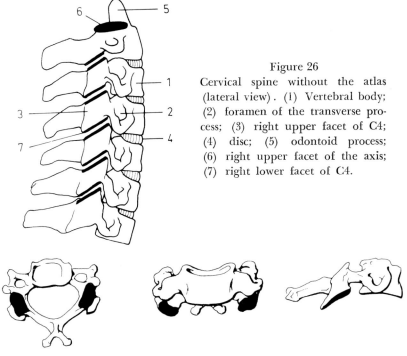

Figure 26

Cervical spine without the atlas (lateral view). (1) Vertebral body; (2) foramen of the transverse process; (3) right upper facet of C4; (4) disc; (5) odontoid process; (6) right upper facet of the axis; (7) right lower facet of C4.

Figure 27. Mid-cervical vertebra and its articular facets. *Left,* upper aspect; *Center,* dorsal aspect; *Right,* lateral aspect.

Two first cervical vertebrae, the atlas (Fig. 28) and the axis (Fig 29) are different from the others. There is no disc between these two vertebrae. The first disc is present between C2 and C3 (Fig. 30).

The cervical spine shows a number of peculiarities which are important to be considered here.

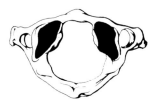

Figure 28. Atlas (view from the top).

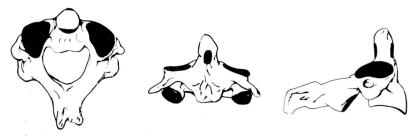

Figure 29. Axis. *Left,* upper view; *Center,* anterior view; *Right,* lateral view.

Articular Facets

Their inclination increases below the axis, the facets of which are almost horizontal, while they offer a plane of 45 degrees over the horizontal for the other vertebrae (Fig. 31). Along the sagittal axis the lower facets are oriented posteriorly and slightly medially. This disposition facilitates movement of gliding in all directions but mostly in flexion-extension.

Spinal Processes

Atlas has no spinal process. The size of the latter increases from C3 to C7. They are oriented almost horizontally and interfere one with another in hyperextension.

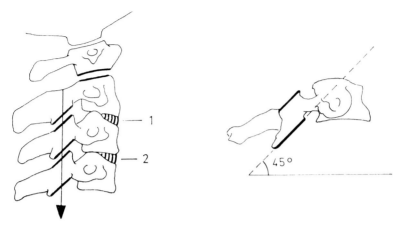

Figure 30. The posterior joint and the first cervical disc.

Figure 31. Inclination of the plane of the facet over the horizontal line.

Palpation reveals that the spinal process of C7 is the only one which clearly protrudes under the skin. It is the only one which is most frequently bifidous.

Uncus

The unci characterize cervical vertebrae from C3 to C7. Located laterally, they determine a saddle form of the upper aspect of the cervical vertebrae (Fig. 32). The lower aspect presents a converse shape, offering an incisure corresponding to the uncus.

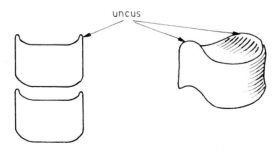

Figure 32. *Left,* frontal section of two cervical vertebrae (bodies) ; *Right,* the saddle shape of the upper aspect of the cervical vertebra.

As is well known it was Luschka (1850) who was the first one to stress this peculiarity of the cervical vertebrae.

Since that time, it has been customary to consider this unco-vertebral area as true joints having articular cavity, cartilaginous layer, and articular capsule. The disc is considered to occupy only the center of the vertebral plate (Fig. 33). Töndury, (1953) however, expressed a different view on this point.

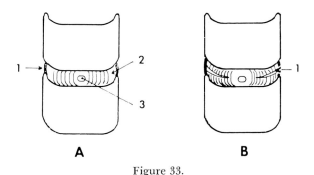

Figure 33.

A, Classical concept of the uncus. (1) unco-vertebral ligament, (2) articular cavity, (3) disc.

B, Concept of the uncus according to Töndury (see text p. 67-68). (1) fissure.

The importance of these articulations is due to the intimate relationship between them and the vertebral artery as well as the sympathetic rami which are present around it. These joints may be the site of an arthrosis with cartilaginous lesions and osteophytes. The latter usually project posteriorly toward the intervertebral foramen where the spinal nerve emerges, being lateral to the vertebral artery (Fig. 34).

In addition, it is often found that the pulp of the degenerated disc infiltrates the very cavity of the uncovertebral joint, which may be the site of an arthrosis. Thus, the union of the posterior osteophytes of unco-arthrotic origin and of the posterolateral discal hernia form a nodule which projects itself into the intervertebral foramen and which de Sèze has called a disco-osteophytic nodule (Fig. 35). Cervicobrachial neuralgia often results from the compression of a cervical root by an osteophyte. This herniation is

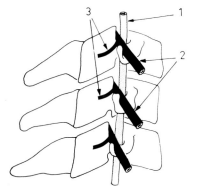

Figure 34. Vertebral artery and spinal nerves. (1) Vertebral artery; (2) anterior branch of the spinal nerve; (3) posterior branch of the spinal nerve.

generally called by the surgeons "hard hernia" in contradistinction with the "soft hernia" formed by a nucleus pulposus prolapsed through the ruptured annulus.

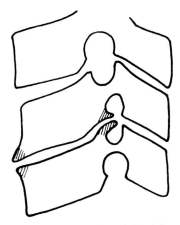

Figure 35. Disco-osteophytic nodule (after de Sèze).

Töndury (Fig. 33) does not accept the notion of an uncovertebral joint (1953); he believes that one deals with a lateral fissure of the disc which appears at about eleven years of age and extends more and more in depth with advancing age, so that, finally, the communication with the nucleus pulposus is established. Thus, the discal pulp may migrate peripherally and contribute to the formation of the disco-osteophytic nodule. The unciform processes derive from the neural arc of the cervical vertebrae. In the *fetus,* one finds collagenous fibers which reach the processes of the adjacent vertebrae. There are no vertebral fissures. The discs are limited by epiphyseal cartilage. In the *newborn* collagenous fibers of the uncal (unciform) process unite with the peripheral layers of the disc and even in children of 6 to 7 years of age, there is no evidence of an unco-vertebral "joint." Cervical disc shows narrow fissures from the age of 9 or 10 only. Töndury (1953) showed by histological studies that these are the results of ruptured collagenous tissue and do not represent true joints. The study of the discs in adults of increasing age shows that this rupture progressively reaches the discal center or may be extended from one side of the disc to the other. Lateral discal hernias are formed in this fashion with a prolapse directed toward the intervertebral foramen, the diameter of which is being narrowed in this way.

Transverse Processes and Vertebral Artery

Transverse processes originate from the lateral mass by two roots which form the transverse foramen (Fig. 36).

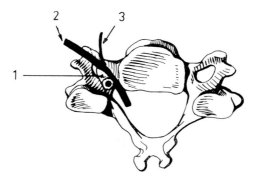

Figure 36. Transverse processes, vertebral artery (1) and spinal nerve with its anterior branch (2) and its posterior branch (3).

Transverse foramen is present in each cervical vertebra. However, it is small for C7 where only the vertebral vein is located. The foramena of six first vertebrae thus form an interrupted canal in which the vertebral artery (branch of the subclavian artery) is located, as well as sympthetic plexus, the vertebral vein and the nerve of François Frank. At the level of the upper cervical spine, this artery makes a detour, as the transverse foramina of the atlas are located laterally to those of the axis. This forces the artery to make an arc with lateral convexity. Then, the artery describes another arc between the transverse foramen and the foramen magnum of the occipital bone, having a lateral convexity (Fig. 37).

One may well imagine the traction to which this artery is submitted as the head moves from one extreme position to another (Fig. 38). It could be shown by arteriography that the circulation *was arrested during a movement of the head in extension with rotation to one side and lateral bending to the other.*

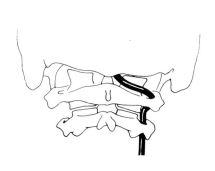
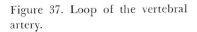
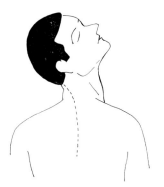

Figure 37. Loop of the vertebral artery.

Figure 38.

In fact, the close contact of the vertebral artery with the moving bony structures of the cervico-occipital joint explains why it can be injured by excessive manipulation of the cervical spine.

As known, severe accidents have been described following manipulation, or even as a result of prolonged extreme positions of the head, including compression of the artery between the atlas and the occiput. In a normal subject, transitory interruption of the circulation in the vertebral artery does not generate any disturbance, as the blood supply of the brainstem is maintained by the vertebral artery of the opposite side. However, the situation is completely different if these arteries have atheromas and if the diameter of the artery on the opposite side is reduced too much. Moreover, the anatomical variations and anomalies are often present in these arteries. Thus, transitory neurological deficits may be induced (vertigo, syncopies, diplopia) in extreme rotation of the head (Kleyn and Nieuwenhuyse 1927).

The complications of the unco-arthrosis or, less frequently, of the arthrosis of the posterior joints may produce segmental narrowing of the artery, responsible for what has been called the "vertebral artery syndrome."

Malformations of the Cervico-occipital Joint

Malformations of the cervico-occipital joint, although often remaining silent, are relatively frequent and may be associated with neurological complications at times revealed or exaggerated by the local trauma.

This is why one should avoid manipulations without a preliminary radiological examination of the subject in whom the neck appears to be too short or in whom the hairline is too low, or the head movements too limited.

The most frequently malformation is the presence of a basilar impression which may be easily revealed by x-rays showing that the odontoid process ascends the Chamberlain line (Fig. 39). This line is drawn on the lateral x-ray picture between the posterior border of the bony palate and the dorsal edge of the foramen magnum.

Another landmark is given by the line of Fischgold on the AP

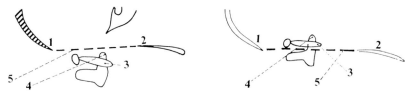

Figure 39. Chamberlain line. *Left,* normal subject; *Right,* basilar impression. (1) Posterior border of occipital foramen; (2) posterior border of the boney palate; (3) atlas; (4) odontoid process; (5) Chamberlain line.

view—the bimastoid line usually goes through the joint between the atlas and the occipital bone (Fig. 40). When there is basilar impression, the atlas-odontoid bony complex is found above this line. Basilar impression may be associated with other malformations: occipitalization of the atlas, nonfusion of the posterior arc of the atlas, stenosis or deformation of the foramen magnum, dislocation of the joint between the atlas and the axis, spina bifida, etc. It is hardly necessary to add that these malformations are associated with those of other nervous and vascular structures and that one should abstain from manipulating these vulnerable structures (see also Godlewski, 1966; Godlewski and Dry, 1964).

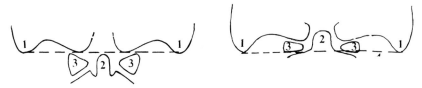

Figure 40. Fischgold line. *Left,* normal subject; *Right,* basilar impression. (1) Mastoid; (2) odontoid process; (3) atlas; (4) bimastoid line of Fischgold.

Range of Motion of the Cervical Spine

The mobility of the cervical spine and its resistance are remarkable when one thinks of all the stresses which are exerted upon it while it supports a large ball of 4 to 5 kilograms, moving in all directions, increasing in certain individuals by additional heavy loads.

The cervical spine is more mobile than any other spinal segment. One should consider the following:

1. The height of the discs in relation to that of the vertebral body: one-third for the cervical spine, one-sixth for the dorsal spine and one-third for the lumbar spine (Olivier and Olivier, 1963).

2. The small anteroposterior and transverse diameters in relation to the height of the vertebral body.

3. The orientation of the facets.

4. The particular geometry of the first cervical vertebrae, atlas and axis, which contribute to the occipitocervical joint.

Flexion-Extension

At the level of the occipitospinal joint, these movements essentially take place in the joint between the atlas and the occipital bone by gliding of the condyle forward and backward over the facets of the atlas, respectively for extension and flexion: 20 degrees for extension; 30 degrees for flexion (Olivier and Olivier, 1963) (Fig. 41).

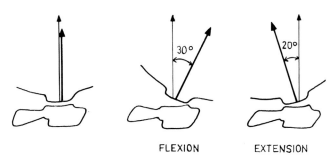

FLEXION   EXTENSION

Figure 41. Movements of flexion and extension between the occiput and atlas.

However, this movement spreads over the joints below and the amplitude of this total movement is great indeed. These movements were studied by many authors, namely, by Raou on cadavers (1952), and by de Sèze *et al.,* 1951, using x-rays of living subjects. Here are the results obtained by de Sèze *et al.:*

	Hyperflexion	*Hyperextension*	*Total*
C2-C3	5°	8°	13°
C3-C4	5°5	10°	15°5
C4-C5	7°	12°	19°
C5-C6	9°	18°5	27°5
C6-C7	6°5	11°	17°5
		Grand total	92°5

Kottke and Mundale (1959) published the following data for 87 subjects between the ages of 15 and 30:

Occiput-Atlas	*Flexion*	*Extension*	*Total*
			20°
C1-C2	2°	9°	11°
C2-C3	8°	3°	11°
C3-C4	7°	9°	16°
C4-C5	10°	8°	18°
C5-C6	10°	11°	21°
C6-C7	13°	5°	18°

Using goniometry, Buck, Dameron, Dow, and Skowlund (1959) report the following averages in young students:

Total flexion 66° ⎫
Total extension 73° ⎬ young males
    ⎭

Total flexion 69° ⎫
Total extension 81° ⎬ young females
    ⎭

The averages of Kottke and Mundale (1959) are as follows:
    Flexion 70° ± 10°
    Extension 75° ± 10°

These averages are derived from a study of young normal subjects.

Lateral Bending

OCCIPITO-CERVICAL JOINT. The range of motion is 15° to 20° limited by stretching the anterior and posterior structures as well as by lateral ligaments (Olivier and Olivier, 1963). Between the atlas and the axis, there is only 5 degrees of motion, which as seen below, is associated with no rotation of the head.

OTHER CERVICAL VERTEBRAE. Lateral bending is limited when it is not associated with other motions. If, however, an associated movement of rotation brings the facet to the same side, the range of lateral bending is increased. As is well known Lovett (1907) claimed that lateral bending and rotation cannot be completely dissociated. One may state that in practice no movement of appreciable amplitude is possible in either direction without these two movements being combined one with the other. In such cases, lateral bending and rotation are directed to the same side. Raou (1952) measured, on cadavers, the maximal amplitude of these movements. He found 30° to 50° of lateral bending for the entire cervical spine, according to different subjects. Kottke and Mundale (1959) found 45° ± 10°. When one actively bends the neck laterally, as much as possible, the range of motion of the middle and lower cervical spine is the same as for its rotation to the same side. The difference between these two motions is due to the upper cervical segment which in the case of lateral bending is associated with the rotation to the opposite side, keeping the face in the frontal plane, while, when one studies the rotation of the entire cervical spine, the upper segment rotates in the same direction as the remaining cervical spine.

Rotation

In the joint between the atlas and the axis the rotation predominates, while the movement of lateral bending and flexion-extension are very limited. However, although the rotation is very pronounced, representing 30° to 35° to each side (half of the total cervical rotation), it is not pure. If one considers the axis being immobile, during rotation, both lateral masses of the atlas glide along the anteroposterior axis, although each of them moves in the opposite direction over the facets located just below. When the head is rotated to the left, the left lateral mass moves backward, while the right one moves forward. Moreover, the orientation of the facets which are markedly convex along the anteroposterior axis results in a lateral bending to the side opposite to that toward which the rotation is effected. This is a screwtype movement (Roud, 1913). If, therefore, one wishes to implicate this joint, one should associate rotation with a lateral bending to the opposite side. This simultaneous lowering of the head during its rotation compensates the effect of torsion of the spinal nerves and the vertebral artery (Olivier and Olivier 1963). Buck and associates (1959) report the following range of motion for the total rotation of the cervical spine: 146° for the young male; 147° for the young female. According to Kottke and Mundale (1959), these figures are 75° ± 10° for rotation toward each side.

Active Movements

Muscular contractions obviously are not able to duplicate the total passive range of motion. For this one should apply an outside force, mobilization or manipulation.

During voluntary movements of extension the muscles splenius capitis and cervicis, as well as the complexus and perispinal muscles (intertransversii and others) are involved. When the scapulae are immobilized, the levator anguli scapuli participates in the action.

Rotation of the head is essentially due to the contraction of posterior recti and obliquus superior and inferior.

Rotation of the neck and of the head to the right is due to the synergetic contraction of the right splenius and left sternocleido-mastoideus.

If the sternocleidomastoideus contracts on one side only, the neck is bent laterally and rotated so that the face is oriented toward the opposite side.

Let us add that EMG studies showed that continuous activity is present in the cervical muscles during the alert state while it subsides during sleep (head-drop) (see Lescure, 1959; Fielding, 1964; Florent and Gillot, 1966).

Applications to Manipulation

Manipulation in flexion and extension at the level of the upper cervical spine involves mostly the joint between the atlas and the occipital bone.

Manipulation in rotation with lateral bending to the opposite side involves mostly the joint between the atlas and the axis, particularly when the head is in extension.

On the contrary, manipulation of the upper cervical spine in rotation with a marked lateral bending to the same side involves mostly C2-C3, since when one induces lateral bending on the same side as rotation, the joint between the atlas and the axis is blocked.

Finally, at the level of the lower or middle cervical spine lateral flexion and rotation are generally performed to the same side.

However, these observations are not valid, unless cervical mobility is normal or only slightly limited; they are not necessarily applicable to the spine with disturbed biomechanics, as for example, in the case of a herniated disc. It is obvious that the movement which may initiate the recovery of cervical mobility may not be comprised of rotation associated with lateral bending to the same side. Such a movement may be possible and useful; however, it may be impossible and noxious. Everything depends upon the modality of discal herniation. As far as we are concerned, it is only the analysis of painful or restricted movements which contain the key to the correct combination of manipulative maneuvers, according to the rule of no pain and free movement.

Examination of the Cervical Spine

Mobility (Figs. 42 to 44)

PATIENT IN SITTING POSITION. One examines the patient first in a sitting position determining the range of motion of flexion, lateral bending, rotation, and extension. One asks him at first to perform actively these movements and then one examines the passive range of motion, the patient being completely relaxed. One notes the tender points and limited movements.

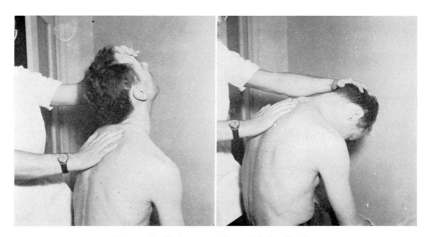

Figure 42. *Left,* extension; *Right,* flexion.

One may accept with Beal and Beckwith (1963) the following:

1. The normal flexion of the neck should permit the subject to touch the sternum with his chin.

2. The normal extension should permit one to look upward along a vertical line.

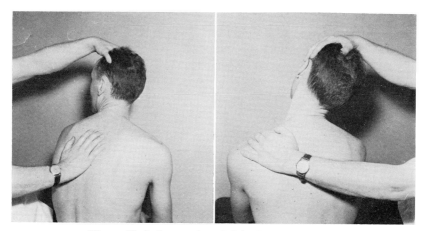

Figure 43. *Left,* rotation; *Right,* lateral bending.

3. The normal lateral bending should permit one to have the ear touching the shoulder.

4. In rotation, the chin should touch the acromioclavicular joint.

PATIENT SUPINE. Examination of the cervical spine mobility is facilitated by the patient's relaxation. This relaxation is best achieved when the patient is supine with his head hanging beyond the table, the physician supporting it with his hands placed

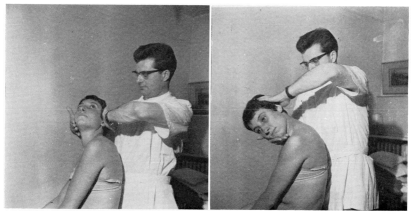

Figure 44. *Left,* combined left rotation and extension; *Right,* combined left rotation and flexion.

Orthopedic Medicine

under the occiput, while his fingers palpate the paravertebral grooves on each side (Fig. 45). This is the method Mennell (1949) advised.

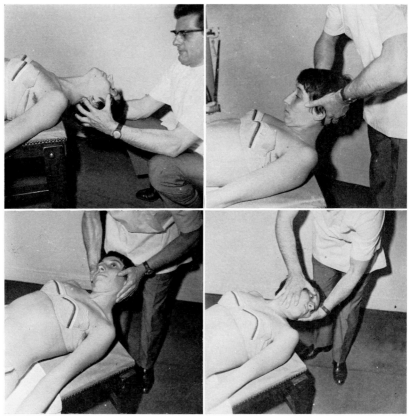

Figure 45. Patient supine, examination of global mobility. *Top left,* in extension; *Top right,* in flexion; *Bottom left,* lateral bending; *Bottom right,* in rotation.

Range of passive movements, particularly those of rotation and lateral bending, is greatest in this position. The physician will evaluate, at first, global movements, then he will try to determine more precisely the level of their limitation—upper cervical region (Fig. 46), middle or lower cervical region (Fig. 47).

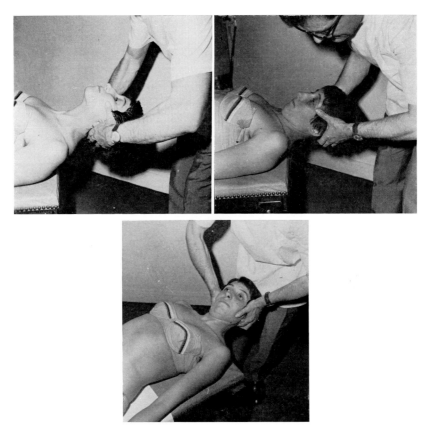

Figure 46. Patient supine, examination of mobility of the upper cervical spine. *Top left,* in extension; *Top right,* in flexion; *Bottom,* in lateral flexion.

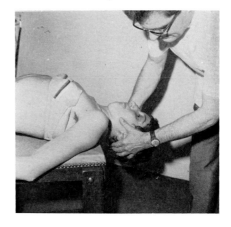

Figure 47.
Extension of the lower cervical spine; the physician blocks the upper cervical spine in flexion.

It is important to look in this position for what Mennell (1949) called a "lateral carrying movement of the neck" (Fig. 48). The hands of the physician remain parallel to each other and he displaces them together, first to the left then to the right, without imparting to the neck any lateral flexion, but moving it lightly to the right or to the left. It is important that the shoulders of the patient and the base of his neck remain immobile and that the line of his eyes rest strictly parallel to the edge of the table. This reminds us of the movement of the Cambogian dancers. The disappearance of this lateral carrying movement may help to localize segmental rigidity. Indeed, according to the location of the physician's finger tips either at the lower, mid or upper cervical level, the local rigidity may be tested. On the other hand, this maneuver may be an excellent relaxing exercise for the patient.

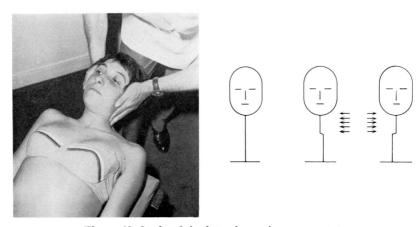

Figure 48. Study of the lateral carrying movement.

There are other maneuvers which permit one to localize a limitation of the segmental vertebral movement. These are those which will be described in the fourth part of this book and which are related to the techniques of manipulation itself.

Segmental Examination

The existence of intervertebral derangement is manifest in certain cases; for example, in a typical case of cervicobrachial neuralgia of radicular origin. However, even then, it is important to look for local signs which may be indispensable for manipulative therapy. The latter, as we know, is based upon the analysis of painful and restricted movements. However, in some cases of chronic conditions, there is an additional global stiffness involving a moderate painless limitation of all motions, masking the presence of a segment vulnerable to an extreme movement in one direction. It is then essential to reveal this minor intervertebral derangement and, most important, to determine the direction in which manipulative therapy may be helpful. We have already shown (p. 55) the essential elements of such segmental analysis. We shall review here only some of the most important signs. The latter, as we know, have no pathogenic significance, and yet their presence suggests that there is some mechanical disturbance which may be susceptible to manipulative therapy. If, in addition, the search for such signs elicits, reproduces, or exaggerates the complaints or the pain of the patient, their importance is all the more suggestive.

Pressure Points

PARAMEDIAN POSTERIOR POINT (Fig. 49). The tender point is unilateral. It is located at one finger width of the median line. It

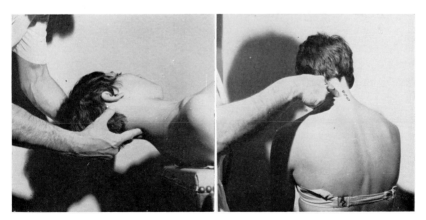

Figure 49. Posterior articular paramedian tender point. *Left,* patient supine; *Right,* patient in sitting position.

is exquisitely more tender than the adjacent areas above and below it and more tender than a symmetrical point. It corresponds
to the posterior articular bony structure, which at this point is en-
circled by the posterior branch of the spinal nerve.

It should be investigated with the patient in supine position,
the neck being completely relaxed, the head being supported by
the hands of the physician who tries to further relax the muscles
of the cervical spine, by rolling the head slightly from side to
side. Then, very gently, probing slightly with the pulp of his
medius fingers on both sides of the line of the spinal processes,
gliding them slowly from the cervicodorsal level toward the occiput, he will try to identify a small area of tissue which appears to
be under tension, having an edematous consistency, offering to
palpation a particular nodulelike formation. If the physician
slightly increases his pressure at this point, he will elicit an acute
pain. This is the "posterior point." If he does not intend to develop this particular skill of examination by palpation, which requires specific training, and which may be quite helpful in manual medicine, he may simply look for a tender point by exerting
pressure over the skin, every centimeter or so. However, the only
ones which offer interest for our present discussion are the tender
points located at one finger width from the median line. Once
this point is identified, one should look for other signs in order to
complete the examination.

AXIAL PRESSURE OVER THE SPINAL PROCESSES. After ruling out
superficial pain of the spinal process due to a simple apophysitis,
easily identified by a superficial rubbing, one will exert a firm and
protracted pressure over each spinal process, particularly at the
level of the tender "posterior point" (Fig. 50). It is appropriate
to repeat this examination with the cervical spine placed in a
normal position as well as in flexion and then in extension.

LATERAL PRESSURE OVER THE SPINAL PROCESS. If one deals with
lower cervical or upper dorsal vertebra, the lateral pressure over
the spinal process, exerted from one side, then from the other may
elicit pain (Fig. 50). The involved segment, responsible for this
pain can be exteriorized by simultaneous pressure in the opposite

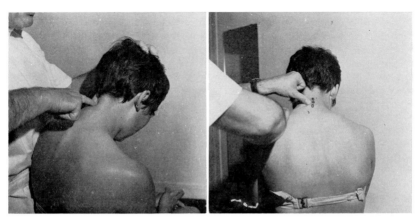

Figure 50. Pressure over a spinal process. *Left,* axial pressure; *Right,* lateral pressure.

direction, made at the level of the adjacent vertebrae above and below the one which is involved.

ANTERIOR CERVICAL POINT. The search for the anterior cervical tender point is very useful at the level of the middle or lower cervical spine, particularly when one deals with atypical pain of the upper extremity which seems to originate from the cervical spine and when one tries to determine which cervical root may be responsible for this pain.

This tender point is located in the anterolateral region of the cervical spine. The patient should be in a sitting position, facing the physician. The latter exerts a moderate pressure with the tip of his thumb directed horizontally (the right one for the left side of the neck and the left one for the right side), thus exploring one level after the other. Only the involved level is really tender, which is easy to check by exploring the opposite side or the adjacent segment above or below the tender point (Fig. 51), particularly when the pressure is maintained for a few seconds when it reproduces the pain or other complaints of the patient. It indicates the involved cervical root, compressed at its emergence from the cervical spine. This is why we call this point the anterior cervical doorbell push-button sign.

It is such examinations, systematically conducted, which permit us to demonstrate in many cases, the cervical origin of the interscapular dorsal pain or dorsal pain of stenotypists.

TENDER SUPRASPINOUS LIGAMENT. Finally, tender supraspinous ligament in the case of involvement of two lower cervical segments may be identified by the "key sign" described previously (Fig. 52).

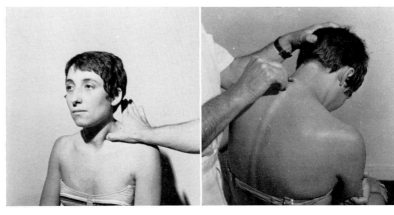

Figure 51. Cervical doorbell push-button anterior sign.

Figure 52. Key sign: pain over the supraspinous ligament.

At the level of middle and upper cervical spine, only the posterior point and the lack of local segmental mobility are easy to identify.

TRACTION AND AXIAL PRESSURE. Axial pressure is applied by both hands pressing the head of the patient. It may temporarily exacerbate the symptoms of cervical origin (Fig. 53). Conversely, and more importantly, firm traction may elicit important information (Fig. 54). It is, we believe, indispensable to try before a treatment by traction is prescribed. The latter will not be attempted before the proof is made that manual traction relieves the patient's symptoms, and it should be avoided if manual traction aggravates them.

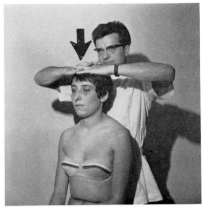
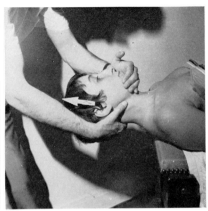

Figure 53. Axial pressure over the head.

Figure 54. Test of manual traction.

Examination of Skin Tissue

Examination of the skin as well as that of subcutaneous tissues should not be omitted. The skin-rolling technique should be used for the search for infiltrated tender areas, particularly if the pressure over them elicits habitual pain from the patient. One should also search for infiltrated and tender areas over the skin of the involved upper extremity (Fig. 55).

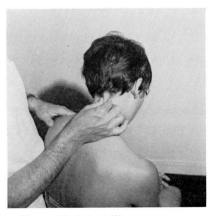

Figure 55. Skin-rolling maneuver.

Manual Muscle Testing

One should also evaluate the strength of cervical muscles, first against manual resistance. In many cases, particularly prior to the prescription of rehabilitation procedures, it is appropriate to evaluate the global strength of the extensors and the flexors of the neck, which one will test selectively. Thus, one will test the extension of the head over the neck (Fig. 56A), the extension of the neck (Fig. 56B), the flexors of the neck (Fig. 56C), the flexors of the head (Fig. 56D), the muscles producing lateral bending of the head (Fig. 56E), and those of head rotation (Fig. 56F).

CERVICODORSAL JUNCTURE
Examination of Mobility

One starts by examining the mobility of the lower cervical spine, patient being first in the sitting position, then supine, his head bending beyond the examination table, using maneuvers described on p. 76. Then one tries to locate the tender segment (see also examination of the mobility of the cervicodorsal junction in a sitting position) (Fig. 57).

Segmental Examination

The following procedure should be carried out for a segmental examination:

1. One searches for tenderness of a spinal process by exerting pressure over them.

a) One should first rule out superficial tenderness of a simple apophysitis by slight rubbing of the skin by the fingertips (Fig. 58) which a few drops of Novocain will make disappear.

b) One will note whether or not a deep pressure, protracted and firm, elicits pain (Fig. 59).

2. Then one will search for a sign of lateral and opposed pressure of the spinal process (Fig. 60) (see p. 82). If a tender process is found, pressure is exerted in the opposite sense over the spinal process located just below it, or just above it, in order to better identify the involved level (Fig. 61) and the direction in which the rotation thus induced is painful.

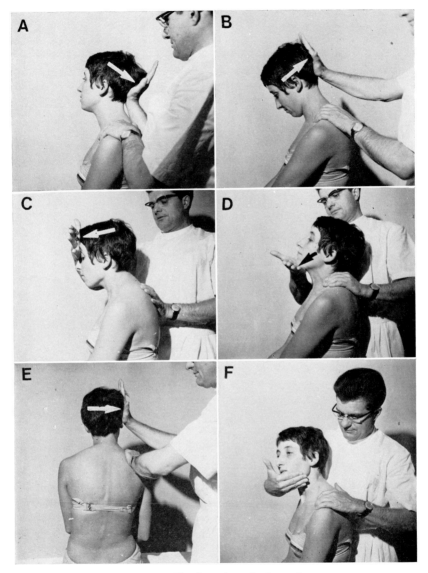

Figure 56. Testing of cervical muscles.

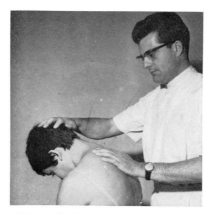

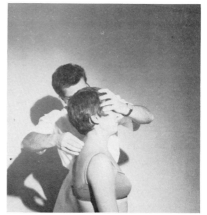

Figure 57. Examination of cervico-dorsal junction in a sitting position. *Left,* in flexion; *Top* right, in extension; *Bottom,* lateral bending.

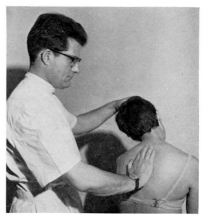

3. The use of a ring pressing over the spinal process may confirm local involvement (Fig. 62).

4. Paramedian tender point located one fingerwidth from the middle line, overlying posterior articular bony structure or "posterior articular tender point" (see p. 81) will be detected by palpation of often associated tissular changes.

5. Finally, a search is made for the anterior cervical doorbell push-button sign, in case of involvement of the last two cervical vertebrae.

6. By using the technique of skin-rolling, one will try to find a paravertebral area of cellulitis which is important to identify if it

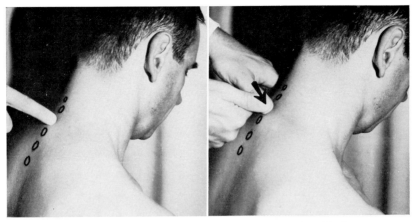

Figure 58. Search for apophysitis. Figure 59. Search with deep pressure over the spinal process.

is unilateral and corresponds to the side of spontaneous pain (Fig. 63).

DORSAL SPINE

The dorsal spine is comprised of twelve vertebrae (Figs. 64 to 66). The vertebral bodies are relatively high in relation to the intervertebral discs. The articular facets are oriented in an almost

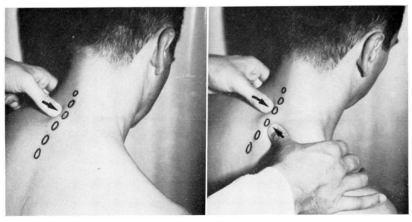

Figure 60. Lateral pressure over the spinal process. Figure 61. Lateral pressure with counter pressure.

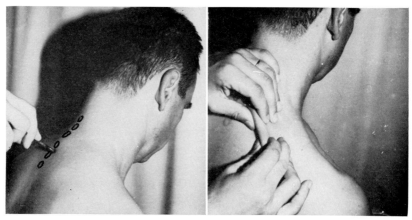

Figure 62. Sign of the key ring.   Figure 63. Skin-rolling technique.

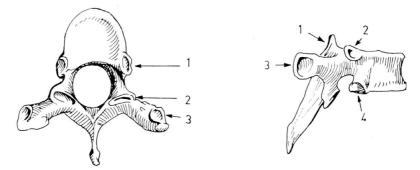

Figure 64. Dorsal vertebra. *Left,* upper view; *Right,* lateral view.
1. Superior articular facet; 2. Superior costal fovea; 3. Transverse costal fovea; 4. Inferior costal fovea.

frontal plane; the upper facet is oriented backward and slightly upward and laterally (Rouviere, 1943). The spinal processes are long with a marked slant downward. The thoracic vertebrae are articulated with the ribs. All these elements restrict the movement of the thoracic vertebrae one over the other. Only their rotation is relatively free, first because of the orientation of the articular facets, and second, because of the fact that the curvature of these facets constitute a segment of a circle whose center is located in the center of the vertebral body. This is true only for the thoracic

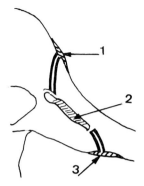

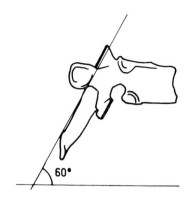

Figure 65 Costal-vertebral joint. (1) Anterior costo-vertebral ligament; (2) interosseus ligament, (3) anterior costo-transversal ligament.

Figure 66. Inclination of the facets over the horizontal line.

vertebrae (Mennell, 1949). This movement, according to Raou (1952), is of the order of 3 to 5 degrees at most, on each side, for each of the first nine thoracic vertebrae and still less for the three last ones. The zone of greatest mobility is TH8-TH9. No significant movement in lateral flexion is possible without an associated movement in rotation in the same direction, for in pure lateral flexion, the lower facet butts against the upper root of the transverse processes of the vertebrae located just below (Rouviere, 1943). Lovett (1907) also states that rotation and lateral flexion cannot be performed separately. According to Raou (1952), lateral bending is of about five degrees for each thoracic vertebra of each side. Flexion and extension are not favored by the orientation of the facets and by the relatively low height of the intervertebral discs. They are on the order of five degrees for each of the successive vertebral levels.

Thus, as a rule, manipulation in rotation of the thoracic spine should be performed in lateral flexion on the same side. For example, right rotation must be associated with right lateral flexion, the spine being placed either in anterior flexion or in backward extension, whichever the case may be. However, there are contraindications to this association based on the study of limitation of movement and the evaluation of the elicited pain.

Examination of Mobility of the Dorsal Spine

Flexion

STANDING. One asks the patient to round his back. The physician observes whether or not this movement is painful, if the curvature of the spinal processes is continuous, or if there is segmental rigidity.

SITTING DOWN. The patient is asked to sit on the table (Fig. 67, left) with his legs hanging down. Then one produces repeated movement of low amplitude flexion followed by relaxation with the heel of the left hand placed over the neck or the highest level of the thoracic spine, while the right hand carefully palpates the spinal processes which must fan out during flexion. It is by this maneuver that one may discover the paravertebral zones of rigidity and contractures.

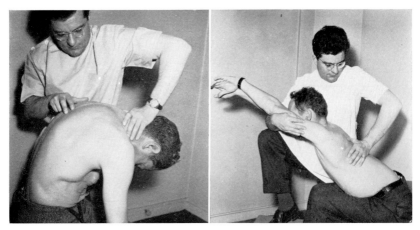

Figure 67. Examination of the mobility of the dorsal spine in a sitting position. *Left,* in flexion; *Right,* in extension.

Extension

STANDING. One asks the patient to turn over backwards and notes whether the movement is painful, limited and/or if it reveals rigid areas of the spine.

SITTING DOWN. The patient sits on the table with legs hanging (Fig. 67, right), with his arms stretched forward and supported by the right forearm of the physician who is standing to the right of the patient. With his free left hand the physician performs successive pressures above the entire thoracic spine while he performs repeated movement of hyperextension, localized at all the segments of the thoracic spine, by slightly elevating his right forearm. This maneuver obviously is painless in a normal individual, in which case the left hand should perceive an elastic resistance at each segmented level.

Lateral Flexion (Fig. 68)

The patient in sitting position with his legs hanging is asked to bend first to the right and then to the left. The physician observes the vertebral curve which should be quite regular and symmetric on each side, and normally, no pain should be elicited. The patient then clasps his hands behind his neck with elbows thrust forward and the physician, in order to evaluate left lateral flexion, places his right forearm on the chest of the patient and grasps the left arm with his hand. He then pulls the arm down and lifts the right shoulder of the patient. This produces a movement of left lateral hyperflexion of the spine.

Note: During this movement the physician should not move the shoulders laterally, as in such cases the lateral bending takes place mostly in the lumbar spine.

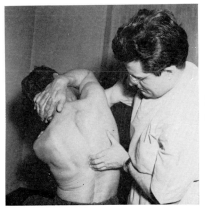

Figure 68.
Examination of the dorsal spine in lateral flexion.

Rotation (Figs. 69 and 70)

The patient is in a sitting position with his arms crossed over his chest. The physician stands behind him slightly to the side to which he rotates. In the figure the rotation is performed to the left. The physician places his left arm in front of the chest of the patient and grasps the right arm of the latter. He pulls the patient toward him, moving the spine in left rotation. This rotation takes place in the thoracic as well as the lumbar spine. However, as is known, the latter is minimal. The physician observes the degree

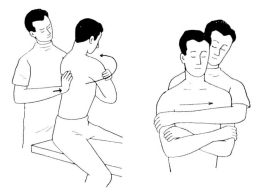

Figure 69. Examination of the dorsal spine in rotation.

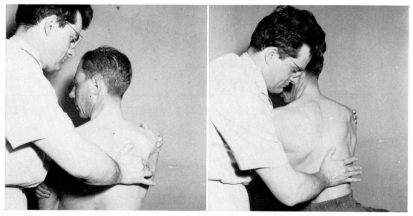

Figure 70. Examination of the dorsal spine in rotation. *Left,* mid-dorsal region; *Right,* lower dorsal region.

of limitation of this global movement and notes whether or not this movement performed in either direction elicits pain. During the second phase of this maneuver, the physician evaluates segmental mobility at each level of the thoracic spine. For this purpose he repeats the same maneuver and effects alternating movement of rotation and derotation. He exerts pressure with his right hand over the right paravertebral region in order to exaggerate the rotation to the left, and vice versa. Normally the hand which exerts the pressure over the spine encounters elastic resistance. On the other hand, nomally, this movement should not elicit any pain. Any localized rigidity or elicited pain or an exaggeration of pain must be carefully recorded.

Finally, the examination should be terminated by the skin-rolling procedure, which may reveal infiltration of the skin and subcutaneous tissues by cellulitis and which may outline a band or an elongated area along the dermatome corresponding to the level of the vertebral derangement (Fig. 71, right). In fact, the areas of superficial tenderness originating from a minor vertebral derangement and an area of cellulitis are often poorly diagnosed and sometimes constitute a disturbing source of errors.

None of these signs, taken by itself, is sufficient to make a diagnosis. However, considered as a total picture corresponding to the same precise level, it may, in the light of additional clinical and radiological information, permit one to make a diagnosis of a minor intervertebral derangement at that level.

Segmental Examination

Segmental examination is conducted as stated on p. 52 in order to reveal the involved segment. Some peculiarities should be considered for the dorsal region. One searches for the "paramedian point" at one fingerwidth from the median line, which is unilateral, precise, elective and circumscribed. The pressure over it often reproduces the habitual pain of the patient. It is associated with tissular changes, cutaneous as well as muscular, which are very localized and which are revealed by careful palpation of the area. These changes should be investigated, the patient being in a sitting position, bent slightly forward, his shoulder drooped, his el-

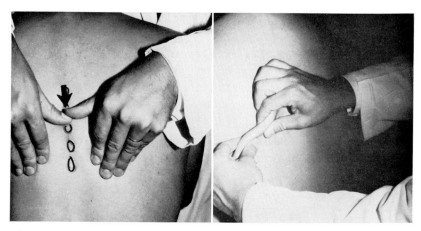

Figure 71. Dorsal spine. *Left,* downward pressure. *Right,* skin rolling test.

bows on his knees. A cause for error to be avoided is as follows: in the dorsal region some tender paravertebral areas, particularly at the mid-dorsal region, may have originated from a much higher level (see dorsalgia). Indeed, the posterior branches of the spinal lower cervical and upper dorsal nerves, once emerged from the spine, descend in the paravertebral groove over three to four segments. In the course of this descent, they give branches to the paravertebral muscles and a cutaneous branch which pierces deep layers and becomes superficial at one to two fingerwidths from the median line. It supplies the adjacent dorsal area. For example, posterior branch D2 emerges at the level of D5 at a point which could be taken for the "posterior articular point," imitating the tenderness of the corresponding posterior articular body structure.

In case of irritation of the posterior branch of a spinal nerve, one may therefore encounter two tender points: the first one at the place where the nerve emerges from the spine and encircles the posterior articular bony structures and the second three or four levels below at the place of emergence of the cutaneous branch, which is usually somewhat lateral to the paramedian point, particularly at the lower dorsal region.

The examination is continued then by exerting pressure over the spinal processes. Superficial pressure due to an apophysitis can be eliminated by injecting a few drops of Novocain, and then exerting a protracted, deep pressure first in the forward direction (Fig. 75), then downwards (Fig. 71, left). One then applies (Fig. 72-73) lateral pressure and counterpressure to the spine (see p. 20), searching for the induced tenderness by pressing toward the right, then toward the left side. For example, if the pressure toward the left side exerted upon a given spinal process (Fig. 72) is effective, one applies simultaneously a counterpressure toward the right side upon the spinal processes located immediately above and below the tender one in order to see whether the induced pain is increased. Thus, the involved level may be better localized.

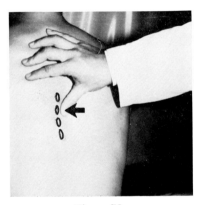 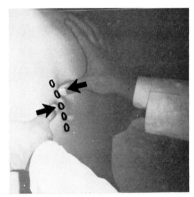

Figure 72.   Figure 73.

If the reciprocal maneuver is painless, a conclusion may be made as to the direction of the direct manipulation, if desirable (Fig. 73). Usually the interspinal ligament is also tender; this is found by applying exquisitely localized pressure by a key ring (Fig. 74).

LUMBAR SPINE

The lumbar spine is comprised of five vertebrae and presents forward convexity (Fig. 76). The discs are high (one-third of the vertebral body height). The orientation of the anterior facets is such that lateral bending is limited and would make rotation impossible if there were not a certain play between them. In fact, the upper facet is flattened in the transverse direction; its medial as-

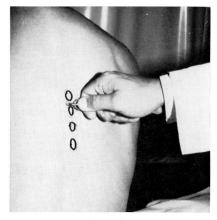

Figure 74.

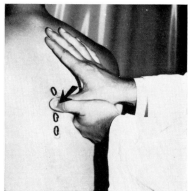

Figure 75.

pect is made of an articular surface having the form of a vertical groove, the concavity of which is oriented not only medially but also somewhat backwards. The lower facet, on the contrary, is

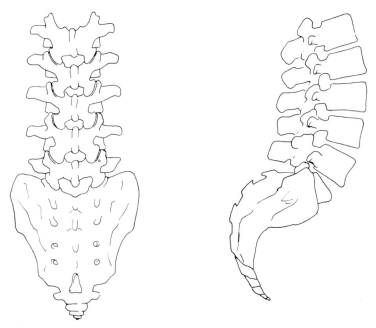

Figure 76. Lumbar spine, posterior *(Left)* and lateral *(Right)* views.

oriented laterally and somewhat forward and offers a convexity forming a segment of a cylinder. It glides in the concavity of the upper facet belonging to the adjacent vertebra located just below (Figs. 77 and 78). However, anomalies are quite frequent (Freudenberg, 1967) (see also Ferrand *et al.*, 1961).

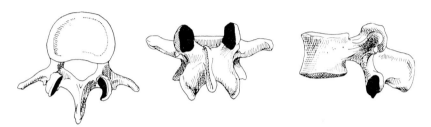

Figure 77. Lumbar vertebra, upper aspect *(Left)*, anterior aspect; *(Center)*, lateral view *(Right)*.

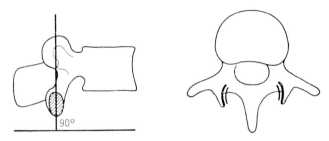

Figure 78. Posterior joints. *Left,* inclination over the horizontal line; *Right,* sagittal plane.

Mobility

Lateral Bending

According to Raou (1952), lateral bending is 20° to 30° on each side.

Rotation

Rotation is very limited, in view of the shape of articular facets (Fig. 78). However, in the cadaver, Raou (1952) obtained for forced movements 7° to 14° on each side.

This rotation is manifest when one examines the spine obtained after recent death. However, it is increased when there is
associated flexion or lateral bending or both. These findings suggest that the lumbar spine had to absorb the large movements of
trunk rotation, this being done progressively segment by segment,
from its upper to its lower end in order to protect the lumbosacral
joint (MacConnail, 1958). From this viewpoint, it is appropriate
to mention that when one considers a given articular system for
the purpose of manipulation, the most restricted physiological
movements are the most important ones. They are often involved
in the articular block, and their liberation predetermines the
possibility of accomplishing the movements of large amplitude
(see also Goldthwait, 1911; Goldthwait and Osgood, 1905).

Examination of Posture

Patient is in an erect position.

1. The dorsal inspection reveals whether or not the spine is
vertical or scoliotic (organically or functionally) and whether the
pelvis is level, judging by the relative position of the iliac crest
and posterior iliac spines (Fig. 79, left).

If one faces the patient, bending forward, one may have a better view as to possible disturbances of the spinal curvature. (Fig.
79, right).

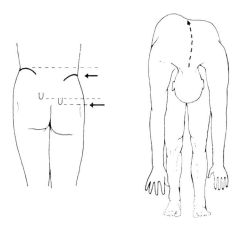

Figure 79. Static examination of the lumbar spine.

2. The lateral view offers information as to the degree of lordosis (Fig. 80) : normal (*a*), exaggerated (*b*), absent (*c*), or replaced by lumbar kyphosis (*d*).

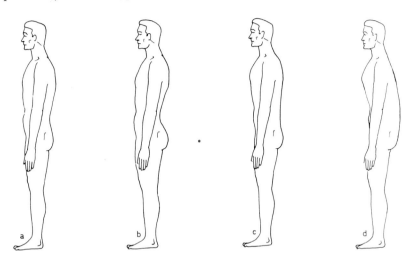

Figure 80. Static examination.

Range of Motion

Active Mobility

1. Patient in an erect position.

a) Bent forward: The patient is asked to bend forward with knees extended and the examiner notes whether or not the lumbar spine flexes smoothly and whether scoliosis, if present, is accentuated, persists, or subsides. The distance between the fingertips and the floor is then measured. It may sometimes be of interest to repeat this maneuver with the patient standing on one leg only—the right one, then the left.

One may conduct the Schöber test as follows (Fig. 81) : One marks two points on the lumbar spine, for example L5 and L1; then one measures the distance which separates them. Normally, this distance should increase while the patient bends forward. If the spine is stiff, the distance remains the same.

Note: Although the distance from fingers to floor is another way of quickly evaluating lumbar flexibility, it may be a source of

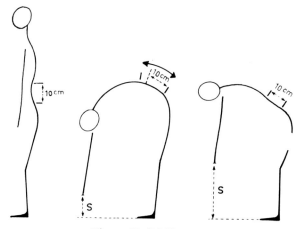

Figure 81. Schöber test.

error. The patient with a rigid spine may still touch the floor with his fingers if his hip joints are exceptionally free and if his hamstrings can be easily stretched.

b) Bent laterally, first to the right and then to the left, the patient shows whether there is a discontinuity of the spine, expressing segmental rigidity (Fig. 82, left) or whether the spinal curvature is normally harmonious (Fig. 82, right).

c) Bent backwards, the patient shows whether or not extension is possible, painful, or limited.

In summary, one seeks to reveal any rigidity, limitation of motion, or pain during each of these motions.

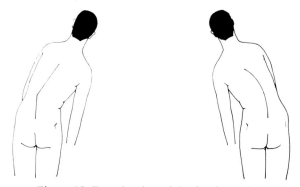

Figure 82. Examination of the lumbar spine.

2. Patient standing, bent forward with hands over a table.

One asks the patient to induce on himself an exaggerated lordosis (Fig. 83, left) or kyphosis (Fig. 83, right). Thus, one may exteriorize anteroposterior rigidity. However, it is often found, particularly in chronic cases of low back pain, that the movement of flexion-extension is free while standing erect, but that the subject is unable, being in this position, to control these movements as if this part of the spine escaped all voluntary control.

Rehabilitation of these patients consists in reeducating these muscles so that their contractions are consciously perceived and controlled.

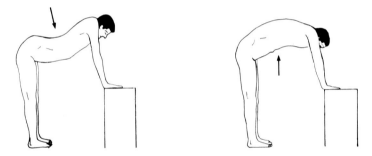

Figure 83. Examination of the lumbar spine.

Passive Mobility

Passive mobility, of course, is the mobility of particular interest in manipulative medicine. Personally, we always examine a patient placed astraddle the end of an examining table, the patient offering the dorsal view to the physician. The latter induces all possible movements of the spine either isolated or in combination one with the other (flexion, extension, right and left rotation, and lateral bending). (Fig. 84).

In order to better evaluate painful and/or limited movements, the physician moves the spine up to the point of "taking up the slack," in each of these orientations. The result is recorded on the star diagram (p. 141).

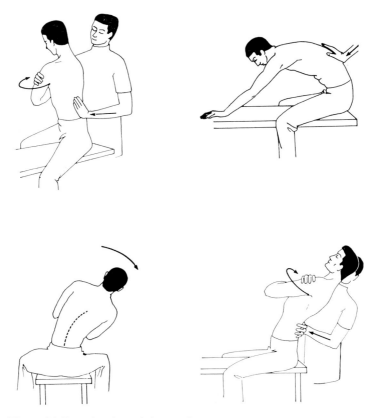

Figure 84. Examination of the passive movements of the lumbar spine.

Segmental Examination

The following is the best position for this examination: The patient is lying prone *across* the table, with, if necessary, a cushion under his abdomen (Fig. 85). A lateral pressure is exerted with the thumb over each of the spinal processes, first to the right and then to the left (Fig. 86, top). If one of them is tender, a search is made for additional information by exerting counter pressure over the spinal process just below it, then over that just above it, to make a more precise localization of the involved segment (Fig. 86, center and bottom). Then one will use a key ring in order to test tenderness of the supraspinous ligament (Fig. 87, right); final-

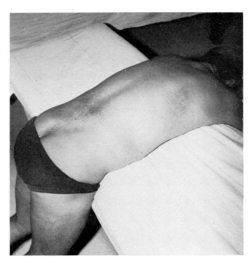

Figure 85.

ly, the degree of tenderness of spinal processes can be determined by direct, protracted, deep pressure, preferably exerted through the thumb of the other hand (Fig. 87, center), after ruling out superficial tenderness due to a simple apophysitis (Fig. 87, left).

If (1) pain by reciprocal lateral pressure over the spinal process, (2) the sign of the key ring, or (3) a paramedian tender point at one fingerwidth from the midline, corresponding to the bony structure of the posterior joint are elicited at the same level, then one may be certain that an involvement of the related intervertebral segment is present.

If clinical history, radiography, and all possible additional tests are in agreement with a minor mechanical intervertebral derangement, such a diagnosis becomes probable.

The direction of restricted and/or painful movements will permit one to predetermine the kind of prescription which will be formulated for manipulation.

Skin Examination

Skin-rolling technique, here again, may permit one to identify tender infiltrated areas, particularly those the pressure of which elicits the patient's habitual pain.

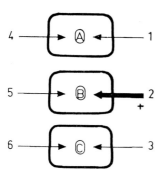

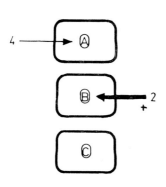

Figure 86.

One exerts successive pressures—1, 2, 3, 4, 5 and 6. In this case, pressure 2 is painful, corresponding to the movement of the vertebra *B* to the left. Then while pressure 2 is maintained, a counterpressure 4, then 6 are exerted simultaneously in order to make more precise the localization of the involved segment.

Simultaneous counterpressure 4 does not change the results of pressure 2.

However, simultaneous counterpressure 6 does increase pain notably. Therefore, the joint *BC* is the one which is involved.

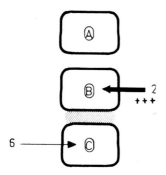

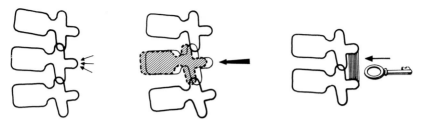

Figure 87. Pressure over the spinal process and its ligaments. *Left,* Superficial rubbing of the spinal process. This rubbing elicits pain if there is apophysitis. *Center,* Deep pressure. In the absence of an apophysitis, the pressure exerted over the spinal process may elicit vertebral or intervertebral pain. *Right,* Pressure over supraspinal or interspinal ligaments may increase pain (key sign).

Examination of Muscles

Some tender points are usually found in the lumbar region and are of great interest for the experienced clinician. Thus, for example, the insertion of the iliolumbar ligament over the iliac crest, posterior and superior iliac spines (unilaterally tender), supratrochanterian point, trochanter point, etc. should be explored.

This examination also comprises that of paravertebral muscles which will be most carefully palpated, searching for contracted and tender muscle fascicles, as well as those of the muscles located in the external iliac fossa. The latter will be particularly well appreciated with a patient in prone position. Exquisite tenderness of these muscles is very often found in chronic lumbalgias and protracted sciaticas. It is by combining an isometric contraction with associated palpation that one may reveal a tender muscle. For example, opposed abduction for the gluteus medius and the fascia lata; opposed internal rotation for the gluteus minimus; opposed external rotation for the pelvitrochanterian muscles; opposed extension for the gluteus maximus (see also Good, 1957).

EXAMINATION OF THE ABDOMINAL MUSCLES. The examination of the lumbar spine should be completed by examining the abdominal muscles, the strength of which controls the stablization of the lumbar spine.

The subject, in a supine position with knees flexed, is asked to raise his head, then his trunk, while his feet are braced. The same movement with superimposed rotation will be used to test the obliques.

Lasegue Sign

The examination of the lumbar spine in a patient presenting a local dysfunction should always be completed by *neurological* examination of the lower extremities (sensitivity, reflexes, and muscle strength). However, among all of the tested signs, the Lasègue sign is the most important as it permits a rapid and convenient measurement of the efficacy of therapy and particularly of the maneuvers of mobilization which precedes manipulations.

At times one may find a *contralateral* Lasègue sign. Thus, in looking for the Lasègue sign on the nonpainful side, one may produce pain when the extremity is raised. This constitutes an excellent radicular sign. It should be differentiated from the bilateral Lasègue sign which is common and of no real clinical value. A true Lasègue sign should also be differentiated from pain due to the stretching of hamstrings. It is known that the hamstrings may become very tender during chronic sciatica.

In the femoral neuralgia one can see an inverted Lasègue sign. With the patient in a prone position, the lower extremity is raised in hyperextension.

Examination of the hip should always complete the testing of the lumbar spine. This examination is both radiological and clinical and should not be considered here in detail.

One should remember that the normal range of motion of the hip is as follows: external rotation, 60°; internal, 30°; adduction, 30°; abduction, 60°; flexion, 130°; and extension, 10° to 20°. We should stress the frequency of the incidence of minor insufficiencies of the hip joint with the femoral head being incompletely covered by the glenoid fossa. This is translated clinically by fatigue and pain, of which the patient complains at the level of the glutel region or in the crotch. This should be looked for very carefully on the x-ray plates.

One should also remember the incidence of pain due to periarthritis of the hip or to chronic bursitis of the gluteus medius. The latter is expressed during examination by a precisely localized, acute tenderness at the pressure of the posterior and superior aspect of the great trochanter. Simple treatment consists of cortisone injection (combined with an anesthetic) into this precise point.

Movement of the Sacro-iliac Joint *(Figs. 88 to 90)*

A movement of *nutation* consists in inclination of the upper sacrum forward, while movement of contranutation is the movement where the upper sacrum moves backwards (Fig. 91) ; an axis around which such movement must be carried out is called "axis of nutation." The position of this axis has been the object of many papers and discussions, particularly among the obstetricians. Some believe that this axis goes through the articular surface, while others believe that it is located behind the articular area. There are also those who deny the presence of a movement of rotation (see Delmas, 1950; Colachis *et al.,* 1963; Ingelrans and Oberthur, 1950; Rotes-Querol, 1954; Sureau, 1949; Weisl, 1954) (see also Part IV, p. 390.)

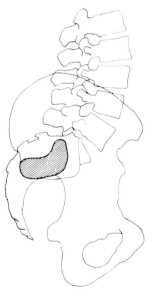

Figure 88. Sacro-iliac joint.

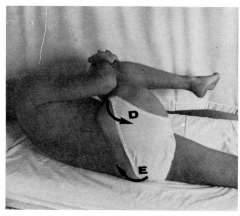

Figure 89. The sacrum being immobilized, the ilac crest may tilt backwards (*arrow D*) or forwards (*arrow E*).

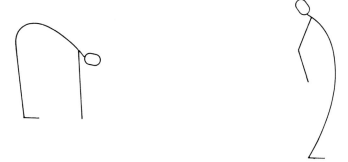

Figure 90. Body movements in which nutation and contranutation occur.

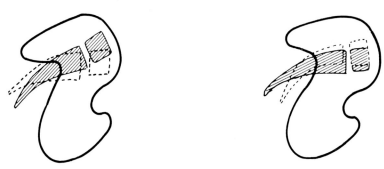

Figure 91. *Left,* movement of nutation; *Right,* movement of contranutation. The broken lines indicate the final position of the sacrum.

PART II

ESSENTIALS OF MANUAL MEDICINE

Chapter 6

History

ALL OVER THE WORLD, there have always been "bonesetters" who were able to reset "nerves" or to replace a small bone or two by applying, at times, correct procedures despite a wrong diagnosis. Their secrets were transmitted from father to son as a part of their practice, a practice cloaked in such mysticism that the operator himself did not know which was the beneficial act in the treatment. The traditional bonesetters do not practice the manipulations that are the object of this book; rather they practice frictions, pressure, and massage of the muscles and tendons which, however, are at times amazingly effective.

It is true that one finds in the ancient treatises certain maneuvers which bear a resemblance to our present manipulations. However, their first systematic use dates from about 1840 when some pupils of Ling from Sweden, as a result of penetrating analytical studies of movements, were led to practice a few forcible manipulations of the spine. The maneuver in Y of Tissié, for example, is a manipulation which permits one to release in some patients a costo-vertebral block with resulting instantaneous increase by several centimeters of the thoracic perimeter in forced inspiration.

The first "osteopaths" (e.g. Still, 1899) developed and classified manipulative techniques which gave birth to almost all the presently used maneuvers. Their mistake, for some time, was to consider these techiniques as a universal therapeutic method. Obviously, this concept has changed even among them. However, although they have abandoned most of the old theories, in particular the pathogenic ones, their manipulation remains a part of a conventional system requiring the use of a particular jargon. They are conditioned by diagnostic palpation so subtle that no objective criteria may be evolved from these practices.

We are not going to discuss here chiropractors, and their publicized "theories." According to Davenport School, all diseases are due to a displacement of the atlas: It was J. B. Mennell (1877-1957) who introduced gentle vertebral manipulations without anesthesia in the domain of traditional medicine. As a professor of physical medicine, he devoted all his life to manipulations. The goal of his life work was to make the art of manipulations a scientific system despite the difficulties encountered in acquiring the art. He studied voluntary and involuntary joint movements with great care and showed conclusively that the involuntary motions were very important in manipulative therapy. The evaluation of these movements was for him a part of the treatment. When one of them was limited, he would restore it by progressive or sudden mobilizations. However, although he described very useful manipulative techniques, he was less explicit as to their indications, particularly in regard to manipulation of the spine. The most important part of his work was related to manipulations of the limb joints. Indeed, he made a great number of remarkable observations and originated many interesting concepts concerning joint pain. Mennell was the first to introduce manipulations in physical medicine and was a true pioneer in this field.

Like J. B. Mennell, we have explored the possibilities of applying osteopathic techniques to manipulative therapy in osteoarticular pathology. We have learned these techniques from M. C. Beal, to whom we express our gratitude. We have analyzed them, determined their indications, and their results, taking into consideration the most recent anatomophysiological data and thus have arrived at a new concept of manipulative medicine and methodology.

Medical manipulation, as we see it, is very different from the system which has been developed in Great Britain under the name of *manipulative surgery*. The most known among manipulation surgeons is Timbrell-Fischer (1944). He uses manipulations under anesthesia for restoring range of motions in joints frozen by "adhesions." Indeed, the manipulative surgeons believe that a number of crippling infections, traumatic as well as "rheumatic" conditions, involve and freeze joint motions by such "adhesions." As soon as their range of motion is limited or lost, a vicious circle sets in and new "adhesions" are formed leading to muscle atrophy and contractures. Mobilization is the best therapeutic tool to use in order to break this vicious circle. Immobilization is the enemy of the joint!

These manipulations aim at the crippling conditions such as coxarthrosis, periarthritis of the shoulder, arthritis and meniscal lesions of the knee, sacro-iliac sprain, and disturbances of plantar arches with tendon "adhesions" rather than, for example, the discogenic disease, or cervicobrachial neuritis.

These maneuvers appear to us as very traumatic and blind, and their results are quite inconsistent. In our judgment, the success of some of these procedures does not justify the price paid in terms of possible complications and accidents.

The book offered here attempts to present a system of manipulations inspired by a personal concept which is very different from that of manipulative surgeons. First, we are dealing with manipulation without anesthesia, conducted in common painful conditions of the spine: essentially regional pain in the neck, upper back, lower back, radiculitis, and the complaints related to mechanical or functional disturbances of the spine. Second, our goal is to apply treatments which are effective as well as harmless and painless to the patient.

Chapter 7

Definitions

MANIPULATION AND MOBILIZATION

MANIPULATION AND MOBILIZATION are terms which are often used interchangeably. They are not, however, synonomous.

Preparation of the Manipulation

Preparation of the manipulation involves positioning and "taking up the slack." Here is an example: A patient is placed on his back. The physician holds the patient's head in both hands as indicated by Fig. 92. He slowly rotates the head to the left. This maneuver involves the neck movement; this is "positioning." However, the operator will soon perceive resistance: He is unable to go any further; he has the impression that he has reached the end of any possible movement, an impression shared by the patient. If he persists and maintains the pressure against this resistance and stretches the soft tissue structures, he accomplishes that phase of the procedure which is called "taking up the slack." In this particular case he does it in left rotation.

Mobilization

Mobilization consists of decreasing the pressure, letting the patient's head return to the midline and then repeating several times the left rotation taking up the slack. We call this procedure, repeated several times, mobilization in left rotation, an elastically flexible movement. Thus, mobilization consists of a series of movements within the normal and usual range of motion without going beyond it.

Execution of the Manipulation

If, after having taken up the slack, the operator adds a very slight motion of additional rotation by a limited and sudden *thrust* effectuated by his right wrist, he has the impression that

116

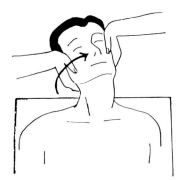

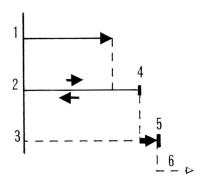

Figure 92. One may define the degrees of joint movements in the following fashion: (1) active voluntary movement (V) of Maximum amplitude. (2) Passive movement (P) which has an amplitude slightly greater than A (mobilization). (3) Finally, manipulation (M) which is a forced movement going beyond the physiological play but not beyond the anatomical play. If the anatomical play is transgressed, a dislocation (L) will follow. (4) 2 minus 1 is additional displacement due to mobilization (P). This is reversible. (5) 3 minus 2 is additional displacement due to manipulation (M). (6) Additional displacement leading to dislocation (L).

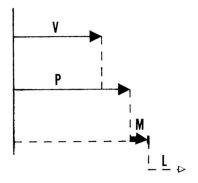

some resistance has been overcome and that the range of motion has increased by some additional degrees. This is associated with a characteristic cracking sound analogous to cracking of knuckles (Fig. 92). This abrupt, brusque, yet precise movement, following taking up the slack of the soft tissue structures, is a manipulation, in this case in left rotation. This brisk maneuver tends to put certain elements of the joint beyond its limits seen during voluntary and habitual movements, but does not transgress anatomical tolerence. This does not mean that it must be brutal nor does it mean the operator has to display great strength to perform it.

In no case should this manipulation be painful; moreover, it must be easy to perform, provided the patient has been placed in the appropriate position and the force applied correctly. In other words, the first phase of the manipulation, consisting of exact positioning, is indispensable. This is a function of the correct choice of technique. It is during the second phase of the maneuver ("taking up the slack") that the operator prepares the movement to be effected in the direction determined by the examination of the patient. This phase is a segmentally oriented traction. Finally, the third phase is the manipulation proper. It is usually associated with the well-known popping sound.

The Cracking Sound

A novice is usually very pleased and the patient satisfied when the cracking sound takes place, as it suggests wrongly that "something was out of place and is now back again." In reality, it simply signifies that the degree of mobilization was sufficient to induce a brisk separation of the articular surfaces. This noise indicates that the manipulation took place, and nothing else. There are cases where the operator may be justified not to go so far as to induce the sound and there are many cases when he must go beyond this limit. The popping is an habitual accompaniment of the manipulation. It is not perceived during passive mobilization having as its goal increasing the range of motion. The cracking sound can be perceived during vertebral manipulations as well as during the manipulation of the extremities. It is possible to induce it in the fingers, feet, etc.; it appears each time one obtains a brief separation of the articular surfaces. In the case of the spine, the posterior or apophyseal joints "pop," not the disc. The cracking sound is due to the stretching of the joint which reduces pressure of the synovial fluid. This causes tiny gas bubbles to form within the fluid. They burst and make noise; the gas is then reabsorbed into the synovial fluid.

Once this cracking or snapping sound is obtained, one has to wait a certain time before it can be reproduced. This "recharging time" is variable from subject to subject and may last from one to several hours.

The cracking sound does not prove that the manipulation has been successful. Any manipulation, good, bad, or useless, may produce such a sound. The most important thing is to elicit it at the level where the manipulation should take place. If, moreover, the latter was executed in the proper direction, then, and only then, has the cracking sound some value: it proves that this region was manipulated. The presence of the sound is not necessary or sufficient; it is simply habitual. A good manipulator should be capable of popping the spine of a normal subject, vertebra after vertebra, without eliciting any pain.

Chapter 8

Nomenclature of Manipulation
and Manipulative Prescription

M ANIPULATION IS A GLOBAL movement which can, in all cases, be broken down into its constituent components, according to each of these spatial planes: (1) rotation, (2) flexion-extension, and (3) lateroflexion.

All manipulative movements can be perfectly defined by these coordinates. One can see from this that there is a great variety of possible maneuvers.

COMPONENTS OF MANIPULATIVE MOVEMENT

Elementary physiological movement of the vertebral column are flexion, extension, lateral inclination, and left and right rotation. Some manipulations can then be practiced according to all these different directions or a combination of them. Manipulation acts on the entire mobile segment: disc, posterior joints, and their interconnecting system. Let us see then what happens in the intervertebral joint during each of these manipulations (Fig. 93). To manipulate an intervertebral joint in extension is to claim that during this maneuver anterior borders of the vertebral bodies

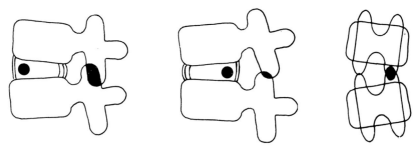

Figure 93. Intervertebral joint movements. *Left,* in extension; *Center,* in flexion; *Right,* in right lateral bending (posterior view.)

separate one from the other, while the intraarticular space of the posterior joints decreases. Flexion is the inverse of extension: the anterior borders of the vertebral bodies come together; the posterior borders separate. The nucleus of the disc slides a little toward the rear and the intraarticular space of the posterior articulations increases. Lateral inclination or lateroflexion, to the right, brings together the vertebral bodies of the right side and separates them on the left. The same movement is made at the level of the posterior articulations. To manipulate in right rotation is to impart a movement such that the right transverse of the vertebra concerned tends to be carried towards the rear in relation to the vertebra below it. It is, in effect always relative to the segment immediately below, that we will describe the manipulative movement.

We thought that it was convenient to represent these movements on a diagram shaped like a star; this diagram is a very helpful part of the report of the results of the examination of vertebral mobility (Fig. 94).

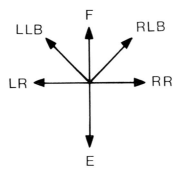

Figure 94. Star diagram. F, flexion; E, extension; RLB, right lateral bending; LLB, left lateral bending; RR, right rotation; LR, left rotation.

Imagine a subject standing with his pelvis fixed. He rotates the trunk towards the right, that is to say that the right shoulder becomes posterior in relation to the plane of the pelvis. It is a dorso-lumbar rotation towards the right.

Take the same patient in the same position, but this time the shoulders are fixed and the pelvis turns. His pelvis should undergo a left rotation in order to reach the same relative position as before: the left hip becomes posterior, while the right becomes anterior. Then again, we may say that we deal with a dorsolumbar rotation towards the right because the rotation of the trunk is judged in relation to the pelvis (segment below), which is considered as being fixed. This is true even if it is an act of rotation on only one vertebral segment or if it is an act of flexion, extension, or of lateroflexion at that level.

It is always by reference, then, to the segment immediately below, considered as *fixed* that we define a position or a vertebral movement.

MANIPULATIVE PRESCRIPTION

If one wishes to precisely define a manipulation so that a brief prescription will permit one to identify it without error, and to reproduce it exactly, one must indicate (1) the level which it involes, (2) the direction of the maneuver, and (3) the technique to be used.

Involved Segment

Most frequently one deals with a precise level: C5-C6, D3-D4, L5-S1, etc.

In other cases, the procedure is less selective and then one identifies it as cervical (C), cervico-dorsal (CD), dorsal (D), lumbar (L), or lumbosacral (LS).

One should complete the prescription by indicating the part of the region to be manipulated: upper (u), middle (m), or lower (l). For example: Cu (upper cervical spine); Dm (mid-dorsal spine); Ll (lower lumbar spine).

Direction of the Maneuver

One must precisely define the maneuver in three planes: frontal, sagittal, and horizontal. Each movement of the spine is a combination of flexion or extension, right or left rotation, right or left lateral bending, as stated previously. Therefore, one shall write:

Flexion	F	Left rotation	LR
Extension	E	Right lateral bending	RLB
Right rotation	RR	Left lateral bending	LLB

If one states that a segment is to be manipulated in right rotation, right lateral bending and flexion, the position of the joint during manipulation is determined, but the direction in which the joint was forced is left uncertain. A manipulation in right rotation applied to a joint set in a right lateral bending and in extension is not equivalent to a manipulation in right lateral bending applied to the same joint, set in the same position (right rotation, right lateral bending and extension).

This is why, in order to identify precisely a manipulation, we prefer to describe it as follows: manipulation in right rotation of a joint set in right lateral bending and extension, if it is essentially in the direction of rotation that one intends to force the movement. In order to be brief, we state: manipulation in *right rotation,* right lateral flexion and extension; in other words, we *underline the dominant* component, corresponding to the direction in which the movement will be forced. Thus, manipulation becomes a precise orthopedic maneuver.

Technique

The level and the direction of the maneuver being thus determined, there remains to be specified the technique to be used.

Thus, the position of the patient will be predetermined:

Supine (sup) (Fig. 95A)
Prone (pr) (Fig. 95B)
Side lying (sl) (Fig. 95C), right (rsl), left (lsl)
Sitting (sit) (95D)
Astride (ast) (95E)

There are, therefore, five basic positions for manipulation.

Then one may specify a particular character of the maneuver. For example: Cervical manipulation—head free; head braced. Dorsal manipulation—sternum braced; knee maneuver, etc.

The following table summarizes all these elements of a prescription, identifying four different maneuvers (Fig. 96).

We are specifying then the region, the level, the component movements (with the dominant direction being underlined), the patient's position and its specific characteristic, if necessary.

Orthopedic Medicine

Region	Level	Direction		Technique Position	Variety
Cervical (C)	Upper (u)	Flexion	(F)	Sitting (sit)	X
		Extension	(E)		
Dorsal (D)	Middle (m)	Lateral	(RLB) or		Y
		Bending	(LLB)	Supine (sup)	Z
Lumbar (L)	Lower (l)	Right rotation	(RR)		
		Left rotation	(LR)	Prone (pr)	
				Right side lying (RSL)	

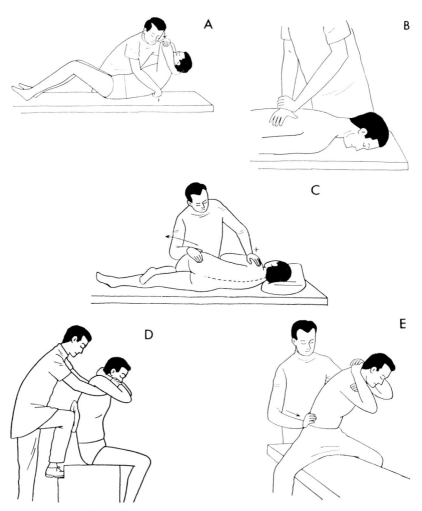

Figure 95. Positions of the patient. *A,* supine (sup) ; *B,* prone (pr) ; *C,* side lying (sl) ; *D,* sitting (sit) ; *E,* astraddle (ast.) .

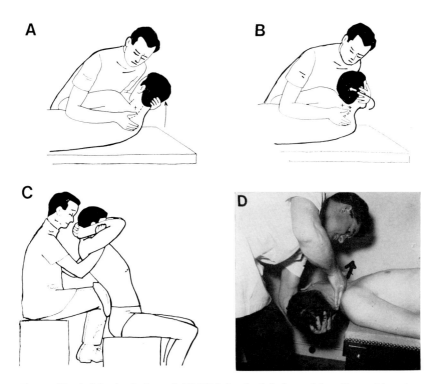

Figure 96. *A*, Manipulation of C6-C7 joint in left lateral bending with spine being in flexion, the patient in the right side-lying position: C6-C7/+*LLB*/RSL.

B, Manipulation of C6-C7 joint with spine in left lateral bending and extension, carried out in right rotation in a patient placed in right side-lying position: C6-C7/LLB + E + *RR*/RSL. If one applies manipulation in left lateral bending on the same patient in the same position, one will prescribe: C6-C7/E+ RR + LLB/RSL.

C, Lumbar manipulation, middle level, in extension will be prescribed as follows: Lm/E/Sit/Knee.

D, According to our terminology, this cervical manipulation will be prescribed as "cervical manipulation in extension and in left rotation of the lower cervical segment." However, for a greater precision, one will prescribe manipulation in left rotation of the spine in extension, since it is in rotation that the maneuver will be forced. The patient being supine, one will prescribe: C1/*E LR*/Sup/head free. With this nomenclature, the maneuver is not described as to its goal, but simply its components, as seen from outside.

Chapter 9

Direct and Indirect Manipulation

W E DIVIDE THE techniques of manipulation into three types: we call the first type direct. In such cases direct pressure is applied on the spine itself. The second type is called indirect as the manipulations are performed indirectly through the natural levers formed by hand, shoulders, pelvis and legs, the spine being moved through their intermediary. The third type is also indirect manipulation, but during this manipulation the operator stabilizes a part directly. We call this type semi-indirect.

DIRECT MANIPULATIONS

These maneuvers are essentially those of chiropractors. They are executed with the heel of the hand; more exactly it is the pisiform which constitutes the point of pressure. The exerted force is brusque, brief, and abrupt. It is applied either at the level of the transverse process (Fig. 97) or the spinal process (Fig. 98). For example: a pressure over the left transverse process of B will impart to this vertebra a right rotation. Simultaneous pressure over the right transverse process of C will elicit torsion between B and C. The inverse movement is obtained by exerting pressure over the right transverse process of B and left transverse process of C. These maneuvers are more difficult to perform than they appear to be. They necessitate a strong pressure which cannot be graded and therefore are dangerous. They are always unpleasant and sometimes painful and they offer only limited possibilities (Fig. 97).

INDIRECT MANIPULATIONS

In contradistinction to direct manipulations, the indirect ones may vary infinitely. They permit one to manipulate in all directions every vertebral segment with a strength which is always possible to grade. They are preceded by the preparatory stages

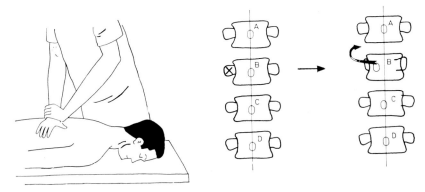

Figure 97A. Direct manipulation. The pressure over the left transverse process of *B* elicits a right rotation of *B* over *C*. However, *C* may also be slightly moved.

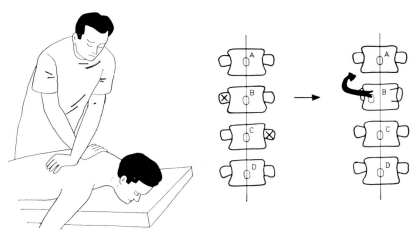

Figure 97B. Direct manipulation with contra-pressure. If the physician exerts a contrapressure over the right transverse process of *C*, the movement of rotation between *B* and *C* is more complete, inasmuch as *C* remains fixated (a dynamic pressure over *C* would produce a movement which would be too violent.)

which we mentioned above—positioning and taking up the available "slack" in the joint. These offer the operator the possibility of executing movements of repeated and measured mobilization obviously superior to the abruptness of the direct maneuvers.

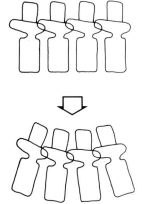

Figure 98
Direct pressure over a dorsal
or lumbar vertebral segment
produces a local extension.

Without considering minute details, here is an example of an indirect manipulation which must be carried out in three stages: (1) positioning of the patient, (2) taking up the slack, and (3) manipulation proper.

The patient is in the right side-lying position, The physician faces him, places his left forearm under the left armpit of the patient and stabilizes with his right forearm the patient's left ischion. This is the positioning (Fig. 99). He pushes with his forearm the left shoulder of the patient to 45° in relation to the plane of the examining table and maintains this position while his right arm exercises the pressure in the opposite direction over the left hemipelvis, thus producing a movement of rotation of the lumbar spine up to the point of resistance, or taking up the slack. Finally, with his left arm maintaining the stabilization of the left shoulder, he abruptly exaggerates pressure over the

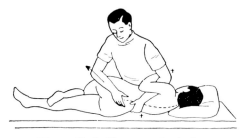

Figure 99. Indirect manipulation.

ischion, thus imparting to it an additional thrust. This is a manipulation. By changing the relative position of the shoulders and of the pelvis, by placing the lumbar spine either in lordosis or cyphosis, by using other points for stabilization, and by modifying the direction of the manipulative forces, it is possible to design various maneuvers according to the needs of the patient.

SEMI-INDIRECT MANIPULATIONS

In order to gain higher precision in localizing different regions of the spine, one is led to practice manipulations which we call semi-indirect. In this type of maneuver, the maneuver of taking up the slack is always accomplished by stabilizing distant points. However, the operator also applies direct pressure to the manipulated segment with his hand, his knee, or his chest. The effort of manipulation upon a taut spine is accomplished either by sudden exaggeration of a distant movement, the knee or the hand applying a counterpressure for localizing the manipulation; or, on the contrary, by exaggerating the local pressure, thus assisting the movement which was primed by the distant taking up of the slack.

Example: the patient sits on a stool, with his hands crossed behind his neck. The physician stands behind him with both hands placed under the armpits of the patient and pulls the forearms of the patient toward him during the manipulation (Fig. 100) while his sternum localizes the maneuver by applying a

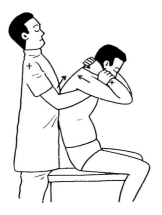

Figure 100. Semi-indirect manipulation.

counterpressure over the spine. We will discuss this technique again below.

THE QUALITIES OF THE MOVEMENT

It is appropriate to mention the following:

1. The manipulation should never result from two movements in the opposite direction. There are many techniques where the operator *appears* to exercise the movements in the opposite direction with each hand. In reality, once the slack has been taken up, one hand must remain immobile, stabilizing, blocking, and restricting any movement; the other hand, and only that hand may be active in executing the sudden additional thrust which is responsible for manipulation. Without this, there would not be any precision, any grading of the latter.[1]

2. The manipulation is not a throwing, propelling movement of appreciable amplitude. One should never start from a neutral position and perform a forced movement from there. One should always bring the joint to a maximal tautening, maintain this position for a short period of time, and only then produce a slight exaggeration of the pressure which is the manipulation. This is the only way to control one's movement precisely and gradually.

3. Manipulation is always a controlled movement, brief, limited, and amortized. When the operator performs this movement beyond the point of taking up the slack, his action is brief, brisk and *measured*. This movement must be limited exactly like the punch of the boxer in which instance the boxer must be prepared to stop the movement immediately upon contact with target. Another example is that of a billiard player who has to strike the ball with a brisk shock which is followed by a slight immediate recoil.

---

[1]In the schematic figures of this book the points of stabilization are indicated by crosses.

Chapter 10

Localization of Manipulations
of the Spine

W E SAY THAT a manipulation may be perfectly defined by its coordinates. It is appropriate now to see how one can apply manipulation to a given level of the spine. To those who are not familiar with manipulations, it may appear absurd to believe that one may act very precisely on a chosen joint of the spine. Nevertheless, it is not only possible but also indispensable in the majority of cases. This problem exists mostly for the indirect manipulations which are almost always manipulations in rotation.

It is undoubtedly necessary to have certain experience and certain dexterity to be able to impose on the patient, by flexible maneuvers, the necessary attitudes and to maintain the correct position during the execution of the maneuver. In order to do so one must take advantage of certain peculiarities of the biomechanics of the spine which permit one to act more selectively on one than another segment by combining different directions of the movement. Indeed, if, for example, a rotation is imposed upon a dorso-lumbar spine of a sitting subject mobilizing his shoulders, the maneuver will affect the low dorsal column at about D8-D9 interspace provided that the spine is in a normal position. However, if one performs the same maneuver with a spine in flexion it will affect a higher segment. When the spine is in extension, a lower segment will be involved. However, in practice, lateral bending is often aiding localization, and, therefore, one may manipulate in extension the lower cervical spine, and in flexion, the upper cervical spine.

Effectively the level of the lesser resistance in rotation varies according to the degree of the associated lateral bending. Lovett (1907) has pointed out that rotation and lateral bending constitute the same movement. If one induces lateral bending at a spinal segment and if secondarily, while maintaining this lateral flexion, one initiates a movement of rotation in the same direction, the rotation tends to be maximal at the summit of the curve formed by the lateral bending. A simple image of this observation may be evoked by comparing this maneuver to the movements obtained with a steel tape measure. Imagine a segment of a tape measure which one immobilizes at the bottom and which one grasps between the thumb and the index finger at the top (Fig. 101). If one rotates the tape, the maximum rotation is observed in the middle; however, if one bends the tape sidewise while rotating it, one can modify precisely the level of rotation. This level is the place of least resistance. A slight lateral bending will localize the maximum change at a higher level than at a pronounced lateral bending.

Thus the point of action of a given maneuver upon the spine varies according to the choice of other coordinates. It is possible, by combining these coordinates, to obtain a localization of the effect upon one or another spinal segment. It is a question of experience. The operator has to impose the movement with one hand while the other controls the level of the spine by palpating the paravertebral muscles, the spinal processes, ascertaining the exact level where the curve resulting from combined movement takes place. The summit of this curve will be the point of least resistance where the action of the maneuver will be localized.

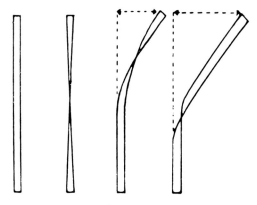

Figure 101.

ELECTIVE MANIPULATIONS

Whatever the dexterity of the operator, this mode of localization in general offers only limited precision. Moreover, the manipulating force applied at a distance may not be sufficient or well controlled. Thus, while retaining this procedure when a semi-precise localization may be satisfactory, one must be able for more elective manipulation, to master the semi-indirect manipulations which we differentiate in two types: assisted manipulations and opposed manipulations (Figs. 102 and 103) .

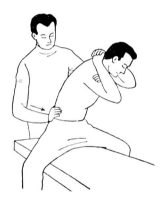

Figure 102. Assisted semi-indirect manipulation.

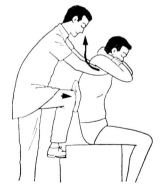

Figure 103. Opposed semi-indirect manipulation.

Assisted Manipulations

This manipulation is designed as was discussed above by combining rotation, lateral bending, extension or flexion, according to the results of the clinical examination, in such a way that the joint to be manipulated is located at the summit of the curve imposed upon the spine. However, in addition, the physician will, during the manipulation, act directly upon this joint by assisting this movement. This direct pressure applied at the level of the transverse or the spinal process of a vertebra just above or just below the level in question (according to different situations) renders this maneuver still more elective. Take an example of manipulation of the dorsal spine when a left forced rotation is desired involving essentially D9-D10 level. The patient is seated astride the table with hands behind his neck. The operator stands behind him and places his left arm under the left armpit of the patient and grasps the latter's right shoulder. Pulling his left hand to the left and backwards, the operator confers to the trunk a rotary movement which will take place at the low dorsal region as we discussed before as there is no extension nor flexion of the spine. However, let us observe now that the operator applies at the same time a pressure with his right thumb at the right transverse process of D9. Then, after taking up the slack, as he exaggerates the rotary movement with the hand holding the patient's shoulder, he simultaneously exercises a brief pressure with the thumb of the other hand over the transverse process. Thus, he increases the movement of rotation by assisting it. This is why we call this technique assisted manipulation. We deal here with an assisted manipulation in left rotation (Fig. 102).

Opposed Manipulations

In other cases it will be necessary to use another type of maneuver in order to obtain elective manipulation. For example, a manipulation in flexion involving essentially D9-D10 is desirable. In this example, we are going to describe a technique of manipulation in which the operator's knee is used.

The patient is seated on a stool, his hands crossed behind his neck. The operator places his forearms under the armpits of the patient and holds his wrists. According to the position in which he places the trunk of the patient and by action of his forearms, the physician brings the subject in a forward flexion and therefore releases his discs posteriorly. In order to make this manipulation act at D9-D10 he produces a general curvature with a summit at that level. Then he applies his knee against the spine at the same level with a little cushion in between (Fig. 103).

He takes up the slack by lifting up the armpits of the patient, then while maintaining firmly the pressure of his knee, he slightly but abruptly exaggerates his traction upwards, at the same time pulling the patient toward him which causes the manipulation associated with the habitual cracking sound. Let us analyze the situation. Figure 104 shows the vertebrae in maximum flexion and the arrow G is the point of application of the knee. Suddenly this movement of flexion is exaggerated while at the same time, the physician pulls the whole spine: the application of the knee opposes the vertebra A to follow the movement. When, by lifting the armpits, the physician flexes the spine, the joint between A and B becomes the one where the maximum of force separating the posterior borders of the vertebral bodies is applied. When the physician exaggerates brusquely the movement of lifting the shoulders and slight traction toward himself he applies a force F which opposes force G of the immobilized knee which maintains the spinal process by pushing it forward and downward. Thus, the knee is a fixed force which opposes the global movement. This

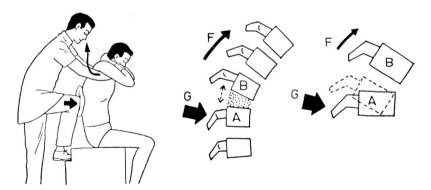

Figure 104.

is called an opposing maneuver. It can therefore be seen that if it is desirable to obtain a movement in flexion between two vertebrae, it is necessary to apply the pressure on the lower vertebra, provided the operator tautens the above segment which is the habitual case. The same type of an opposed maneuver may be used for the manipulations in rotation (Fig. 105).

If we deal with a maneuver in extension, things are essentially different. At the beginning, the operation will be the same: positioning in extension, application of the knee, taking up the slack, then a brief thrust in extension. However, if one considers what is going on at the level of the joint in question, one can see that the knee should be applied against the upper vertebra rather than the lower one as the pressure of the knee exaggerates in this case local hyperextension which then makes this maneuver an assisted one and not an opposing one (Fig. 106).

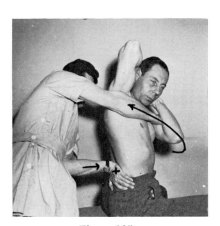

Figure 105.

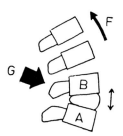

Figure 106.

Chapter 11

Personal Method: The Rule
of "No-Pain and Free Movement"

RATIONALE

THE CHOICE of the manipulation in each individual clinical case is the most important aspect of manipulative therapy and yet, it has not been considered in the past in the same way as we have. No objective criterion has been proposed in order to predetermine the type and the direction of the maneuver to be carried out. Osteopaths and chiropractors did make some suggestions which have been rejected by medical doctors.

In practice even the proponents of the osteopathic school are not slaves of their diagnostic system and are flexible enough in the exercise of their art not to apply an unreasonable technique. The gentleness of their techniques and their ability to choose one out of a great variety at their disposal makes up in efficacy of their treatment, for the inadequacy of their diagnostic procedures. It is obvious, however, that one should evolve a rationale of manipulating techniques which is acceptable to medical doctors. We believe that we have developed a personal method which responds to such a requirement.

Even though a trained practitioner, on the basis of his experience by trial and error, may arrive at the choice of a preference maneuver, it is evident that in each case where manipulation is indicated, there are useful maneuvers and those which are either indifferent or dangerous. The problem, therefore, is to select the former and to avoid the latter. Yet no methodology proposed in the past allows one to clearly make this distinction, so that one may worsen the condition of a number of patients.

A few years ago when we investigated these procedures, we came to the conclusion that one should proceed in exactly the opposite direction to that which appeared to be logical and was indeed, a general rule. Instead of finding the best method of palpation or choosing the best radiological technique in order to detect "vertebral displacement" and then treat them accordingly, we have tried to determine the kind of maneuver which would be most helpful in each individual case. We proposed to avoid any preconceived pathogenetic consideration and to limit ourselves to the objective signs which would not allow any discrepancy in their evaluation. We assumed the following:

1. The minor intervertebral derangements were not sufficient to be detected radiologically except in a very few exceptional cases.

2. Palpation is not sufficient to provide information concerning a faulty position of a vertebra.

3. Even if palpation were adequate from this point of view, it would not be conducive to determining the direction in which manipulation should be carried out.

For these reasons we systematically studied the elementary movements of the involved spinal segment in each case susceptible to manipulative treatment.

We determined which of these movements were free and which ones were either limited or painful. Because we intended to proceed analytically we had to choose only unidirectional techniques which made our task somewhat more difficult, inasmuch as most available techniques were multidirectional. Proceeding in this fashion, we could confirm on thousands of manipulations our first impression, namely, that the most useful maneuver was the one carried out in the direction opposed to that which was painful or restricted or which elicited other complaints from the patient. We called the rule to follow, on the basis of our long and well justified experience, the rule of "no pain and free movement."

Let us take a simple example. If a patient has a traumatic torticollis which prevents him from moving his head to the left, but leaves the head free to rotate to the right, it is, contrary to what is generally believed, by turning the head to the right that one performs the manipulation which will improve the head rotation *to the left*.

In practice the situation is usually much more complex, since each vertebral segment may be moved in six different directions: flexion, extension, right lateral bending, left lateral bending, rotation to the right, and rotation to the left. Manipulation will be conducted according to either the combination of directions opposite to those which are restricted or painful, or successively in each direction which remains free. If a movement is painful or blocked, one should assume that there is a conflictual situation. If one tries to overcome this conflict, one may possibly succeed in breaking adhesions in some cases, but then one takes a risk of irritating the tissues involved and of worsening the disturbance.

This rule of no pain and free movement expresses therefore the therapeutic belief of never forcing a movement which is painful or one which may increase other complaints of the patient for which treatment is carried out. The essential therapeutic movement should be free and carried out in a direction opposite to the one which is restricted.

One should, therefore, select a maneuver which not only is free of pain but also *performed electively in the opposite direction to the painful motion,* hence, the necessity of choosing precise techniques, as to the direction of manipulation, adapted to each individual case. It means that we should condemn any technique which is essentially multidirectional and which prescribes systematic manipulations to the right and to the left. It is fortunate that the vagueries of the standardized techniques now in use not only decreases their efficacy but also attenuates their possible noxious effects.

During certain global manipulations, even though the maneuver is carried out in rotation in the direction which is painful or restricted, a simultaneous application of traction and flexion or lateral bending in the direction which remains free may make it tolerable for the patient or at least does not aggravate his condition.

Some practitioners manipulate the cervical spine in bilateral rotation associated with a very pronounced manual traction. The rotation which can be accomplished under such conditions is very limited; it does not reach the threshold of pain on the restricted side and is not fully efficacious in the direction which remains free. It is the traction which represents in such practices, the most useful therapeutic component, yet not sufficient to totally reduce the block. On the other hand, such a traction may be noxious at the level of the upper cervical spine, where the maneuver of rotation and lateral bending should be carried out completely but using only the tips of the fingers with the greatest possible skill.

At the level of the lumbosacral spine, the standard manipulations are often symmetrical movements of torsion, the patient being in a side-lying position. As practiced most often, these maneuvers constitute combined traction in flexion and moderate rotation. They are not truly painful, unless the flexion is blocked or the rotation is not at all possible, from the beginning of the movement; otherwise, they are neutral and of mediocre efficacy.

We insist that manipulations should be carried out at the involved level, although its effects are distributed at the levels just above and just below the involved one. Perfect control of the technique and the precise ability to manipulate at the useful level greatly increases favorable results of the maneuver if it is appropriately directed. The number of complications increase considerably if the maneuver is directed inappropriately.

Only precise maneuvers, correctly diagnosed and directed will be regularly efficacious and free of complications.

APPLICATION OF THE RULE OF NO PAIN AND FREE MOVEMENT

In practice two different cases should be considered:

1. There is limitation of movement due to simple stiffness. When testing range of motion, one does not meet with any marked resistance; no pain or other complaints are elicited. In such a case, a manipulation in the direction of a limited movement does not offer any serious problem and, therefore, our rule is not applicable.

2. A more frequent case is the presence of several directions in which the movement is limited or blocked. When testing the range of motion, one elicits pain and, therefore, the rule of no pain and free movement should prevail.

Indirect Manipulations

The practical application of this rule is derived from an analysis of the range of motion, painful or free at the segment to be treated. We apply essentially indirect or semidirect maneuvers. We have already indicated their advantages. An additional one is to use them as a technique of the examination, so that a listing of free motions at a precise vertebral level may be compiled. Prior to the description of regional techniques, we will indicate the methods of examination which appear to us as being the best.

The result of this examination involving the elementary components of the movement will be made much more clear and be much better visualized if one uses the star diagram which we have developed with Lesage (Fig. 101, left). This diagram represents a star with six rays indicating six directions of the range of motion: flexion, extension, rotation to the right and to the left, and right and left lateral bending. We indicate painful movement on this diagram by crossbars placed on the rays representing the corresponding direction, one, two, or three bars, according to the degree of pain (Fig. 107, center).

one bar = slight painful limitation of movement

two bars = moderate limitation

three bars = severe painful limitation

One may make this diagram still more precise in the following way. If the movement is limited at the beginning of the range of motion, one places the bar near the center of the star; if it is limited at the end of the range, one places the bar far from the center of the star (Fig. 107, right).

Thus on this diagram (Fig. 107, right):

1. Extension is markedly limited at the onset of the movement (three bars near the center of the star).

2. Rotation to the right is moderately limited (two bars at the middle of the corresponding ray).

3. Right lateral bending is only slightly limited at the end of this motion (one bar near the arrow).

If there is only restriction of the movement, but no pain, one may use x's instead of the bars.

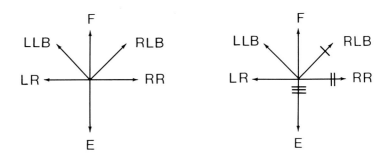

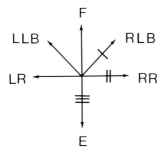

Figure 107. Examples of star diagrams. F, flexion; E, extension; RLB, right lateral bending; LLB, left lateral bending; RR, right rotation; LR, left rotation.

An Example of the Application of the Star Diagram

The application of our rule permits one to determine precisely the useful maneuver. In a case of left sciatica with antalgic attitude to the right and kyphosis (Fig. 108), for example, we will write that right lateral bending is free. Left lateral bending is restricted and painful. Rotation to the right is free. Rotation to the left is painful. Extension is impossible. This is expressed by this figure. Manipulation may be done only in *Rotation to the right,* on a flexed spine, placed in right lateral bending. This maneuver will be totally painless and, according to our almost daily experience, very efficacious and useful.

There is a possibility that the movements in all directions

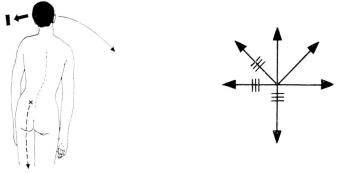

Figure 108.

are painful (Fig. 109). Then one places bars on all the rays of the star: manipulation is impossible to carry out.

In other cases, only two directions are free. These usually are poor indications for manipulation. In practice, only when three directions are free should one consider manipulative therapy, a notion which cannot be overemphasized.

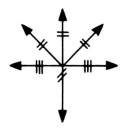

Figure 109.

Direct Manipulation

We use this technique very rarely and feel that its indications are quite limited. They are, however, not totally useless but should be performed flawlessly. Here, also the rule of no pain should be applied.

One should remember that the following maneuvers should be carried out:

1. Globally, by exerting pressure over the spinal processes, thus, becoming maneuvers in extension. They are, therefore,

advisable only if extension is free and if the pressure and "taking up the slack" are painless.

2. When one intends to rotate an intervertebral joint, one should remember that the physician should exert the pressure with the heel of the right hand over the left transverse process of one vertebra and with the heel of the left hand over the right transverse process of the vertebra just below the first one. As the pressure is maintained with this second hand, he exerts a sudden thrust followed by an immediate release with his right hand, thus performing rotation to the right. This sudden thrust should, of course, be preceded by the phase of "taking up the slack."

We have already discussed (p. 52) the technique of segmental examination of the spine. Let us consider a case with an intervertebral derangement between B and C, which is susceptible to manipulative therapy.

The examination reveals that a pressure to the left exerted over the spinal process elicits pain (Fig. 110, left). As one maintains this pressure, one exerts another pressure in the opposite direction, over the spinal process of vertebra C. This increases induced pain (Fig. 110, center left), while the pressure exerted to the right over B and to the left over C is painless (Fig. 110, center right).

Manipulation will, therefore, consist in exaggerating the latter movement (1) pressure over the right transverse processes of B and (2) counterpressure over the left transverse process of C (Fig. 110, right).

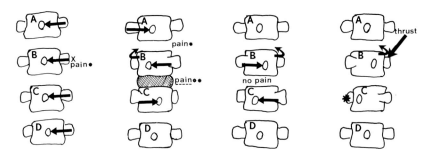

Figure 110.

Thus, the rule of no pain and free movement permits one to (1) indicate or contraindicate the treatment, (2) determine the maneuver to be carried out, and (3) condition the execution of this maneuver.

When manipulation hurts the patient, and yet brings about an improvement of his condition, it may signify that secondary coordinates of the maneuver were poorly determined while its primary component was correctly chosen.

When there is a moderate limitation of the range of motion by simple stiffness, without being associated with pain, while one takes up the slack, it may be possible to manipulate progressively in the restricted direction, if this maneuver remains painless.

It should be shown that it is possible to manipulate a normal spine in all directions at any level without eliciting any pain. Those who wish to use therapeutic manipulation should be able to carry them out painlessly on a normal subject. If not, one should not undertake this therapy.

One should add that the use of postural tests (p. 185) is an excellent precaution in order to avoid the accidents related to disturbance of vertebral circulation.

Chapter 12

Protocol of Therapeutic Sessions

T HE COURSE OF TREATMENT varies essentially with clinical cases. Nevertheless, some general rules need to be observed. The first one is that the "correct use of manipulation depends first of all on the diagnosis" (Mennell, 1964). Any vertebral pain requires a clinical and x-ray examination and in some cases, laboratory tests. One should remember the following:

1. Not all pain originating in the spine whether local, segmental, or projected requires *manipulative therapy*. Therefore, a precise diagnosis should be made before the decision in favor of manipulation is justified.

2. An inflammatory, tumoral, or infectious lesion of the spine may be manifested for the first time only after effort or an awkward movement. It would be a grave mistake to miss the correct diagnosis.

3. The treatment by manipulation is not irreplaceable. Undoubtedly, it may be very tempting because of its elegance and the rapidity of its therapeutic effect which is at times immediate. However, it should not be applied unless it is properly executed. It is better to choose another treatment than to risk a poor manipulation (primum non nocere). Only when all these conditions are satisfied should a treatment by manipulation be used.

MANIPULATIVE DIAGNOSIS

Manipulative diagnosis involves premanipulation testing and examination of the tissues.

Premanipulation Test

Once clinical diagnosis is established and the indication for manipulative treatment is considered, one should envisage technical possibilities of such treatment and the way it may be carried out.

The premanipulation test will consist of an analysis of the range of motion and pain involved in the elementary movements of rotation, flexion, and lateral bending. The results of this analysis will be transcribed over the star diagram and the rule of no pain and free movement will determine the answer to this basic question:

Should one manipulate and if one should, which technique should be selected? We have already indicated the type of the regional examination which is carried out on each patient.

Examination of the Soft Tissues

One should systematically examine the skin and subcutaneous tissue. The physician rolls the skin between the thumb and index finger of both hands, as with a cigar, without decreasing the pressure, all along the paravertebral grooves (Fig. 111).

This skin-rolling maneuver may be used, not only over the paravertebral grooves, but also over the entire back, the extremities, etc., whenever one is treating a painful part. One should not neglect abdominal or precordial regions. How many useless tests and treatments, as well as erroneous diagnoses have been practiced only because this simple maneuver was neglected, and thus, a localized infiltrating "cellulitis" was not recognized.

In the case of the spine, it is most frequently at the level of spontaneous painful areas (but not always!) that one will find two or three vertebral segments involved, associated with an acute tenderness elicited by the skin-rolling maneuver. The skin at this level appears thickened and having a nodular consistency, while above and below this level, it appears to be normal.

These cutaneous tender infiltrations often show a distribution following the posterior branch of the spinal nerve. (Fig. 112).

Sometimes these infiltrations disappear after manipulating which deblocks the corresponding vertebral segment. In other cases, they persist and the patient continues to complain about a painful part.

The Muscles

As previously stressed, one should examine muscle tissue, particularly in the paravertebral groove, subscapular fossa, and lateral

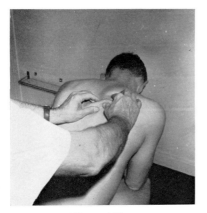
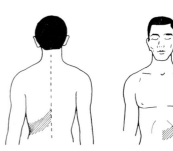

Figure 111.   Figure 112.

gluteal regions. One finds there indurations, which may or may not disappear following manipulation. If they do not, one should treat them locally.

THE MANIPULATIVE SESSION

A manipulation session, and we mean a session and not an isolated action, should always be preceded by a particular type of examination, which we have already mentioned and which aims at the choice of the proper maneuver to be used. This examination consists of the determination of the limitation of the range of motion and painful movements, the exact location of the direction in which such a limitation is observed and a minute search for the tender points; not only those which the patients tell the physician about, but also those located in the muscles which have to be effectively relieved by the appropriate maneuvers of relaxation or decontraction and the paravertebral tender points which the patient is unable to localize. The physician after having completed the clinical and premanipulative diagnosis will then start the manipulation proper. He places the patient in the desired position and then begins to perform slow and rhythmic movement of *decontraction,* which will permit him at the same time to evaluate the quality of the patient's muscles, their tone, and development (one should beware of using too strong a maneuver with patients who have muscles of poor quality as these patients are prone to develop excessive generalized pain). It is also necessary to detect the presence of deep contractures which were not apparent at the beginning of the examination although other contractures may start to disappear under the influence of this type of petrissage which is the maneuver of decontractions. These maneuvers performed slowly, amply, steadily, uninterruptedly, never hurting the patient, have a definite sedative effect and are able by themselves to bring about a notable improvement. It is not rare to improve and sometimes cure a sciatica solely by the massage of the external iliac fossa and particularly of the gluteus medius (Fig. 113); also the decontraction of the supraspinal fossa and of the rotators of the scapula may often have a favorable effect upon a cervicobrachial neuralgia (Fig. 114).

A repeated examination of the range of motion, which may show a possible gain, will be followed by the maneuvers of mobilization which will permit one to better evaluate the limitation of movement. These mobilizations will be performed in all directions which remain free. These movements of mobilization have to be slow, sustained, elastic, and continuous. They will be repeated a dozen times in each direction, particularly for those that are successful. Finally, a new examination of the painful and limited movements (some of which have been already improved) will be followed by the manipulation proper, three or four ma-

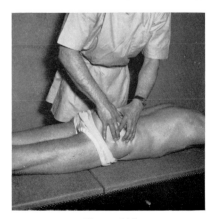
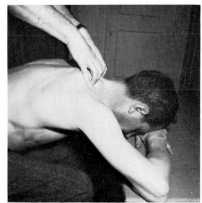

Figure 113. Figure 114.

neuvers only, aiming at an improvement first of the least limited movement and then progressively at deblocking the most limited ones. During the first session in an acute case or when dealing with a stiff spine, it is better not to manipulate at all and to be limited by a mobilization. One should not be too persistent with the latter even though they may be painless, as during the first session one does not know the sensitivity of the tissue and one may elicit violent reactions even after a mild treatment. We have already seen in a preceding chapter that the maneuvers should be conditioned by the rule of no pain and one should never force a movement which is blocked. The freezing maneuver is always oriented in the opposite direction to that of the limitation of the range of motion. Take for example the case of acute cervical pain where the examination has shown that the right rotation is limited and painful, the right lateral bending is limited and painful, the extension is limited and painful (Fig. 115).

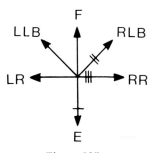

Figure 115.

Although the left rotation, left lateral bending, and flexion are free and painless; one finds a tender point over C6, for example. It is possible that a simple maneuver centered over C6 and performed in flexion, left rotation, left lateral bending, will bring about a sudden total improvement. However, in most cases, it appears to be preferable to divide the movement into several stages. The following is the proper way to conduct the treatment in the example above, according to our technique of "consecutive movements."

It is a good habit to mark with a cross the degree of the movement limitation. In this particular case we can write:

Right rotation	+++	(very limited)
Right lateral flexion	++	(limited)
Extension	+	(slightly limited)

(See star, Fig. 115).

One will act then in the following manner: first, free the least limited movements, in this case the extension by manipulating in flexion (Fig. 116) which one may associate with a slight left rotation. The extension being freed, the examination shows:

Right rotation	+++
Right lateral bending	++
Exension	Free

(Fig. 117)

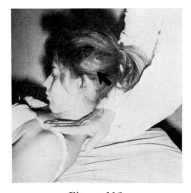

Figure 116.

One will be able to manipulate then in left lateral flexion and left rotation. One will start both the progressive mobilizations, using, if necessary, an extension which has just been freed: left rotation upon the spine in left lateral bending and extension (Fig. 118). Finally, a maneuver in left lateral bending on the spine in left rotation and in flexion is performed (Figs. 119 and 120). The movement will be perfectly free when the manipulation in right rotation, right lateral bending, and in extension can be performed painlessly. Then it may be the last maneuver of the

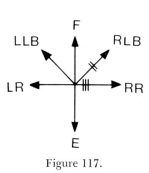

Figure 117.

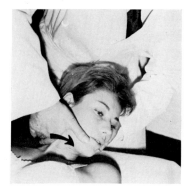

Figure 118.

last session. In general, it is not advisable to apply this maneuver at this time. It is preferable to wait for a few weeks and sometimes to omit this last maneuver. Thus, in a given case, it is always possible to include in a rigorous way the precise maneuver to be performed. If no maneuver can be conducted without pain, in other words, if the movements of flexion, extension, right and left rotation, and right and left lateral bending, are limited or painful, no maneuver should be performed. The manipulation is *con-traindicated* in such a case.

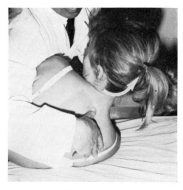

Figure 119.

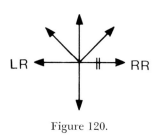

Figure 120.

REACTIONS TO TREATMENT

Diffuse Pain

Postmanipulative diffuse pain is usual after the first session. It is generally moderate and relieved by aspirin and hot baths. It lasts 6 to 48 hours and is observed in 40 percent of cases. Only in exceptional cases is it violent. Usually, it does not recur after the following sessions and when it does, its intensity and duration are more limited.

Transitory Exaggerations of the Original Pain

These are quite frequent even after a successive manipulation with good results. After the manipulation one can witness a complete and immediate disappearance of the pain which may be permanent or transitory. In the latter case, an attenuated pain recurs in the following days which requires a second manipulation. In other cases, a few hours following the treatment after the disappearance of pain, it recurs with greater intensity being associated with diffuse aching and lasting 6 to 24 hours, to disappear again, this time for good.

Finally, another variety may be observed: the patient has the impression immediately after the manipulation that the gain was slight or nil. However, the following day or the one after, he feels a great improvement of the painful phenomena sometimes after manifesting a reaction to the treatment. In some long-standing cases it may happen that the improvement is seen several days after the manipulation.

The reactions are frequent and violent in those cases where the sympathetic nervous system disturbances are most prominent. This is an excellent sign. Whether we deal with postmanipulation diffuse pain or a temporary exaggeration of the original pain, the rule with very rare exceptions is that one should never conduct a second session of manipulations before the reactions generated by the first one are extinguished.

These reactions occur usually only after the first session; they are generally attenuated after the second, and they occur rarely after the third. If the reactions recur after each session, the treatment should be discontinued and the diagnosis reconsidered. On the other hand, one will disregard the diffuse pain which occurs several days after the maneuver in a segment of the spine other than the one which was manipulated. Piedallu (1947) attributes this diffuse pain to a state of progressive reorganization. One should not confuse the transitory exaggerations of the original pain, which are quite inevitable, with the exaggeration of the pain due to the poorly conducted manipulation or those that were erroneously indicated and which are the aggravation of the patient's condition. In the former case, the patient does not suffer during the session; he is improved afterwards; there is always a free interval between the session and the reaction which generally occurs after 6 to 18 hours and during which the patient feels better or at least does not feel worse. On the contrary, if we deal with an exaggeration of the pain due to a poor execution or poor indication of the maneuver, this pain occurring immediately following the manipulation and without any free interval will rapidly increase in intensity. Moreover, while in the former case, the reaction will last 24 to 48 hours, in the latter, the pain may persist days and possibly weeks and will resist all therapy. It is evident that if the reactions are observed mainly after the first manipulation, the aggravation may follow every session.

Functional Reactions

Besides the painful reactions, there are functional reactions. These may be immediate, almost instantaneous. It is common to observe that after even the slightest manipulation, the patient perspires profusely over the trunk and axilla. This recurs during each session whether they are separated by a few days or a few months. This simply shows the action of the maneuver over the sympathetic nervous system and should not modify in any way the course of the treatment.

Much more rarely one may observe episodes of a generalized tremor which cannot be ascribed to fear or nervousness of the patient. The patient has, for several minutes, violent trembling and at times, chills immediately following the vertebral maneuver particularly in the case of a cervicodorsal manipulation. During the hours which follow the lumbar or lower dorsal manipulation, one may sometimes observe abdominal bloating (meteorism) with or without associated diarrhea. The menstruations are often affected, the manipulation precipitating an early onset and heavy flow. One of our patients whose neck was manipulated four times in a month for a periarthritis of the shoulder had each time the same evening menstrual bleeding lasting four days, analogous to the normal menstruation. When seen again, one year later, three times in a month for a cervicobrachial neuralgia, she had each time a menstrual period lasting four days. It is not rare to see during a 24-hour period following a manipulation session, that a patient has an epigastric painful crisis, sometimes abdominal or pelvic. These crises may be of great intensity lasting for several hours, particularly in patients who have complained of such symptomatology during their illness. This reaction generally signifies the disappearance of this symptomatology and may be permanent.

In exceptional cases (one to two patients out of a thousand) the first sessions of manipulation, whatever the reason for which they have been conducted, elicit a true "sympathetic storm" with fainting, palpitation, cold perspiration and also nausea, lasting from 24 to 48 hours.

This is not related to any error in technique and it is not a contraindication of this treatment. The following manipulation which is done about ten days later may not elicit any violent reaction and in general results will be excellent, as will the patient's general health. As a matter of fact, the patient may find that he is relieved of other mild functional disturbances. It is self-evident that these reactions are observed in patients with an unstable autonomic nervous system, and one should warn these patients that such a crisis may occur.

REPEATED SESSIONS OF MANIPULATIONS

The manipulative treatment is sometimes remarkable by its instantaneous quasi-miraculous results: acute lumbago may be immediately cured; the painful and blocked back of a patient subject to chronic lumbago may instantaneously become free and painless (the patient being able to touch his feet), the sciatica immediately improved.

However, it would be erroneous to believe that if the manipulation is not immediately effective, treatment should be suspended. One should not always expect an instantaneous result. However, in addition, next to the immediate cures which are not rare, it is common to find an improvement during the first session. For example, the Lasègue test may show a change of some degree and the patient reports a change for the better. If the manipulation is easy to perform at the first session, one always obtains a definite gain. This gain may be maintained or not, but it is always present. On the other hand, if the spine is very stiff and a satisfactory manipulation is difficult, one should wait for a session when the manipulation can be conducted in an easy way (the third usually for a chronic case) in order to formulate a decision as to its efficacy. The prognosis will be good if this session brings about a definite improvement. One should never perform a second session before the reactions from the first one are completely extinguished. It is never rewarding to manipulate too much or too frequently. For example, in a sciatica it is not wise to conduct the session at more than five-day intervals. One session per week is good timing for treatment of a crisis of chronic lumbar pain or of the painful scoliosis. Treatment will consist of from three to six sessions. In addition, it is advisable to repeat the treatment from time to time (1 to 3), dependent upon the case as a maintenance treatment which should particularly include rehabilitative exercises.

Different subjects do not react to, nor tolerate the treatment by manipulation in the same way. The pyknic type tolerate the frequent and intense treatment better than the asthenic who are poorly adapted to this mode of treatment. For the latter type, one should limit oneself to the most useful maneuvers and space them as much as possible. Without this, the manipulations may result in a true painful vertebral syndrome with false transitory improvements following the sessions which tend to perpetrate this situation.

Aged patients derive great benefit from mild mobilization; it brings about for them a greater range of motion and causes the disappearance of mild disturbance due to the paravertebral contractions maintained by the segmental stiffness. It may be surprising to find that certain senile spines may be considerably improved by a few delicate movements, that appear to be illusory while both clinical and x-ray examinations may lead one to believe that the patient is beyond the reach of manipulative therapy.

A common complaint is that the results of the manipulative treatments are not durable. This is sometimes true, although there are many cases when good results can be maintained despite the apparently poor conditions of the patients: poor posture, insufficient musculature, important discal changes.

The result depends on the correctness of the choice of treatment and the quality of its execution, in other words, upon the operator. This point which seems to be evident needs to be strongly emphasized, however, for it is generally believed that once a segment is popped, all has been accomplished. There is a world of difference between selective manipulation and forced mobilization lacking in precision. There is also a world of difference between well-conducted manipulative treatment in well-timed sessions, well-graduated, and progressive sessions and few sessions of repeated popping every two or every eight days. If the maneuver has not been sufficiently precise and complete, the resulting improvement obviously has little chance of continuing. Also, if the manipulator disregards the presence of a static imbalance, for instance the presence of one shorter leg, or if one neglects to decontract the vertebrae segment above or below the painful area, the improvement will not last. This "reharmonization of segmental movements" is a major point during the treatment by manipulation which should not be limited to the painful segment only. When this reharmonization is obtained, the quality of the therapeutic results is generally such that it leads certain manipulators to completely neglect the rehabilitative exercises which are, however, indispensable for a spine lacking good muscles or good balance. Indeed, muscular insufficiency, poor muscular synergy, and lack of muscular control are mainly responsible for spinal fragility, and it is against this situation that well-designed exercises are aimed. It is only when one cannot prescribe such exercises that the patient will be condemned to wear a brace in certain cases of recurrent lumbar pain.

Let us stress again the necessity of performing one to three maintenance sessions per year in certain conditions such as cervical arthrosis in which there is a usual tendency of recurrence of stiff necks.

Chapter 13

Indications for Manipulative Therapy

W E SHALL discuss clinical indications and related problems in more detail in Part III of this book. Let us here simply outline the major aspects of this discussion.

The indications of manipulations are reversible mechanical derangements of the intervertebral joint whether they are discal, disco-articular, articular, or resulting from the segmental vertebral stiffness and also from the painful symptoms which they cause.

It is proper to state at the very onset of this chapter that there is no irreplaceable therapy. It is certain that there are cases where manipulation alone may cure or improve the patient. However, these are not the most common cases. Most frequently, other therapies may achieve the same result. *It is better not to manipulate than to manipulate incorrectly:* the cure, then, is worse than the disease. What is irreplaceable in the manipulative therapy is the rapidity of the results—at times, instantaneous, generally requiring two to three sessions, only in exceptional cases more than six.

We are going to briefly review the principal indications of manipulations. We will consider in detail the most important ones during the third part of this monograph. It is sufficient to mention here that the greatest merit of vertebral manipulation is to call attention to the vertebral origin of certain diseases and the existence of many cases of projected pain which may lead to a diagnostic error.

CERVICAL REGION

The cervical region offers to the manipulator a wide field of action. However, although it is easy to accomplish a forced mobilization of the neck by right or left rotation, it is difficult to apply precisely the maneuver to a specific segment in a given direction, especially when one deals with the high cervical region. Thus, the results vary a great deal with the correctness of the technique used and with the operator. The acute torticollis is a good indication but it is often better to treat it by the maneuvers of decontraction and mobilization rather than by abrupt manipulations. The *cervicobrachial neuralgia* is also a good indication; it may be improved very rapidly, sometimes instantaneously. It is one of the rare afflictions where it may be of interest to associate traction to the manipulation. The *cervical painful syndromes:* cervical post-traumatic pain or pain associated with cervical arthrosis with a resulting stiff neck, always react well to manipulations. The manifestation of the Barré Lieou syndrome constitutes an excellent indication of cervical manipulations. Let us review briefly the elements of this syndrome which was called "syndrome sympathique cervical posterieur": (1) headaches; (2) otolabyrinthic syndrome—subjective dizziness and vertigo, nausea, buzzing in the ear; (3) visual disturbances—dancing spots before the eyes and stinging sensation; (4) laryngeal phenomenon—voice changes, feeling of constriction, feeling of a foreign body; (5) psychic manifestations—anxiety, "emptiness of the head," and memory disturbances. All of these symptoms are rarely seen together. However, they are observed in isolation as different constellations. We are going to return to this syndrome later on.

If one judges the results obtained by cervical manipulations, one must conclude that the headaches of cervical origin are the most frequent ones among common headaches. They constitute a good indication of manipulative treatment which improves them rapidly and consistently. These indications are found both in subjects with an arthrosic cervical spine and in younger patients without arthrosis. It almost always involves unilateral supraorbital headaches, more rarely Arnold's neuralgia. The *vertigo* of cervical origin is also associated with a tender point with localized contracture in the inferior occipital fossa. One then deals most often with dizziness rather than with true vertigo. This vertigo is very frequent and good results obtained by manipulation of the high cervical spine are numerous. Conversely, manipulations performed in the direction of the blocking increase these complaints, or may even elicit them. The *acroparesthesias* of cervical origin react very inconsistently to manipulations. Those which involve a precise dermatome seem to react more consistently than the global acroparesthesias. It is evident that the acroparesthesias due to the compression of the median nerve in the carpal tunnel by tenosynovitis of the flexors are generally not influenced by the cervical maneuvers, although in our experience we have had a few cases when cervical manipulation was effective. Obviously, one should not overlook the diagnosis of other paresthesias originating in the spinal cord. When *scapulohumeral periarthritis* is acute, it is justifiable to treat it by rest, application of ice, administration of anti-inflammatory agents and not by manipulations. However, it is different in the case of a painful shoulder of the chronic type. Two cases should be considered: (1) There is no limitation of movement: there may be an involvement of one or several tendons (supraspinatus or biceps, most often). The cervical spine often plays a role in these cases, inasmuch as low cervical manipulations permit one quite often to bring about rapid success, sometimes immediately. (2) There are limitations of shoulder movements. If these limitations are global and if arthrography shows a contracted capsulitis, there is no hope for cervical manipulations. However, there are a certain number of painful shoulders with a more or less limited range of motion which are occasionally relieved instantaneously by cervical manipulation. This, of course, raises the interesting problem of pathogenesis.

The cervical column is almost always involved in head traumas. Also, the classical subjective syndrome of head trauma is often due to vertebral sprains and in these cases the manipulation constitutes a treatment of choice which consistently improves these patients whose complaints are often not taken seriously.

DORSAL REGION

The painful syndromes of the dorsal spine—the dorsal pain of malposture, the pain of scoliosis, and the dorsal pain secondary to muscular effort—are very good indications for manipulative therapy. As we shall see below many cases of back pain are of cervical origin (Maigne, 1964). A certain number of patients complaining of *precordial pain* suffer from an intercostal neuralgia or from sprained ribs or segmental pain in the D1 dermatome, and it may be influenced by appropriate manipulation. Some cases of *thoracic pain* may be due to neuralgia of the intercostal nerve related to vertebrodiscal chronic sprain or to the posterior or anterior costal sprains, afflictions which react well to manipulations.

LUMBAR REGION

Acute Lumbagos

Acute lumbago is undoubtedly the affliction which has contributed most to the reputation of manipulation. This is due to the fact that it is always impressive for the patient and for the doctor to obtain an immediate improvement of acute pain associated with a manifest functional deficit. It is also because certain lumbagos are easy to improve even by manipulation lacking in precision. Most of the patients are very rapidly and often instantaneously cured, although there are some types which react less well.

Chronic Lumbagos

Treatment by well-conducted manipulations gives very appreciable results in the chronic lumbagos. It does not appear that one is able to formulate a good or bad diagnosis on the presence or absence of x-ray signs: osteophytosis, discal degeneration, discal pinching, or the static disturbances—hyperlordosis or a flat lumbar region. In all these cases, the percentage of successes and failures remains approximately the same. Lescure reports 75 percent of good results after a month of treatment, which appears to us to be correct, in other words, after two to six manipulations. However, the manipulation, which improves occasionally for a certain time, generally does not bring about a durable result unless the static disturbances are corrected, including the plantar arches through appropriate rehabilitative exercises.

Common sciatica is considered in France as always being of discal origin (which is not always correct). The *discal sciatica* constitutes an excellent indication for manipulations. Almost always there is a notable improvement even during the first manipulation. In 25 percent of cases this is a complete improvement. In 75 percent of cases, very good results are obtained after one to five treatments, in other words, after one to twenty days of treatment by manipulative therapy only. The age of the sciatica is not a bad factor; one does not seem to find significant differences between results obtained in recent and long-standing cases. The latter, however, seems to react better and more rapidly than the former. It has often been said that manipulations should be reserved for recent cases of sciatica in young patients. However, according to our experience the results of manipulation are rather less favorable in subjects of 20 to 30 years of age than in those between 40 and 50.

THE COCCYX

The pain of the coccyx following a fall or after a delivery are cured consistently after one to three sessions. This is not the case in nontraumatic afflictions which often fail to respond to treatment.

THE RIBS

Most often one deals with costo-vertebral sprains of the false ribs. They cause numerous errors of diagnosis. They may be secondary to some attempts of the trunk rotation or to the direct traumas. They induce intense pain at the acute phase somewhat analogous to that of lumbago, but usually without notable contraction. The pain is located in the lumbar fossa radiating toward the groin and acutely intensified by certain movements and sometimes by respiration. These spasms may be confused with an attack of kidney stones if the notion of an initial effort is not clearly present or they may be taken for a fractured rib if the trauma was violent. The pain may decrease in intensity and become a chronic one, returning periodically, being caused by poor posture or certain movements. A simple maneuver which we call a "maneuver of the rib" is sufficient to confirm the diagnosis and may bring about an immediate improvement. We will study in detail these sprains which are almost always overlooked.

FUNCTIONAL DISTURBANCES

Patients manipulated for lumbar pain frequently report that their habitual constipation disappears or that certain digestive pains are suppressed. Others report that they have no more palpitations after mobilization of their neck. Obviously, it doesn't seem rational to systematically treat all these autonomic nervous system disturbances by manipulations. However, if the usual remedies are not successful and if the clinical signs call attention to the spine, then a therapeutic trial is acceptable provided the diagnostic examination was well performed and that no contraindication to manipulation was found. It is well known that a number of patients suffering from asthma are helped by costal vertebral deblocking, and Lescure (1959) has described a syndrome of a false asthma in infants responding remarkably to manipulations.

Occasionally, a case of facial pain cured by cervical manipulation may be observed. Some claim successful treatment of Basedow's disease occurring after cervical trauma (Riederer & Rettig, 1955, published such a case following chiropractic treatment). We may also mention that occasionally we could cure or improve mastodynia and several times pseudo-ulcers in patients with dorsal pain. However, it is well known how uncertain one is on these grounds and how important it is to wait for a systematic and exhaustive experimentation before drawing significant conclusions. One should keep in mind that there are painful syndromes which are of spinal origin but which are erroneously diagnosed. In certain cases manipulation may suppress them.

Later on we will discuss in more detail the principal indications of manipulative therapy (see also Cyriax, 1964; Cecile *et al.,* 1966; Lescure and Renoult, 1966; Lescure, Trepsat, and Waghemacker, 1953; Licht, 1960; Maigne, 1953, 1955, 1960, 1965, 1966; Maitland, 1964; Maitrepierre, 1959; Mostini, 1960; Renoult, 1965; de Sèze, 1955; Terrier, 1958; Waghemacker, 1962; Wilson and Ilfeld, 1952; de Sèze, Robin, and Levernieux, 1948; Waghemacker, 1965).

Chapter 14

Contraindications

Sᴏᴍᴇ ᴄᴏɴᴛʀᴀɪɴᴅɪᴄᴀᴛɪᴏɴs are *absolute*. They are related to the nature of the disease. It is self-explanatory that the vertebral fractures and pain related to inflammatory tumoral or infectious diseases constitute an absolute contraindication. As pointed out before, these diseases may be recognized for the first time at the occasion of an effort made by the patient or by a trauma. This means that treatment by manipulation is justified only when a precise diagnosis has been formulated correctly on the basis of both clinical and radiological examination and, if necessary, laboratory tests. It is very important to have excellent x-ray pictures as the poor ones are more dangerous than none at all. A poor x-ray of the neck in a patient having trauma may overlook a fracture of the odontoid or the atlas.

In addition to these definite contraindications there are others which are *less absolute,* such as the pain of *Scheuermann's disease* which in its acute period is generally aggravated by manipulations. The stiff back which is characteristic of the sequelae of this disease, on the contrary, may be improved by delicate, prudent, and progressive mobilizations. One should never attempt abrupt manipulations or a compressive direct manipulation upon such a back.

Other contraindications are not related to the disease, but to a given clinical case, for example, a case of cervicobrachial neuralgia or of sciatica where no movement is possible without eliciting pain. It is also the case of intense dorsal pain where mobilization in any direction is painful. In these cases, only sedative maneuvers involving the muscles may have a favorable effect. An arthrotic spine quite stiff, a senile spine, or an osteoporotic spine should not be "manipulated," if one considers by this term a simple abrupt brief movement. On the contrary, these cases may derive benefit from mild, progressive, and repeated mobilizations.

Everything in manipulation is a question of grading and adaptation to a given case. It is important to be able to use all the possibilities of manual treatment. A physician should not limit his therapy to manipulation only. It would be ridiculous to overlook chemotherapy and other possibilities of physical medicine of which physical manipulation is only one type. It would also be erroneous to believe that the manipulative method consists only in popping a vertebral segment in the correct direction. The manipulative treatment involves many more nuances and a simple maneuver barely sustained, practiced with a single finger applied to the sternocleidomastoid muscle is sometimes sufficient to improve a torticollis that has not responded to twenty maneuvers. Thus, complexity of the manipulative therapy depends upon the grading of the maneuvers: at times one should only slightly graze the surface in the maneuver; in other cases, one must press firmly. The nuances, the subtleties, truly cannot be practiced by those who have not become masters of their hands and techniques and who have not applied these treatments during a long and meditative training. The manipulation is more than an act; it is a method.

Lescure (1951) has stressed the possibility of reharmonizing segmental vertebral mobility by using manipulative therapy. When there is a segmental vertebral stiffness, the segment located above it must carry an additional burden; the areas of overfunctioning are located just above the area of physiological immobility (lower lumbar area, lower cervical region) . However, corresponding phenomena are observed above the segments of pathological stiffness. The maintenance of harmonious mobility is the best natural protection of the spine. The technique of manipulation must therefore be most subtle and perfect, as the mobile segments will have a greater tendency to be affected than the segments which are pathologically stiff.

This is to say that there are contraindications of manipulations related to the manipulator himself. He should be not only a physician, but a physician trained in the area of osteoarthritic pathology. He should be highly trained and be able to adapt his technique to his abilities.

Diagnostic error is another trap. Among different ambushes, one should cite spinal cord tumors and vascular pathology of the cord which may manifest themselves at the beginning by pain and parasthesias. Psychoneurotic patients may be considered as those manifesting Barré-Liéou syndrome (1925). An insufficiency of the vertebrobasilar circulation may cause grave errors of diagnosis. One should inquire as to the "drop attacks" and search for pyramidal, cerebellar, and visual field defects. Most of the reported incidents are related to vertebrobasilar accidents. One should always apply the postural tests (see p. 185). Another ambush is related to poor quality of x-ray pictures. In one case, only tomographs could reveal a fracture of the atlas. This is also the case of vertebral metastases.

However, those who intend to help their patients may consistently improve some of them by adopting a certain number of techniques and by adapting them to their patients. One should also advise beginners not to be too enthusiastic by their first spectacular success, as it may lead them to use this therapeutic method poorly or too often, although they may possess only its rudiments. Manipulative therapy is certainly tempting by the rapidity and elegance of its action, but it is only rarely irreplaceable and it is better to use more classical techniques than to manipulate poorly and make the patient worse (see also Depoorter, 1966; de Sèze, 1955; de Sèze and Thierry-Mieg, 1955; de Sèze *et al.*, 1948).

Chapter 15

Accidents, Incidents, and Abuses
of Manipulations

W HEN THE indication of manipulations is well justified and when they are correctly executed, no accident occurs, or the incidents are very rare. The quasitotality of accidents due to manipulations are produced by unskilled and unsophisticated manipulators or because of a diagnostic error.

DRAMATIC ACCIDENTS

Dramatic accidents are not exceptional in the hands of the ignorant, the literature continually citing a wealth of new cases, and it is probable that their number will increase day by day in proportion to the increase of those nonphysicians who try to practice manipulation. At the basis of all the dramatic accidents, some of which are fatal, there is only one cause, that of an error in, or an absence of, diagnosis. In a case of brutal manipulation of the cervical spine of patients suffering from Pott's disease, metastasis, osteoporosis, or a fracture, sudden death or quadriplegia may result from a forced manipulation upon a dorsal or lumbar spine rendered fragile by an organic disease. These are the most frequent examples of the dramatic accidents.

However, in addition to these accidents, due to a gross error of diagnosis, attention was recently directed to the possibility of postmanipulative vascular accidents: thrombosis of the vertebral artery, basilar trunk, or of the posterior-inferior cerebellar artery (Wallenberg's syndrome) which was fatal in three cases, the fourth one having survived as per the report of Schwartz *et al.,* (1956). Complications appeared immediately following the manipulation. It was a case of chiropractic manipulation, therefore a powerful one involving the high cervical spine. The course was favorable after several months. A case reported by Ford and Clark (1956) is particularly striking. A young bacteriologist found his wife holding her head with both hands, turning it from left to right. She explained to him that her neck was a little stiff and that these small movements of the head were helping her. The bacteriologist complained also of some stiffness of his neck and asked his wife to move his head in the same fashion. He suddenly died from a thrombosis of the vertebral artery following a slight neck rotation.

Such accidents are exceptional, in view of the great number of manipulations which are carried out, correctly or incorrectly, every day. There is probably less than one death of this nature out of several tens of millions of manipulations.

When a rotation and hyperflexion of the upper cervical spine is performed, there is an arrest of the circulation in the vertebral artery on the opposite side. If there is in addition a vascular anomaly preventing a normal blood supply, the circulation within a part of the brain is deficient. Indeed, one can observe the, Wallenberg syndrome in workers who have to maintain their head in a faulty position (extension and lateral bending).

An important precaution is to maintain the head of the patient for several seconds, prior to any cervical maneuver, in a position preparatory to manipulation. Should the patient complain of vertigo or nausea, or should he exhibit any nystagmus, one should not administer manipulation. It is possible that an anticoagulating therapy urgently applied could favorably modify the course of these complications—one more reason to claim that only physicians should practice vertebral manipulations. (see also Boudin *et al.,* 1957; Grossiord, 1966; Held, 1965, 1966; Herbert and Fenies, 1959; Fisher, 1943; Benassy and Wolinetz, 1957; Toole, 1960; Klein and Nieuwenhuyse, 1927).

SERIOUS ACCIDENTS

Serious accidents are not rare in the hands of ignorant and unskilled manipulators. They are due to faulty technique: the poorly applied lever, a forced manipulation applied in the wrong direction, etc. These manipulations may result in a severe exaggeration of the original affliction such as torticollis and sciatica lumbago that become rebelliously hyperalgic. A case of torticollis may be transformed into a cervicobrachial neuralgia, a lumbago into a severe sciatica, a mild sciatica into a paralytic sciatica, and this may happen during the session itself. However, in exceptional cases, an unfortunate maneuver not necessarily poorly executed, may sever a herniated disc and drive it into the intervertebral foramen, forcing a surgical intervention. *Fractures of the ribs* with no displacement, although being most frequently seen by unskilled operators, may also occur to knowledgeable practitioners as the osteoporotic ribs of aged patients may be extremely fragile to pressure exercise in certain directions. More frequent and often responsible for persistent pain are the sprains of the ribs produced by poorly adapted maneuvers. We can cite among rare complications the occurrence of purpura following a manipulation (Tomlinson, 1955). We also observed one such case.

INCIDENTS

Incidents of poor results of manipulation occur frequently if the manipulator lacks experience.

The poorly executed manipulation may generate all the symptoms usually treated by these maneuvers. Thus, the maneuvers upon a cervical spine may elicit rebellious headaches, vertigo, visual disturbances, buzzing in the ear, briefly all the *symptoms* of the Barré-Liéou syndrome (1925) and which constitute an excellent indication for manipulative therapy. It is frequent to find patients complaining of cervical, lumbar, and dorsal pain originating during a manipulative session without having suffered from it previously. In some cases this might be a very mild incident caused by a somewhat exaggerated maneuver and easy to correct during the next session. However, more often than not we may deal with vertebral, costo-vertebral, or rebellious sprain which was created by a maneuver associated with a poor stabilization and which was wrongly directed. The complications caused by forced maneuvers are often difficult to treat. One should use more patience and apply very delicate and progressive movements, as these patients have already been made fearful and distrust any maneuver.

There is no therapy that does not present some risk and in

certain particular cases the gestures which are usually harmless are capable of producing dramatic consequences. This is particularly the case in manipulations of fragile and senile spines where these gestures are no longer harmless if the technique is not such that it allows their exact grading. It is necessary to repeat, however, that the grave accidents are extremely rare in relation to the number of performed manipulations. They exist, however, and physicians must be sure of the diagnosis before using this active therapeutic tool. The serious incidents are not rare in the hands of practitioners lacking experience. In the same hands, the incidents that are slight, although annoying and painful, are very common; however, they are fortunately self-terminating. The trouble is that the patient is left with a prejudice against this therapy which is so useful and effective. Thus, the beginner should be prudent: *no worker should attempt to treat difficult cases with these delicate techniques.* The well-conducted maneuvers of mobilization will give them more satisfaction and less trouble than the practice of elective manipulations which are quite difficult. (see also Lescure, 1954; Licht, 1960; Lievre, 1953; Oger, 1964; Rageot, 1966; Rieunau, 1961, 1966; Rubens-Duval, 1958; de Sèze, Kahn, Thierry-Mieg, and Renoult, 1966; Simon, 1966).

ABUSES OF MANIPULATIONS

There is a considerable number of patients being "manipulated" repeatedly and needlessly under most childish pretenses. Such was a case of a little girl who had a left leg shorter than the right one, with equinism and absent fibula and whose neck was manipulated by a chiropractor for one year in order to affect her thyroid, the "gland of growth." The parents did not want to terminate the treatment because, indeed, this leg gained two centimeters in length, despite the fact that the other leg also showed evidence of growth (at the age of 7!).

We (Maigne *et al.,* 1965) often emphasized what Lescure calls "obsessional psychosis of vertebral displacement" (1951). Undoubtedly, an increasing number of more or less qualified practitioners push their patients in this direction: "I had four displaced vertebrae which were put back in place but one of them doesn't hold well." It is very difficult to fight this prevailing idea of the displaced vertebrae. Even if one spends a great deal of time explaining to a patient that one has not replaced his displaced vertebrae, that a vertebrae is not usually displaced and that one simply "de-wedged a discal fragment" or "rendered more flexible his spine," it does not prevent the patient who comes back later on from telling you, "You have put back my fifth lumbar which was displaced." When this is limited to terminology, it is not too serious and is merely irritating, but it may become more serious when certain patients are truly haunted by this image of displacement which leads them to ask to be manipulated by more or less qualified practitioners until one day one of them will cause a vertebral or discal sprain.

Chapter 16

Mode of Action of Manipulations

ALTHOUGH ONE MAY KNOW correctly the indication of treatments for manipulations and one is able, as shown here, to choose in each given case a maneuver to perform, one must confess that their mode of action escapes us in most cases. One observes that manipulations improve the radicular pain of sciatica or cervicobrachial neuralgia and that they render more flexible a stiff spine and relax paravertebral muscles. One also notes that they elicit sympathetic and vasomotor reactions and that they improve some disturbances of the autonomic nervous system. Conversely, they are able to provoke such disturbances or to intensify them.

When manipulations are indicated and successful, it seems evident that they modify a reversible osteo-disco-ligamento-muscular disturbance and that they elicit a useful vasomotor reflex. *However, we can know the mode of action of manipulations only if we know the mechanism of the painful syndrome which is treated by them.* It is quite evident that we cannot invoke the same mechanism of action in a case of an immediate improvement of coccygeal pain (by touching the coccyx only) or a case of Arnold's neuralgia (there is no disc between C1 and C2) or a case of sprained rib (by touching the rib only) or in a case of sciatica. A particular mode of action must correspond to each particular case. *What remains common is the restoration of mobility of the treated joint, mobility which was nil or limited in certain directions.*

Manipulation is applied only to those joints in which certain voluntary or involuntary movements are limited. In addition it is necessary that the movements contrary to those which are blocked be free and that their mobilization be painless. Otherwise, it is not possible to perform a manipulation according to the rules which are spelled out above and experience shows that such manipulation is not desirable.

First, one may ask oneself what is the *mode of action of ma-*

nipulations upon a normal spine. We call a normal spine a column in which no movement is limited or painful and no vertebra nor any paravertebral region is tender or a site of a spontaneous pain, the x-ray pictures obviously being also normal. If one performs cervical manipulation on a person with a normal spine, this maneuver should not be followed by any reaction. Occasionally, however, one may observe an immediate axillary transpiration and nothing else. One may, therefore, assert that, practiced upon a normal spine, manipulation should not elicit any particular phenomena, any more than manipulation deblocking a meniscus performed on a normal knee should elicit an incident (see also Chrisman, *et al.*, 1964).

In a more general way one may state that manipulations imply (1) mechanical effects, (2) reflex action, either somatic or vasomotor, and (3) psychological effects.

1. *Mechanical effects.* These effects have been considered primarily in the past. It is known that a knee manipulation may liberate a blocked meniscus and thus instantaneously relieve pain and discomfort. The knowledge of discal pathology permits us to conceive an analogous mode of action, resulting in the reintegration of a discal fragment into the nucleus pulposus (see details below). We are proposing a hypothesis in which most of the minor vertebral derangements are due to a fragment of the nucleus pulposus blocked in a fissure occurring in the annulus fibrosus (dorsally, ventrally, or laterally). This blocking of a discal fragment is not painful in itself but it disturbs the functioning of a corresponding mobile segment and induces pain in one of its elements (posterior joint, ligaments, etc.). By liberating the blocked fragment one permits restoration of normal functioning of the segment.

One may also invoke the liberating action of manipulations in cases of impingement of the posterior joint facets, a pinching of a nerve twig or of an articular villosity (Junghanns).

Finally, a manipulation may act, as does any other joint mobilization, by increasing the range of motion limited by periarticular tissue reactions. In certain cases, it may break "adhesions" discussed by certain authors (e.g. T. Fisher). It should be understood that even in a case of a classical sciatica the mechanisms discussed below may be operational in part.

2. *Reflex action.* In any vertebral derangement there is some muscle contracture and abnormal tenderness of a ligament or joint capsule. These changes are secondary to mechanical disturbances but may outlast them, thus maintaining a pain-generating vicious cycle. A manipulation which stretches involved structures produces a sudden traction of contracted muscle and other elements of the joints. It thus stimulates the corresponding proprioceptors and induces a reflex action. This mechanism has been stressed by Liberson. Such a mechanism may thus break the vicious cycle.

3. *Psychological effects.* It is appropriate to stress that psychological effects are no more operational in manipulative therapy than in any other therapy presently used in treatment of minor vertebral derangements and in many other fields of medicine. The psychological value of a manipulation depends primarily on the manner in which it is used by the practitioner. When one relieves the suffering of a patient with sciatic pain, it is difficult to consider psychological action alone to be operational in the manipulative treatment.

DISCOGENIC DISEASES

The explanation of the mode of action of manipulation cannot be formulated without the actual knowledge of physiopathology of different symptoms or disturbances relieved by them. To abolish radicular pain or sympathetic disturbance by manipulation of a spinal segment, the range of motion which is limited, does not tell us of the exact mode of this action. In order to know what was changed, the exact nature of the affliction which produced the treated disturbances must be known.

It is through the work of de Sèze (1955, 1961; de Sèze *et al.,* 1962; de Sèze and Welfling, 1957) that we know the role played by the intervertebral disc in the sciatica and in the lumbago and thus we may understand the mode of action of manipulations in these cases. This knowledge will help us to better interpret successes and failures and to better formulate the indications. If a manipulation improves a sciatica due to a discal compression, one must assume that it suppressed a conflict between the disc and the root. We may formulate three hypotheses: (1) the manipulation forced the herniation to reintegrate the central cavity of the disc; (2) it forced it into a "silent zone"; (3) it extracted still more the fragmented hernia which became a foreign body mobilized in the epidural space and which is destined to be resolved. On the other hand, the discal hernia disturbing the physiodynamics of the joint is associated with vasomotor changes and reflex contractures which are also effected by manipulations.

As an example, we will see in the light of the work of de Sèze (1941) in regard to discal sciatica and the antalgic attitudes, how one may explain the action of manipulation in these cases. This will permit us also to incidentally check the justification of the empirical usage of our "rule of no pain." We saw indeed that according to the manipulative procedures which we offer in this book, in the final analysis the maneuver is determined by the antalgic attitude. Hypothetically, such mechanism will be considered in a case of left L5 sciatica with a crossed antalgic attitude and in a case of left S1 sciatica with a direct antalgic attitude.

Left L5 Sciatica with a Crossed Antalgic Attitude and Kyphosis

The root is compressed by a discal fragment which is located laterally to it. The intervertebral space occupied by the involved disc therefore gapes to the left and backwards. The manipulation will be aimed first at increasing this gaping by putting the lumbar spine in a right lateral bending and anterior flexion and by bringing this segment into right rotation. Indeed, left rotation is not only painful, but it also increases the conflict between the disc and the root; while on the contrary, right rotation removes this discal fragment from its contact with the root, the exaggerating of the discal gaping to the left and backward favoring the reintegration of the herniated fragment into the discal cavity (Fig. 121).

Left S1 Sciatica with a Direct Antalgic Attitude

The left root is compressed by a discal fragment which is located medially to it. The disc gapes to the right. The manipula-

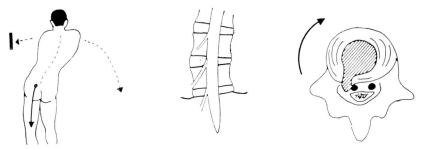

Figure 121. *Left,* Patient is suffering from a left L5 sciatica with a crossed antalgic attitude. Lateral bending is impossible to the left but is free to the right. Extension is impossible. *Center and Right,* The root is compressed by a discal fragment located laterally. The root is driven medially. The black arrow *Right* illustrates the direction of the manipulation in rotation.

tion will therefore, be performed beginning with a maximal lateral bending to the left. This is the most important point. This movement exaggerates the discal gaping. It is by rotation that the conflict between the disc and the root may be suppressed. This movement of rotation in a case of S1 sciatica with direct antalgic attitude is not always oriented in the same direction as that of lateral bending as was the case in L5 sciatica. The examination will lead the operator to perform this rotation either in the same direction as the lateral bending or in the opposed direction. In the former case, it is almost an absolute rule that the extension is free and therefore the positioning will be done in extension (see example chosen for Fig. 122).

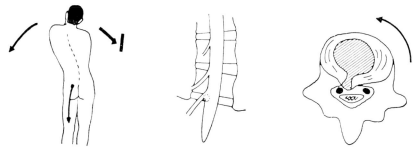

Figure 122. Patient is suffering from S1 sciatica with a direct antalgic attitude. The black flesh *(Right)* illustrates the direction of manipulation in rotation in this hypothetical case.

PART III

CLINICAL APPLICATIONS

Chapter 17

Headaches of Cervical Origin and Migraine

 FREQUENTLY, CHRONIC COMMON HEADACHES resistive to treatment may be cured by cervical manipulation. This brings us to considering the important role played by minimal disturbances of the cervical spine, either in causing or in contributing to persistent common headaches so difficult to treat. It is important to note that, conversely, one of the common complications of poorly executed cervical manipulations is the occurrence of persistent headaches, which has all the characteristics of headaches amenable to correct manipulations.

It is obvious that the cervical origin of a headache should not be considered unless all the organic causes (neurologic, ophthalmologic, vascular, allergic, those related to sinusitis, or toothache, etc.) are ruled out. One should not neglect psychological factors which are so important but which often play only a triggering role hiding real etiology.

Although there are cervical headaches which are caused by important changes of cervical structures, recently studied by many investigators (particularly related to disturbances of circulation involving the vertebral artery), one should not expect that in the case considered here significant lesions will be found characterized by specific x-ray pictures. Without therapeutic proof of the effectiveness of manipulation and counterproof provided by the exaggeration of headache if the manipulation is poorly executed, one might overlook the minor characteristic signs which should lead one to suspect the implication of the cervical spine.

These headaches usually start following a cervical trauma. However, the trauma may have occurred previously or be of only minimal intensity. The headache may be exaggerated by certain positions particularly when the patient is in bed with his head resting in a poor position on the pillow. It may occur only at night or only in the morning. It may be triggered by additional factors; that of a cold draft on the neck, indigestion, menstruation, or most commonly by frustrations. This triggering factor which frequently remains the same in a given individual may lead the patient to believe that the gall bladder or ovaries are involved if the dysfunction of these organs coincides with the headaches and treatment relieves the symptoms. Let us consider the following case history selected from hundreds of analogous cases.

> *Mrs. D., age 42.* Since the age 32. Mrs. D. has complained of violent headaches in the right supraorbital region, associated with nausea, usually lasting from 3 to 4 days, occurring a week before onset of menstruation but occasionally following exposure of the neck to draft or after a frustrating experience. After numerous consultations and therapeutic trials, the most successful treatment consisted of injections of 10 mg of progesterone the twenty-first day of the menstrual cycle. This treatment reduced the headache to a tolerable level. However, after suspension of the treatment, the headache returned with the original intensity. We were impressed by the *consistency* of the topography of pain (the headache being always localized in the occipital region or the right supraorbital area). It was relatively easy to find that there was a limitation of the mobility of the upper cervical spine in right rotation and lateral flexion. There was also a tender point well localized to the right of the base of the occiput. Pressure on this point elicited nausea and the onset of the headache. X-rays were negative. Three sessions of manipulation suppressed the local signs. The patient was examined six years later and reported complete absence of headaches following these manipulations. The patient rememberd at this time that a few months prior to the headaches, she had fallen from a bicycle and suffered minor cervical pain but had quickly forgotten it.

TOPOGRAPHY OF CERVICAL ORIGIN HEADACHES

Occipital and Supraorbital *(Fig. 123, top)*

The most characteristic symptoms of the headache of cervical origin (when all other causes are ruled out) is the *consistency* of its topography. In 90 percent of cases the headache is localized in the supraorbital and occipital regions on one side. Very rarely is it bilateral. Spread to the supraorbital region is rarely absent. However, the occipital pain may be either minimal or nonexistent (left diagram). More rarely the pain is retro-orbital with an irradiation toward the nose.

The intensity of the headache is variable, at times minimal

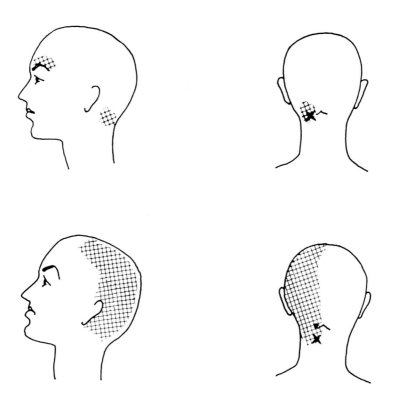

Figure 123. Headaches. *Top,* An occipito-supraorbital headache. An habitual headache of long duration having always the same topography, on the same side. It is very frequently of cervical origin susceptible of being relieved by appropriate manipulation. *Bottom,* Arnold's neuralgia.

and relieved by aspirin, at other times violent and accompanied by nausea. The incidence is also variable; it may occur at prolonged intervals or be present daily, often at the same hour. For instance, it may occur on awakening in the morning, diminishing during the day and reappearing in the evening as a result of fatigue or certain postures.

Such a clinical picture, particularly when present for a certain time in a patient free from other organic signs, focuses the attention of the physician on the high cervical spine.

Occipital Neuralgia

At times pain is strictly occipital unilateral or bilateral. In some cases it radiates toward the mandible.

Arnold's Neuralgia *(Fig. 123 bottom)*

In some cases, the headache has all the classical characteristics of Arnold's nerve neuralgia; occipital pain almost always bilateral, spreading toward the forehead but never reaching it. Treatment by manipulation may also be successful in these cases.

EXAMINATION OF THE CERVICAL SPINE

The examination is carried out on the patient in supine position with his head extending beyond the table using the technique described previously.

The examination is aimed at (1) the tissues of the suboccipital region, (2) the mobility of this region, and (3) the effect of pressure and traction.

Mobility

The mobility of the occipitovertebral region is carefully evaluated in flexion, extension, rotation, and lateral bending. The examination is performed separately for each of these movements and then globally, combining several movements in the same trial; for example, lateral bending, ipsilateral rotation, extension carried out as a combined maneuver on each side, then lateral bending, contralateral rotation, and extension on the right and on the left.

This examination aims at detecting a limited mobility in one direction.

Palpation

Palpation of the superficial tissues may often show a greater tenderness on the side affected by the headache than on the non-affected side. This tenderness is tested by a combined pinching and rolling of the skin.

The deeper tissues and particularly the suboccipital muscles may be contracted. At times the palpation reveals fibrous cordlike fascicles on the side of the headache. Most particularly the presence of a precise tender point may be found two fingerwidths from the midline in the suboccipital fossa at the base of the occiput. This point is particularly evident during the attack of headache although it may persist permanently in a patient with chronic headaches (Fig. 124).

In some cases pressure exerted against this point, when the head is moved in the direction of decreased mobility, elicits a painful irradiation over the supraorbital region. During the attack, the injection of Novocain at this point may decrease or suspend the attack temporarily.

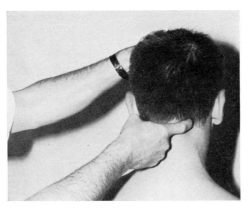

Figure 124. A search for tender points in the suboccipital fossa. It is also helpful to look for them with the patient in a supine position.

Postural Testing *(Fig. 125)*

The positioning of the high cervical spine in the direction of diminished mobility during 40 to 45 seconds often elicits headache (particularly during the period of the attack) while moving the head in the opposite direction brings relief. In addition, manual traction applied to the head for a half minute or so may relieve the headache during the attack while pressure of the head downward with both hands of the physician may either elicit or increase the pain.

Postural testing is an important precaution for eliminating

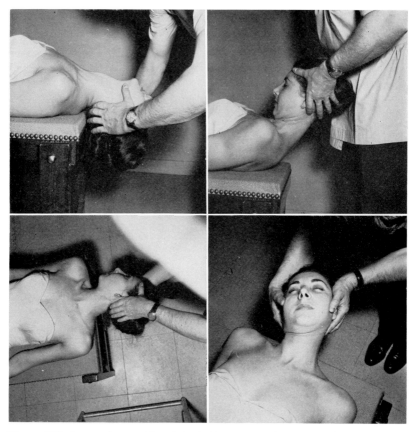

Figure 125. Postural test. *Top left,* in hyperextension. *Top right,* in hyper-flexion. *Bottom left,* in lateral bending. *Bottom right,* in rotation and hyper-extension. These maneuvers are identical to those which are used in order to analyze segmental mobility or to those used in manipulation. However, their execution is different: These maneuvers are "maintained" in extreme positions, so that the physician may find out whether or not they elicit the patient's complaints, for example a headache or a vertigo, etc. In no case should manipulation be effected without these diagnostic precautions at the level of the cervical spine, and, especially, in no case should the cervical spine be manipulated in the direction in which postural tests reveal head-aches or vertigo.

disturbances of the vertebral artery circulation, the cause of the only real manipulation accidents, the other mishaps based mostly on errors of technique or diagnosis.

X-ray Examination

One should not expect to find important characteristic radiological signs. In cases where x-rays reveal positive findings, the latter may also be found in a large number of individuals with no symptoms. Moreover, these findings persist after the patient is relieved from his headache following manipulation.

However, if the x-ray findings are very pronounced, manipulation of the cervical spine may be contraindicated. This seldom occurs inasmuch as our maneuvers are very gentle and are performed with the tips of the fingers.

PATHOGENESIS

Following a successful treatment by manipulation, all the signs of the physical examination disappear as the headache is relieved.

It seems difficult to understand the connection which may be present between the supraorbital pain that occurs in the area of the trigeminal innervation on the one hand and the suboccipital region pain on the other. And yet, if, following skin anesthesia using the method of Kellgren, a concentrated saline solution is injected in the suboccipital region exhibiting the usual tenderness, the usual supraorbital headache may be elicited. Although this constitutes proof of a connection between the neck and supraorbital regions, it does not seem to offer a rational explanation of the clinical findings. The following quotation from Lazorthes (1966) provides an explanation: "the lower end of the afferent nucleus of the trigeminus nerve fuses with the upper end of the dorsal horn, so that the first two dermatomes are common with the area supplied by the fifth nerve. Some nerve twigs arising from C1 and C2 participate in the skin innervation of the supra-orbital region (personal communication) .

TREATMENT

It is not rare to find a painful reaction following the first manipulation, particularly in a patient with chronic headache.

Two to four sessions are necessary in an average case, and four to six in more difficult cases. The maneuvers should be very selective, precise, and limited. They are preceded by prolonged maneuvers of relaxation and mobilization.

A follow-up examination is indicated every two or three months for three or four times, particularly in case of chronic headache. If there is a discogenic disturbance of spine mobility or the presence of low cervical arthrosis, or local or general noncorrectable static dysfunction, "maintenance" manipulations are indicated two or three times a year. In most cases, results are long-lasting. Our statistics show favorable outcome in 75 percent of cases.

In cases where the involvment of subcutaneous tissue is pronounced, particularly when the skin is sensitive to pinching and rolling, massage following mobilization of the spine is prescribed, improvement being obtained only when the entire region becomes mobile.

Manipulations constitute the most convenient and expeditious treatment of these painful states. This direct therapy allows us to reveal the vertebral etiology. It may be associated with physiotherapy, radiotherapy, and sometimes local injection, provided that these therapies aim at the high cervical spine and, specifically, suboccipital tender points. The use of these additional treatments may be of great value in certain cases.

Although these cervical headaches responding to manipulation should not be overlooked, one should not ascribe all headaches to the cervical spine. One should particularly be cautious in the case of recent onset of headaches, which, when predominant in the occipital area, may constitute a symptom of a posterior fossa tumor. Also cervical headaches may be due to occipital localization of Pott's disease, staphylococcic osteoarthritis, cervico-occipital malformation, cervical tumor, etc., in addition to possible psychogenic causes.

ATYPICAL FACIAL PAIN

Cervical manipulation often relieves certain types of unilateral facial pain with temporo-orbital topography. They occur by paroxysmal episodes, often having a certain rhythmicity, and are associated with the increase of lacrimal and rhinal secretions. They are often considered of vascular origin and their relationship to migraine is frequently stressed.

At times this is a facial pain having a strong sympathetic component. The pain is prolonged, and often radiates toward the temporomaxillar joint and the mandible. The patients are most often referred by dentists or oral surgeons who could not identify the syndrome of Costen or relate the pain to any local pathology. If vertebral examination shows a very vivid tenderness of the posterior articular bony structure at the level of C2-C3 on the same side, and if radiological signs are not present, manipulation may be successful in many cases and the pain subsides (see also Galmiche and Lenormand, 1951; Thierry-Mieg, 1959).

MIGRAINES

The True Migraine

The true migraine may be defined as a syndrome involving paroxysmal headaches lasting for hours with a unilateral predominance with nausea, pallor, and sometimes initial visual disturbances. Onset is before the age of thirty in individuals with family history of migraine.

It should be noted that most patients with true migraine may have headaches at times on the right side and at times on the left. *Defined in this way the migraine is never relieved by cervical manipulation.* However, there are patients in whom migraine may alternate with headaches of cervical origin. In such cases, it is not rare to find the latter disappear as a result of manipulations while the former remain uninfluenced.

The Migraine of Cervical Origin

Besides the true migraine there is "cervical migraine" which presents an interesting problem. Bartschi-Rochaix (1947) described a migraine syndrome of cervical origin. The osteophytes and inflammatory reactions related to their formation, according to this author, cause the angiospasms in the area supplied by the vertebral artery. This pathogenesis is generally accepted.

For Taptas (1953) cervical discal pathology essentially influences the preganglionic fibers of the white rami communicants, connecting the cervical sympathetic chain to the cerebrospinal nervous system by way of the five distal cervical roots. The irritation of these structures elicits vasomotor changes in the whole carotid system extra as well as intracranial.

Here, we would likely make the following observations:

1. Common cervical headaches have most frequently supraorbital localization; they may be associated with nausea which in certain patients can be very severe and thus present a pseudomigrainous character. The headache *always occurs on the same side* and there are signs involving the high cervical spine. Moreover, manipulations usually have a favorable influence on these headaches while the ergotamine tartrate is ineffective in these cases. Therefore, these headaches do not have a true migrainous character.

2. Occasionally, however, the character of these headaches may be frankly migrainous, being preceded by scotomata and presenting a clinical course similar to that of a migraine. They might even be sensitive to ergotamine tartrate and terminate in vomiting.

According to our experience, cervical origin may be suspected if the headache is localized always *on the same side* during every paroxysmal episode. The history of cervical trauma having occurred before the onset of the attacks is also extremely important. One must look for signs of cervical dysfunction (generally at a lower level than in the case of the headaches discussed above), usually between C4 and C7. One should try to elicit the signs of an intervertebral disturbance at that level (tender posterior paravertebral point, pain resulting from pressure over the spinal process in vertical and lateral directions) and to study painstakingly the segmental movements, successively tautening the spine in different directions. Postural tests must be applied maintaining tautness for thirty or forty seconds in each direction. This maneuver often elicits the onset of the attack or nausea. This is a critical component of the diagnostic procedure and a very good precaution to take in cases of circulatory disturbances in the vertebral circulation.

Finally a therapeutic trial of manipulation should be done with a rigorously precise technique in order to solve the diagnostic and etiological problem.

The following is an example of cervical migraine of traumatic origin.

Mr. X, operator of a windmill, forty-three years of age. Four years ago, a sack of flour fell on his head. He did not lose consciousness but complained of cervical pain for several weeks. The pain completely disappeared except in movements of extreme right rotation and hyperextension. However, only a few weeks later, migrainous attacks associated with vomiting appeared always on the right side. No family history of migraine, asthma, or eczema was found. These attacks increased in frequency and intensity. Repeated neurological examinations remained negative.

The x-ray pictures showed a slight abnormal cervical curve (disappearance of cervical lordosis and the beginning of a discogenic disturbance, C6-C7 with a moderate diminution of the intervertebral space). EEG was normal; vertebral angiography was not done.

Clinical examination showed definite signs of an intervertebral disturbance, C6-C7, with limitation of movements to the right side. Taking up the slack with the spine in hyperextension, right lateral flexion, and right rotation, maintained for about forty seconds, elicited the onset of migraine. After four manipulations, the patient was completely relieved. He has not suffered from headache since.

Chapter 18

Posterior Cervical "Syndrome" of Barré and Liéou and Subjective Syndrome of Head Trauma

SUBJECTIVE SYNDROME OF HEAD TRAUMA

W E HAVE CONSIDERED cases of headache of cervical origin. However, these headaches may be associated with other complaints which contribute to a syndrome which was described by Barré of Strasbourg and his pupil, Liéou (1925), under the name of the "sympathetic posterior cervical syndrome." At that time they attributed the etiology of this syndrome to an irritation of sympathetic fibers by arthrosis (Barré, 1926). However, for some time these authors abandoned the notion of the "sympathetic" nature of this syndrome which has been attributed to the involvement of the vertebral artery. We are not going to consider pathogenesis of this syndrome. We shall only discuss the clinical observations from the viewpoint of manipulative medicine.

These symptoms are usually present in patients over 50 years of age, having some stiffness of the neck due to arthrosis, in whom a faulty position on the pillow or a prolonged fatigue, as well as any other minimal disturbances are sufficient to elicit a minor intervertebral derangement in such a spine (where the small joints lose their free play). Besides, as we shall see in the next section of this chapter, cervical traumas may induce analogous disturbances in a normal spine.

A faulty prolonged posture at work or even during a period of inactivity may also be responsible. We have even observed that such intractable headaches are relieved by the use of a heel lift in a patient in whom one leg is shorter than the other by less than one inch. Often the symptoms disappear after a spontaneous favorable movement or following a warm shower or after taking aspirin. However, they often persist and then spontaneous regression is rare. One should mention the aggravating role of cold and draft as well as psychological factors. The latter may dominate the picture and become the most important therapeutic problem. The difficulty in diagnosis is, at times, distressing, in view of the identity of the symptomatology described by Barré and Liéou and those found in neurotic individuals. It is important to be able to differentiate in an anxious or depressed patient what is due to cervical etiology (arthrosis or cervical trauma) and what is due to the somatization of a neurotic "delusion" (Barbizet, 1957, 1958). The presence of unilateral symptomatology, of the headache, in particular, the presence of definite cervical signs consistent with the topography of complaints, favor cervical etiology. In cases of doubt, a trial treatment by manipulation may be indicated, provided that a precaution is taken to rule out vertebrobasilar arterial insufficiency, which may be first manifested by the same symptomatology.

Postural tests and the rule of no pain constitute the elements of prudence which are very appropriate in manual therapy of the cervical spine.

Elements of the Syndrome

Following is a list of complaints associated with the syndrome:

1. Headache: The symptomatology is the same as described in the chapter on headaches.

2. Vestibular Troubles: The patients complain of trouble in balancing; they hesitate going across an open space, as they feel they may fall down or give an impression of being drunk; more frequently they complain of having vertigo, almost always resulting from head rotation or its extension over the neck. At times it is a true rotatory vertigo. Labyrinth testing is only slightly positive; in most cases, there is labyrinthine hypoexcitability. Spontaneous nystagmus is rare. At times there is positional nystagmus of quite a special type, induced by head rotation (Aubry, 1964). On the other hand, electronystagmography provides the physician with more precise information (see p. 200).

3. Auditory Troubles: Diminution of hearing, tinnitis, ringing, roaring, whistling sounds, etc.

4. Visual Disturbances: Visual fatigue, sensation of dust in the eyes, dancing points, etc.

5. Pharyngolaryngeal disturbances: Hoarseness, at times aphonia, pharyngeal paresthesia (illusion of a foreign body).

6. Vasomotor and Secretional Disturbances: Hot flashes, perspiration; alternation of the paling and flushing of the face. Nasal hypersecretion, tearing, or conversely, decrease of lacrimal, salivary, or nasal secretion.

7. Psychic disturbances: They are very common so that many of these patients are considered neurotic. They complain mostly of mental fatigue, difficulty in concentration, loss of memory, depression, anxiety, etc. Although it is quite possible that neurotic personality favors a progression of these disturbances, they often appear without any antecedents pointing in this direction. It is appropriate also to stress that they may appear following head trauma and may disappear after cervical manipulation.

These symptoms only rarely appear all together. Their combinations and intensity are variable in each individual (see also Braaf and Rosner, 1962).

Examination of the Spine

The examination of the spine is conducted as described previously (see chapter on headaches). One seeks to determine in which position of the head or neck the symptoms are induced or enhanced, such as vertigo or perception of roaring or whistling. The postural tests should be carried out most carefully (see p. 185). One determines which maneuver decreases the symptoms. It is in the direction of such maneuvers that manipulation will be oriented.

Manipulations of the upper cervical spine are very subtle and difficult to perform according to the coordinates prescribed by premanipulative testing. Yet, manipulation poorly applied, or involving the wrong segment is of no help. If it is too extreme, it may result in irritation of the tissues. If directed in the incorrect sense, the patient's condition may be seriously worsened and one should wait several weeks before the situation may be corrected (with great difficulty) using a maneuver which is usually not easy to perform under such conditions.

Therapeutic Results

Excellent results may be achieved as far as headache and vertigo are concerned, much less satisfactory as to the spontaneous perception of roaring in the ear and still less as to spontaneous perception of whistling in the ear. Visual fatigability is usually much improved, as well as pharyngolaryngeal disturbances. We treated three singers who had difficulty with high notes following cervical trauma; they recovered their normal voices following a few treatments by manipulation. The results are also excellent concerning mental symptoms. It is for this reason that one is tempted to consider the importance of psychological factors in manipulative treatments. Although these factors should not be underestimated, they should not be overstressed. This reasoning does not seem to be more valid than in the case of any other medical therapy, which is often still more impressive from the patient's point of view. It is well known that psychological effects depend more upon the personality of the physician than upon the type of therapy which he applies. It is also appropriate to state that the proportion of neurotic patients varies with the type of recruitment of patient population.

The reader will find detailed techniques of treatment in Part IV of this monograph.

CERVICAL TRAUMAS

A number of cervical traumas increase in direct proportion to the number of car accidents (Feld, 1954).

However, here we are interested in those traumas in which no motor deficit or radiological abnormality are present, not those which offer serious neurological or orthopedic complications (see Blanc, 1964).

These patients complain of the cervical or dorsal intractable pain, of "cervical fatigue," whenever they carry a load. They do not tolerate certain occupational postures. This pain is associated with different manifestations of the Barré-Liéou syndrome diversely combined one with the other. At times radicular signs or those of the tennis elbow or those of tendinitis around the shoulder or even those of a restrictive capsulitis may complete the clinical picture.

The accident does not need to be severe in order to generate cervical trauma. Using the brakes when the light suddenly turns red and when the neck is too relaxed is enough to cause trauma. The neck may be projected backwards even though not violently. The head, which weighs five kilograms and is balanced over the cervical spine, being supported by only two small articular surfaces no greater than a thumbnail, is also thrown backwards pulling the cervical spine with it. In addition, a sudden reflex contraction of the flexors of the neck occurs with a certain delay. We shall not describe all the details of the mechanism of the production of these whiplash injuries, as they are still very controversial and subject to innumerable papers. Grossly, we should differentiate the traumas in flexion, often associated with dislocations or even fractures of vertebrae, from traumas in extension usually free of any radiological sign.

It is easy to imagine that the joint injuries are not the same if during a collision, or any other accident, the head is directed along the axis of the impact or if the head is rotated or if the impact is directed laterally. In the final analysis, it is the result of the injury which is important.

If the radiography of the cervical spine is grossly negative, one still should pay attention to little signs, such as segmental rigidity, changes or inversion of the curvature, slight misalignment of the odontoid process in relation to the lateral masses of the atlas. It appears to us that the latter represents a compensation of a slight cervical scoliosis often found after cervical trauma. There is a rotation of the atlas over the axis, not, as a result of a subluxation, but simply to counterbalance the antalgic cervical scoliosis which appears below these vertebrae, since the eyes must remain horizontal. The convexity of the facets contributes to this appearance of false pinching and of a false misalignment. These changes, secondary to the trauma, persist most often even though the patient, as a result of the manipulative treatment, is free of his troubles and the spine recovers its painless flexibility and resilience. We may mention the interest of tomography of the upper cervical spine in case of such traumas which at times may reveal a hidden fracture, suggesting the importance of a complete neurological examination.

The resistance to therapy and the duration of these disturbances plus the repercussions which they have upon the activity of the patient almost always makes one suspect the presence of either malingering or neurotic personality. Such conclusions are all the more tempting, since there is always a certain psychological element, more or less pronounced, that seems to constitute an integral part of the problem. However, if this situation at times requires a consultation of a psychiatrist, the psychological factors often become rapidly attenuated when the patient's pain subsides.

Indeed, this pain frequently originates from a "minor intervertebral derangement" of the cervical spine. On should look for it most carefully, analyze it, and find an appropriate treatment.

Chances that the neck pain is of organic nature are all the more great if it has consistent topography, being exaggerated, diminished, or reproduced by precise diagnostic maneuvers. One seems to elicit exquisitely precise tender points capable of reproducing or simulating the habitual pain; one finds them at the level of skin projections of the posterior articular bony structures; by the axial pressure over the spinal processes (investigated with the spine extended and flexed) or by a lateral pressure on the anterior cervical point which may reproduce habitual pain (interscapular pain, pain radiated down the upper extremity, or in the shoulder). One should then evaluate muscle strength against manual resistance: first extensors (head over neck; head and neck over the dorsal spine), then the lateral muscles and the rotators. One should palpate muscular masses in order to detect tender areas, the presence of which may elicit projected pain. For example, by pinching the muscle between the thumb and index of the lower part of the sternocleidomastoideus one may elicit ipsilateral frontal headache which constitutes the habitual complaint of the patient. This search for "trigger points" is most important for the prescription of the appropriate treatment which at times may be quite simple, yet effective (injection of Novocain; spraying; massage). One should know the trigger points which have been studied with such precision by Travell (1955).

One should carefully palpate supraspinal and interspinal ligaments, inasmuch as the tenderness of one of them may be responsible for intractable cervical or dorsal pain which otherwise is poorly localized.

Manipulation, well selected and correctly conducted, often constitutes an appropriate therapeutic solution. It should be quite specific, never global, and *never systematically bilateral* so that reactions of the patient to one or the other maneuvers can be evaluated with precision. The maneuvers of relaxation, as well as mobilization, are always indicated, and they should be gentle and discrete. Manipulation should be relatively sparse: one or two maneuvers per session, the latter scheduled only once a week, at least at the beginning.

A warning is in order to those who lack perfect mastery of the subtle cervical techniques. One should learn to effectuate these with the fingertips. One should know how to grade them with precision and adjust them in the right direction. Nothing is more difficult than to correct an aggravated neck condition as a result of poorly prescribed manipulation which is done incorrectly. And yet, of all possible treatments, manual therapy is without any doubt the one which may be of greater help to the patient, if associated with other therapeutic means at the disposal of a physician. Moreover, it permits him to analyze precisely segmental movements of the spine, and judging by the direct responses of the patient to the performed maneuvers, to be able to approach most appropriately the biomechanical disturbances of the neck and their consequences (see also Mennell, 1966; Raney, 1951; Raney and Raney, 1948; Raney, Raney, and Hunter, 1949; de Sèze, Godlewski and Barbizet, 1952; Seligmann, 1963; Toole, 1960; and Wolinetz, 1963).

HEAD TRAUMA

Subjective complaints of patients following head trauma (syndrome of Marie) contain many elements of the Barré-Liéou syndrome. As stated above, the syndrome of Marie concerned subjective disturbances of patients secondary to skull fractures. It is well known that many heated discussions are related to subjective syndromes. Psychiatrists have a tendency to relate them entirely to psychological causes. It is true that psychological elements in such clinical pictures are always marked. Anxiety is often observed as well as pronounced physical and mental fatigue, loss of libido, fear of aging, etc. These patients collect many medical certificates justifying their absence from work. It is often accepted that this syndrome is due to brain lesions or disturbances although the emotional factors should never be minimized in such patients.

However, there is one important observation which is often neglected in these patients, namely, the quasi-constant presence of the cervical involvement which is practically never considered in such cases and which one usually rules out on the basis of an x-ray examination. Yet, head trauma can hardly fail to involve the neck, which is so mobile and so vulnerable. Even if the cervical spine, because of its elasticity and flexibility, escapes being fractured or dislocated, it is the frequent site of traumatic microinjuries initiating a variety of complaints (Barré-Liéou syndrome, neck, dorsal, or interscapular pain, etc.) which can be revealed by a careful examination and which are so favorable affected by manipulative therapy. Their persistence, their apparent refractoriness, only increases the anxiety of the patient. Each patient having a history of head trauma should be considered as a potential carrier of neck traumas. Manipulative medicine may be of great help to such patients, even in cases of chronic disturbances.

Doctor Feld (1954), a neurosurgeon, has called attention to these disturbances of cervical origin; he attributed them to slight misalignment of the atlas and the axis which he considered to be a subluxation, just as chiropractors did. We do not believe that these findings (often present in patients following head trauma, but also in those who had no history of such a trauma) are direct-

ly related to the patient's complaints and that they are real subluxations. At any rate, they often persist without any change even
after the patient improves, following manipulative treatment
which also renders the spine flexible and free of pain or stiffness
(see Isemein and Perdrix, 1960; Isemein and Ramis, 1957;
Koupernik, 1964; Roge, 1964) .

OBJECTIVE PROOF OF THE EFFECTIVENESS OF MANIPULATION

While favorable results of manipulation in patients with lumbago or sciatica are discussed only as to the frequency of their occurrence, it is quite different in the case of the Barré-Liéou syndrome, which is now considered related to the vertebral artery
insufficiency.

The use of manipulative therapy in these cases is often criticized by those who have not practiced manipulative medicine. Many
clinicians deny the organic value of these complaints which, according to them, should be treated by sedatives and psychother-
apy, despite a great number of failures with such therapeutic man-
agement. No one should deny the importance of psychological
factors in such cases. Sometimes they alone are present. Such is the
syndrome of "Atlas" described by Alajouanine and Nick (1948)
(see also Alajouanine, 1957, and Alajouanine *et al.*, 1958) . However, as stated above, the frequently observed beginning of these
symptoms following a minor trauma, their improvement by
manipulation, their aggravation or even irritation by directing
manipulation in the wrong sense, are all important considerations
which should not be ignored.

We owe to Waghemacker (1965) the first elements of objec-
tivity in evaluating this treatment. It is well known that information obtained from the labyrinthine tests is quite limited in such
cases, whether one uses classical tests either the caloric or rotary
techniques (which, in addition, are not without danger to patients
with head or cervical trauma) . Vertebral angiography is not without complications and is often difficult to interpret.

A needed method has been found which provides as precise
information as possible without danger for the patient. This

method of evaluating the therapeutic effects consists of recording electrical potentials originating from the moving eyeballs. One amplifies these potentials expressing nystagmic movements. The patient is placed in an electrically controlled rotary chair which allows one to differentiate different components of the nystagmus as all sorts of stimuli are applied to the vestibular apparatus. Once the record of spontaneous nystagmus (if present) is made, with the subject at first keeping his eyes opened, then closed, one applies a test of acceleration and deceleration. This method permits one to obtain a strictly post-rotational response by imparting to the subject a subliminal speed of rotation, without eliciting any vestibular response during the rotation itself. The nystagmus is recorded at the same time as one makes a notation as to the duration of the subjective vertigo experienced by the subject. Thus, we obtain for each speed of rotation, two elements of the subject's response: one corresponding to the duration of the nystagmus (objective vertigo) and the other corresponding to the duration of the vertiginous sensation perceived by the patient (subjective vertigo). Repeating this test for different speeds of rotation one obtains two tracings—one corresponding to the nystagmus and the other to the sensation of vertigo. It may be stressed that it is not the speed of rotation which stimulates the inner ear, but acceleration or deceleration.

In order to record the corresponding curves, one should note on the vertical axis the durations of the post-rotational nystagmus (expressed in seconds) as a function of the speed of the chair rotation indicated on the horizontal axis (expressed in number of turns per minute or in degrees per second).

Normal nystagmogram thus obtained has the following essential characteristics:

1. A threshold appearing between 1 and 2 turns per minute.
2. A slope of about 45°.
3. An essentially linear relationship.

Thus, one may study on these tracings changes obtained under different pathological conditions. We will simply state that there are different types of curves depending upon different lesions, in particular there is a curve which is characteristic of the involve-

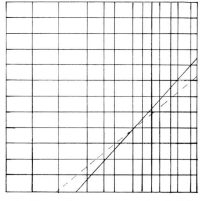

A. Normal nystagmograph. Solid line-normal nystagmas. Interrupted line-normal sensation.

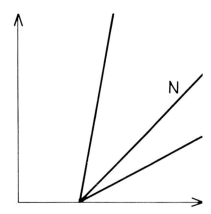

B. Variations of the slope (increased or decreased).

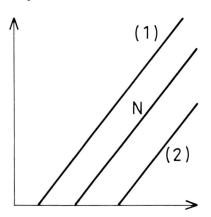

C. Variations of the threshold. (1) hyperreflexia; (2) hyporeflexia.

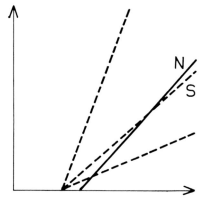

D. Modification of the nystagmograms (subjective) (interrupted lines).

Figure 126. Nystagmograms (schematic).

Horizontal scale: Speed (in turns per minute.)

Vertical scale: Duration (five-second units) of the evoked nystagmus or of the sensation of vertigo.

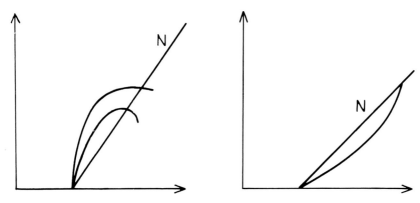

Figure 127. Two typical examples of clinical modifications of the nystagmogram. *Left,* cervical syndrome; *Right,* Meniere syndrome.

ment of the vertebral artery. One should also stress an interest in comparing the objective nystagmus with the recorded sensation, which is an important diagnostic factor and which may reveal participation of psychological components. Decroix *et al.* (1965) studied in this way the effect of manipulations on forty patients with a syndrome of vertebral artery (most often following trauma). They found that treatment by manipulation was truly effective as it tended to normalize the obtained tracings. Subjective improvement usually followed the objective improvement and concerned all the components (vertigo, headaches, etc.). The interest of this study is considerable as it brings proof of the following:

1. The reality of the patient's disturbances.
2. The role of the cervical spine.
3. The justification of manipulative therapy.
4. The satisfactory results which it induces almost exclusively.

This demonstration is very timely, since the belief is still quite prevalent that results obtained by manipulation are mostly imagined by manipulators or are only of psychogenic nature, as if these clinicians had exceptional psychotherapeutic abilities. Needless to say, when incidents with this therapy occur, the method itself is incriminated rather than incorrect prescription or unskilled performance.

Figure 128.
Three Examples of the Cervical Syndrome

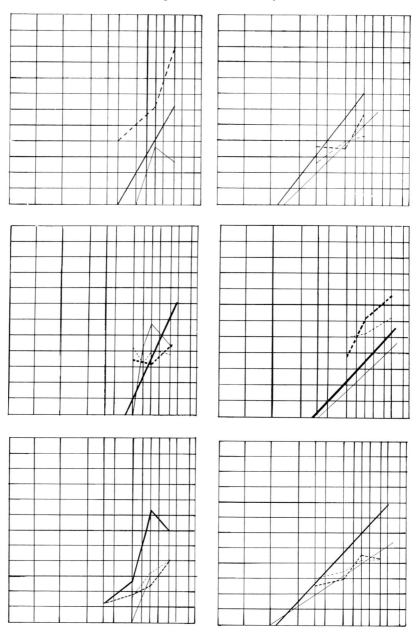

Case 1

Case 1: SD 42 years of age. Traffic accident. Loss of consciousness for 15 minutes or so. Remained dazed for several days. During subsequent weeks: pronounced neck pain, with no radiological abnormalities; then the appearance of vertigo often during rotation and lateral bending to the left as well as during hyperflexion and hyperextension of the neck. Treatment four months after the accident, four manipulations; disappearance of vertigo and neck pain; persistence of physical and mental fatigue as well as complaints of decreased memory.

Left nystagmograms: Before the treatment increased threshold on both sides, a bell-shaped curve on the left side (fine line; heavy line, right side).

Right nystagmograms: After treatment essentially normal tracings.

It is to be noted that the tracing of sensation is only slightly modified on the right side although one finds a minimal sensation on the left. (Dotted line curve of sensation right and left.)

Case 2

Case 2: BR, 35 years of age, cervical trauma: while driving stopped at a red light and projected backwards. Headaches, radicular neuralgia, left C6 which subsided. However, persistence of occipital headache with pharyngal paresthesias and vertigo when the neck is hyperextended in rotation and lateral bending to the left. Treatment started three months after accident consisting of three manipulations: all symptoms disappeared.

Left nystagmograms: Before treatment both threshold and slope are very high. Bell-shaped curve on the left side.

Right nystagmograms: After treatment: Threshold and slope almost normal; normal curve.

Case 3

Case 3: LG, 28 years of age, for the past six months: Neck pain as well as pain in the shoulders, fatigue, physical and mental, noise in the ears, nausea, headaches, vertigo with rotational sensation when head is hyperextended or during change of position. All drug treatments ineffective. X-ray shows cervical kyphosis, and moderate arthrosis. No history of trauma. Examination shows limitation of motion in rotation and lateral bending to the right as well as in extension of the upper cervical spine.

Treatment: After four manipulations, the neck pain disappeared completely as well as the vertigo, headaches, nausea and noise in the ear. There is still a marked fatigability.

Left nystagmograms: Before treatment, elevated slope and bell-shaped curve on the right side. Elevated threshold and curve in plateau on the left.

Right Nystagmograms: After treatment: Normal thresholds and slope. Normal curve. (Note: A curve of sensation shows before and after treatment, the presence of central factors.)

We are reproducing the following in Figures 126, 127, and 128:

1. A normal tracing and different types of tracings which are commonly observed in different conditions.

2. Three examples of cervical syndrome before and after treatment consisting of five manipulations. We are grateful to Doctors Decroix and Waghemacker for permitting us to publish these tracings (see also Klein and Nieuwenhuyse, 1927; Richard, Girard, and Dupasquier, 1948) .

Chapter 19

Limitation of Mobility of the Cervical Spine

CERVICAL OSTEOARTHROSIS

IN ADDITION to the limitation of range of motion of posttraumatic etiology, one should consider (1) chronic osteoarthosis and (2) acute torticollis.

Chronic Pain in Cervical Osteoarthrosis

Neck pain and particularly limitation of the range of motion are the most common and trivial manifestations of cervical osteoarthrosis (Hubault, 1962). The patient experiences increasing difficulty in turning his head in order to look behind him. Often this limitation of range of motion is associated with pain elicited by poor posture, draft, or cold weather. Pain may radiate toward the occipital region or the shoulders. It is not rare to find that the referred pain alone may elicit major complaints, as in the case of pain limited to the interscapular region, proved to be of cervical origin (see p. 255). These stiff necks are often infiltrated by "cellulitis" at the level of the cervicodorsal junction, particularly in female patients. This cellulitis improves when the neck recovers its flexibility, following the treatments. However, in order to subside completely, it should be treated by additional massage by superficial petrissage; otherwise these skin infiltrations may prolong intractable pain. The therapeutic results of manual therapy cannot be judged by the radiological examinations of the spine. In some instances of advanced osteoarthrosis one may achieve excellent results, with the spine recovering almost normal range of motion, while in other instances with only slight radiological abnormalities, therapeutic results may be more limited. When the *osteoarthrosis involves posterior joints* the results of manipulations are less satisfactory and take longer to obtain. In such cases one should not use manipulations that are too brisk, but rather those that are flexible, elective and exerted with a steady progression. The treatment of paraspinal muscles is very important, and consists of deep gliding massage along the long axis of the spine, and limited movements in the perpendicular direction.

One should abstain from any manipulation treatment during an acute inflammatory phase of osteoarthrosis. If one has any doubt as to the cause of the pain, either mechanical or inflammatory, one should consider the rhythm of the painful manifestations in order to be guided by this information for the choice of treatment modality. When there is an exacerbation due to inflammation, "taking up the slack" by prolonged efforts along the elementary components of the range of motion will elicit pain in all directions. It is obvious that one should also abstain from cervical manipulation in inflammatory arthritis, for instance, rheumatoid arthritis or pelvic spondylitis. In such patients, pain is elicited in all directions; and, therefore, manipulations are contraindicated by our rule of no pain and free movement.

Therefore, a preliminary test quite limited and benign will give maximal information as to the probability of therapeutic success of such treatment. If mobilization is easy to perform and brings relief from the very first minute and a reasonable increase of mobility, the prognosis is excellent. If it is laborious, yet when applied steadily does not elicit pain, the treatment should be continued. However, if the test of "taking up the slack" in a laboriously protracted fashion elicits painful resistance, manipulations are not advisable. In the majority of cases the treatment is possible and induces rapid beneficial results upon the mobility of the spine, the pain, and other complaints of the patient. Such effects, therefore, make the manipulative treatment of cervical osteoarthrosis most helpful. It is good practice to repeat "maintenance" treatments of one or two manipulations twice a year. A program of selected exercises to be performed daily also contributes to the therapeutic results (see also Soum, 1962).

Acute Pain: Acute Torticollis

Sometimes a simple forced movement in rotation to the non-painful side instantaneously relieves a "microtraumatic" torticollis. However, most frequently the manipulative treatment of the acute torticollis is not so easy and only precise and careful maneuvers may be immediately successful.

The maneuvers of progressive decontraction and those of muscle relaxation are generally helpful. One should indeed avoid too abrupt movements which may make the patient worse. One should not forget that certain cases of torticollis are due, not so much to mechanical causes, but to a virus infection inasmuch as one can see at times a true epidemic of torticollis in a community.

Obviously, one should not manipulate such patients. However, once the acute phase has subsided, there may be persistent stiffness, a limitation of movements, even some pain, and then manual therapy may become quite effective.

It is at the level of the cervico-occipital junction that most of the instances of torticollis commonly seen in medical practice originate; however, a block at the midcervical region may also occur (see also Jacquemart and Piedallu, 1964).

Congenital Torticollis

Jacquemart and Pledallu (1964) have reported good results in sixteen cases of "obstetrical torticollis."

Chapter 20

Cervical Radiculitis

T HIS NEURALGIA is characterized by pain along the upper extremity due to an irritation caused by compression of a nerve root (C5-C8) at the level of the cervical spine. It results in most instances from mutual unco-disco-radicular interference (de Sèze *et al.,* 1949, 1951). The relative importance of mechanical (uncodiscal) and inflammatory (radicular) factors is variable according to different clinical cases. The pain constitutes almost the entire symptomatology. It may be present along the entire dermatome corresponding to the involved root or be limited to a small area: the epicondyle, a finger, etc. The patients almost always complain simultaneously of an interscapular pain which often precedes the radicular symptomatology. It may be extremely acute or moderate, or occur only during certain movements of effort, coughing, or laughing. It is usually increased when the patient is in bed and alleviated by certain movements, for example placing one's hand behind the head. This, in fact, is a position when the roots of the brachial plexus are relaxed.

DIFFERENT CERVICAL SYNDROMES

One may consider different radicular syndromes (Fig. 129).

C5 Syndrome

Characteristic topography of pain and, at times, objective sensory changes: anterior aspect of the shoulder, occasionally extending down to the lateral aspect of the elbow.

Characteristic motor disturbances involving the deltoid, supraspinatus, teres minor, and occasionally biceps.

C6 Syndrome

Characteristic topography of pain and, occasionally, objective sensory changes in anterolateral aspect of the shoulder, lateral

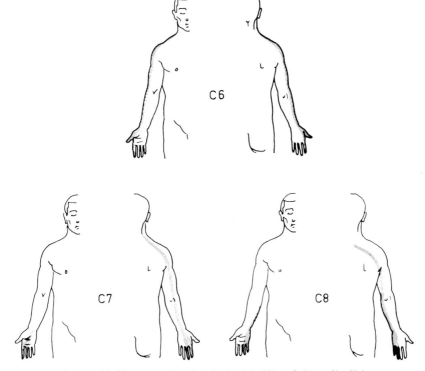

Figure 129. Topography of pain in C6, C7 and C8 radiculitis.

aspect of the upper extremity down to the thumb (included).

Reflex changes, at times, absence or decrease of the bicipital and brachioradialis reflex.

Motor disturbances and atrophy: biceps, brachioradialis, flexors of the first three digits, thenar eminence.

C7 Syndrome

Characteristic pain topography and, at times, objective sensory changes: cervicodorsal junction, posterior aspect of the shoulder, arm, forearm, dorsum of the hand, index, middle finger and, at times, the fourth finger; reflex changes at times, decrease or absence of the triceps jerk.

Motor disturbances and atrophy: triceps, extensors of the wrist, extensor communis.

C8 Syndrome

Characteristic topography of pain, and possibly, objective sensory changes: medial aspect of the arm, forearm, wrist and the fourth and fifth fingers.

Reflex changes, at times, decrease or absence of the pronator reflex.

Motor disturbances and atrophy; hypothenar eminence.

Such are radicular syndromes of the upper extremity. Objective findings are present in only half of the cases (Barbizet, 1958). Reflex changes are not often seen and the motor changes are present in still fewer cases. The diagnosis is usually easy. One should be able to differentiate these syndromes from the ones related to peripheral nerve injuries (involvement of the median nerve in the carpal tunnel, the ulnar nerve in the epitrochleo-olecranon groove or in the canal of Guyon, for example). One should not forget the syndrome of Pancoast-Tobias (irritation due to a tumor of the lung apex) or the tubercular lesions of the apex treated by pneumothorax. Cervicobrachial neuralgia may result from a vertebral tumor or from spondylitis, or from a neural or an intramedullary lesion (syringomyelia).

Spontaneous resolution of the benign cervicobrachial neuralgia is usual but may be too long and the pain may be too distressing. Thus, manipulative therapy when effective, may be quite helpful (see also Degenring, 1966; Keegan, 1944 and 1947; Lacapere, 1933, 1950, 1954; Thierry-Mieg, 1963).

EXAMINATION OF THE NECK

Range of Motion

The range of motion should be studied with the patient in a sitting position first, then supine with the head beyond the edge of the table in a maximal relaxed position. The result of this test should be reported on the star diagram.

Manual Traction (Fig. 130, left)

The patient being in a supine position, the physician grasps the occiput and the chin and maintains traction for one minute

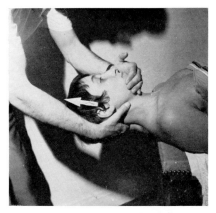

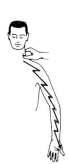
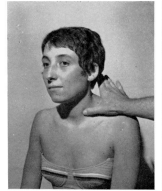
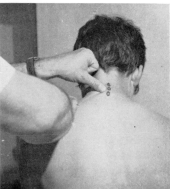

Figure 130. Examination of the neck. *Top,* Test of manual traction; *Lower left (diagram and photo),* Anterior doorbell pushbutton sign; *Lower right,* lateral pressure over a spinal process.

or so; he then asks the patient whether this maneuver decreases his pain in the shoulder or in the upper extremities. Obviously if this maneuver exacerbates the pain, any manual or mechanical traction should not be used.

SEGMENTAL LOCALIZATION

Segmental localization may be derived from the analysis of pain topography if fingers are involved. If not, the posterior and anterior tender points which were described above will have to be explored.

The posterior point (see p. 81) is located one fingerwidth from the midline, in the paramedian groove, at the level of the projection of the bony structure of the posterior joint. When it is painful, it is generally but not always tender on the involved side.

The anterior doorbell pushbutton sign is investigated on the anterolateral aspect of the neck (Fig. 130, lower left) with the physician's thumb maintained in a horizontal position, the doctor facing the patient who is in a sitting position. This investigation which we conduct systematically permits us to reveal the cervical origin in most instances of benign dorsalgia: a slight pressure exerted over the emerging ventral root reproduces or exaggerates the pain or parasthesias experienced by the patient. When the sensory topography is not clear, this examination contributes to the segmental localization.

AXIAL PRESSURE OVER THE SPINAL PROCESS

Axial pressure over the spinal process, or better, in the case of the lower cervical region, lateral pressure over this process (Fig. 130, lower right) permits one to analyze more precisely the level of the intervertebral block. The related findings contribute to the determination of the most elective manipulative maneuver. One should also use a lateral pressure over the spinal process with contrapressure exerted over the spines of the contiguous vertebrae (p. 82). *Interspinal pressure* will be applied also on the patient in a sitting position, the head being hyperflexed. The interspinal pain may be seen in discogenic diseases responsible for neuralgia. However, one should keep in mind the possibility that the interspinal ligamental pain alone may be responsible for the cervical pain or referred to the posterior aspect of the shoulder or to the upper extremity. In such cases the anterior doorbell pushbutton sign is absent. However, the supraspinous ligament is very tender and its irritation by a subcutaneous needle reproduces the referred pain which can be controlled by a few drops of Novocain-cortisone mixture. It is still better to inject sclerogenic substances into the supraspinal ligament (Hackett, 1956; Barbor, 1966; Le-Goaer, 1960, Troisier, 1962, 1966).

THE ROLE OF MANIPULATIONS IN THE TREATMENT OF CERVICAL RADICULITIS

In many cases of cervical radiculitis manipulation is rapidly effective. In the *hyperalgic* forms when the neck movements are absent, one should not manipulate. The treatment of choice is immobilization of the neck in a rigid collar or even in a cast. Anti-inflammatory medication or the ganglionic blocking agents are very effective, and sometimes an infiltration of the stellate ganglion is advisable. In some cases, however, maneuver of relaxation, or a gentle mobilization in the direction of the movements remaining free can be beneficial. Only one maneuver of gentle manipulation should be carried out at each session, provided that it remains pain-free.

Note: Manipulations at times are effective if centered on D3-D5 where spontaneous pain and pin-pointed tender areas may be present. Pressure on this area reveals brachial pain. In such cases brachial pain does not show a radicular topography, but rather resembles a sympathetic involvement. Conversely, many interscapular neuralgias are improved by manipulation of the lower cervical spine (see p. 255). In cases of pain of *average* intensity, manipulations will be exerted in the direction of free movements. The treatment must be conducted with particular gentleness. In the cervical spine more than in any other region, elective and gentle manipulations are effective. Thus a therapeutic session should be conducted as follows (after the direction of free movements have been identified) :

1. *Maneuvers of relaxation* of the cervical region and of the supraspinal area as well as scapular muscles immobilizing the scapula, are to be effected very slowly (see Fig. 140, p. 000).

2. *Mobilizations* along the free directions are to be performed preliminary to three or four manipulations which will be carried out.

3. *Manipulations,* depending upon the results of preliminary testing and the information acquired during mobilization, will be carried out as follows:

a) In rotation in the nonpainful direction, being associated with either extension or flexion.

b) In lateral bending only or associated with flexion or extension.

c) In rotation and lateral bending.

This protocol is obviously given only as an example, as the program of the session and the combination of maneuvers will change from one patient to another. Let us consider a case of neuralgia of C8 segmental origin on the right side. Each maneuver is followed by a search for painful movements which show improvement and thus permits one to choose the next maneuver.

TREATMENT OF CERVICAL RADICULITIS

Example

Examination shows that the patient has a radicular cervical neuralgia on the right side (C8) (Fig. 131).

Preliminary testing shows the following (Fig. 132):

1. Right lateral bending is very limited and painful.
2. Right rotation is limited and painful.
3. Extension is limited and painful.

The patient will therefore be mobilized in left rotation, then left lateral bending, then in flexion. A series of 10 to 15 move-

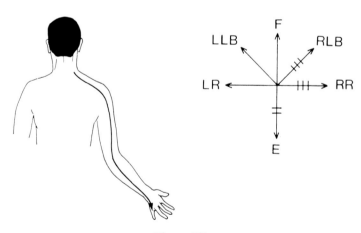

Figure 131.

ments each as represented in Figures 133, 134, and 135 will be carried out. Then one will effectuate the following:

1. A global manipulation in cervicodorsal flexion (Fig. 136).

2. A manipulation in left rotation with the spine bent forward (Fig. 137).

3. A manipulation in left lateral bending and forward flexion (Fig. 138).

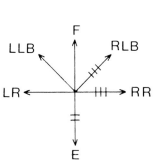

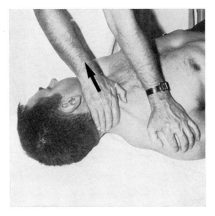

Figure 132.   Figure 133. Mobilization in left rotation.

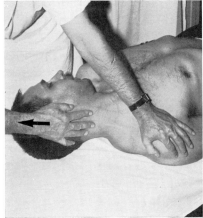

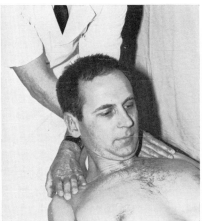

Figure 134. Mobilization in left lateral bending.

Figure 135. Mobilization in flexion.

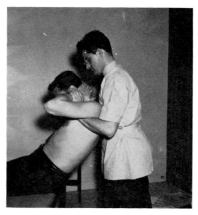

Figure 136. Global manipulation in flexion.

Let us add that massage by petrissage of the supraspinal fossa is an important phase of the treatment of the cervical radiculitis (Fig. 140).

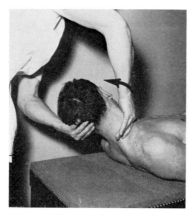

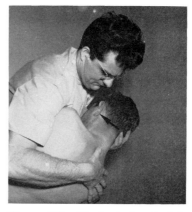

Figure 137. Manipulation in left rotation, the spine bent forward.

Figure 138. Manipulation in left lateral bending, the spine bent forward.

Another example:

In another case of right cervicobrachial neuralgia the examination may show the following (Fig. 139) :

1. Right rotation is very limited and painful.
2. Right lateral bending is very limited.
3. Flexion is limited and painful.

Figure 139. Another example of a right cervicobrachial neuralgia. Here, extension of the spine is no longer painful, but the flexion is. The maneuvers will, therefore, be different from those of the preceeding example (see Figures 140-143).

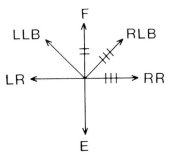

Manipulation will be effected as follows:

1. In left lateral bending (Fig. 141).
2. In left rotation, with the spine in extension (Fig. 142).
3. In left lateral flexion and extension (Fig. 143).

These directions may be combined in different maneuvers from that indicated in the above example (see also Cailliet, 1964; Lacapere and Maigne, 1957; Peillon, 1959; Serre and Simon, 1964; Thierry-Mieg, 1966; Troisier, 1960).

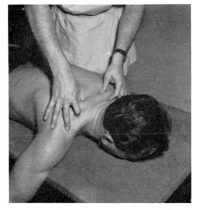

Figure 140. Massage by petrissage of both supraspinal fossa, a maneuver of relaxation.

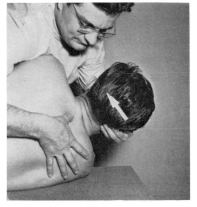

Figure 141. Manipulation in left lateral bending.

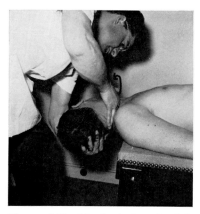

Figure 142. Manipulation in left rotation with the spine in extension.

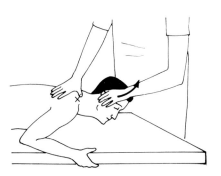

Figure 143. Manipulation in left lateral bending and extension.

Manipulation and Traction

It may be advantageous, at times, to combine a treatment of manipulation with treatment by traction. The low cervical region without any doubt is the one where traction is most helpful. When effected alone, its results may be comparable to those of a manipulation. In every other segment it induces much slower improvement which is less consistent. There are regions such as the upper cervical one or the dorsal one where the effect of traction is minimal. Traction may be used either simultaneously with manipulation (Cyriax, 1960; 1964) or independently.

Manipulation with Traction

This is done in case of manipulations in rotation under traction. The physician grasps the occiput and the chin of the patient, bends backwards with his arms outstretched, applying to the cervical spine a progressively effective traction and, provided that this maneuver is free of pain, will effectuate a manipulation in rotation in the nonpainful direction.

We prefer to effectuate this manipulation with traction with the following personal technique (Figs. 144 and 145) : A belt hangs in front of the physician and then is placed under the

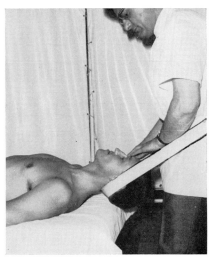

Figure 144. The physician uses a belt (width, 6 to 8 cm) which passes behind his back and under the occiput of the patient. He maintains the forehead of the patient as he bends over backwards in order to effect a progressive cervical traction which he may perfectly control without any fatigue.

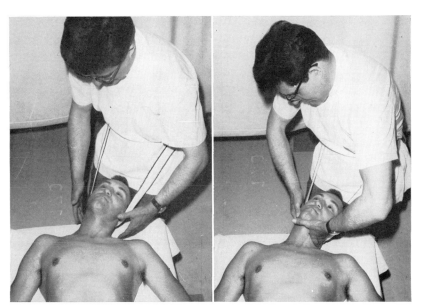

Figure 145. With the same technique, one may effectuate manipulation under traction. The physician may impose a right or left lateral bending by moving laterally (left) and exert a manipulation in rotation (right) upon the spine position in such fashion.

occiput of the patient lying supine on the table. The doctor, bending backwards, then effects the manipulation which he is able to control. His hands are free to palpate the paravertebral grooves and thus to evaluate the action of the traction upon the muscles and to initiate the manipulation at the most appropriate movement. Obviously, the patient is asked from time to time about the effect of this maneuver upon his pain and only those which reduce the pain are effectuated.

Mechanical Traction

If the manual test is favorable, one may associate with manipulations cervical traction with the patient lying supine on a tilt table, the head of the patient being held either in a Sayre's traction device (Fig. 146) or by our own apparatus (Fig. 147). The latter has the advantage of not using the chin of the patient for traction. It, therefore, permits one to avoid an inconvenience for those patients with dental prostheses or for those whose temporomaxillar joints are tender. Moreover, the patient may open his mouth and talk, which may reduce his anxiety. This apparatus should be well adjusted; if not, it may glide over the skull of certain patients who lack posterior convexity or in whom occipital prominences are not developed.

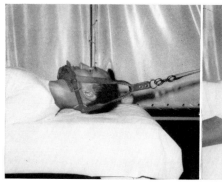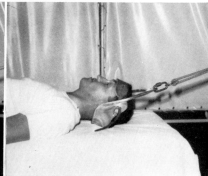

Figure 146. Mechanical traction with Sayre's collar.   Figure 147. Mechanical traction with the author's apparatus.

Chapter 21

Painful Shoulders

Sнoulder pain is often related to cervical spine pathology. Lacapere (1950) used to say that in a painful shoulder "the shoulder
is nothing, the neck is everything." Cervical manipulations may
constitute a true therapeutic test, and when they are effected because of minor mechanical derangement of the lower cervical
spine, this statement is often and somewhat unexpectedly confirmed. It is obvious that manipulations do not solve all the
therapeutic problems raised by a painful shoulder. However, a
favorable effect, sometimes obtained instantaneously, is helpful
not only from the therapeutic, but also from the pathogenic point
of view (see also Denis, 1952; DePalma, 1957).

EXAMINATION OF THE SHOULDER

It is important to examine the cervical spine in all cases of
painful shoulder. A search for the anterior doorbell pushbutton
sign, reproducing spontaneous pain (see p. 83) is of great help.
Its localization will focus the attention of the physician upon this
area, and following an x-ray examination may lead to cervical
treatments.

Examination of the shoulder will be carried out at first by a
study of the following:

1. Range of active motions:
   Place the hand behind the neck.
   Place the hand behind the back.
   Abduction
   Flexion
2. Range of passive motions
3. Movements against resistance.

The physician resists different movements effected by the
patient. It is to Cyriax (1960) that we owe the introduction of

this type of manual muscle examination with the purpose of test-ing muscle or tendon tenderness. In a case when all movements are painful, one may conclude that there is an involvement of the joint capsule. One examines in succession internal and external rotation; abduction; adduction, extension (retropulsion), and flexion (antipulsion).

SHOULDER MUSCLES

Combined action of several muscles is necessary for the satis-factory functioning of the shoulder (Fig. 148). Some of the muscles are stabilizers; others are prime movers (Codman, 1934; Inmann and Saunders, 1944, 1947). Briefly, one may summarize their actions as follows:

Abduction: Deltoid; supraspinatus.

Adduction: Teres major, latissimus dorsi, pectoralis major, teres minor.

External rotation: Infraspinatus; teres minor

Intĕrnal rotation: Subscapularis and also pectoralis major, teres major, latissimus dorsi

Flexors: Anterior deltoid; clavicular head of pectoralis major, coracobrachialis.

Extensors: Posterior deltoid, teres major, latissimus dorsi.

Testing them against resistance (Cyriax, 1960; Troisier, 1962) permits one to determine which muscle is involved (Figs. 149 and 150). We add to this examination a direct simultaneous palpation of the muscle which permits one to reveal some tenderness to pres-sure which is not shown by the test of opposed resistance. For ex-ample, one often finds that palpation of the contracted infra-spinatus elicits exquisite pain, while the contraction alone may be pain-free. Massage and infiltration of tender points will relieve the patient. It is also desirable in certain cases to add traction of the muscle. For example, it is not sufficient for the examination of the biceps to make it contract against resistance to flexion and supina-tion of the forearm. It is also important to palpate the muscle and its tendons simultaneously and then apply traction upon it by forc-ing the forearm downwards and backwards (see Fig. 151).

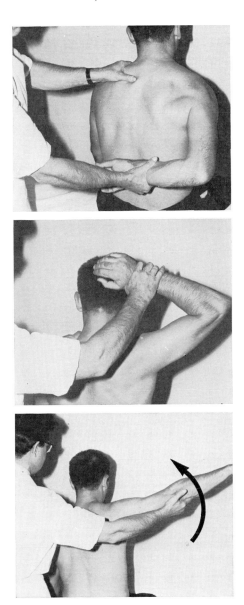

Figure 148. Three major movements of the shoulder. *Top,* Internal rotation and adduction: place the hand behind the back. *Center,* External rotation and abduction: place the hand behind the neck. *Bottom,* Abduction.

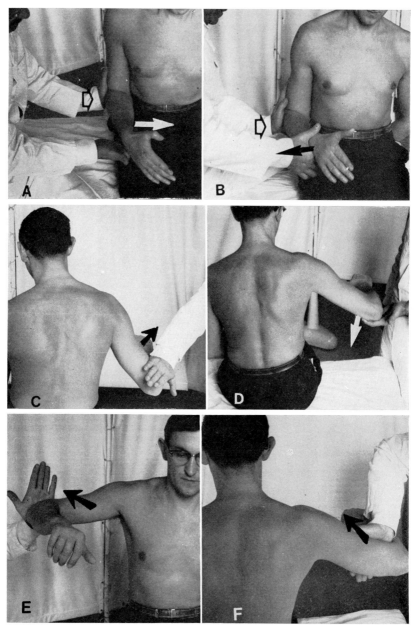

Figure 149. Examination of the shoulder by the study of resisted motion. *A,* resisted internal rotation; *B,* resisted external rotation; *C,* resisted abduction; *D,* resisted adduction; *E,* resisted extension (horizontal arm); *F,* resisted flexion (horizontal arm).

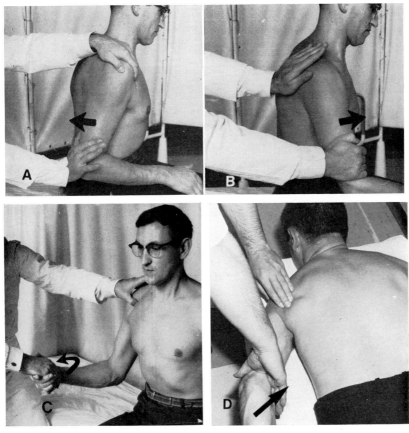

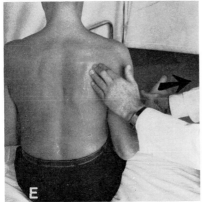

Figure 150. Examination of the shoulder by the study of resisted motion (continued). *A,* resisted extension (vertical arm); *B,* resisted flexion (vertical arm); *C,* resisted supination (palpation of the bicipital tendon); *D,* resisted extension (palpation of the latissimus dorsi and teres major); *E,* resisted external rotation (palpation of the infraspinatus).

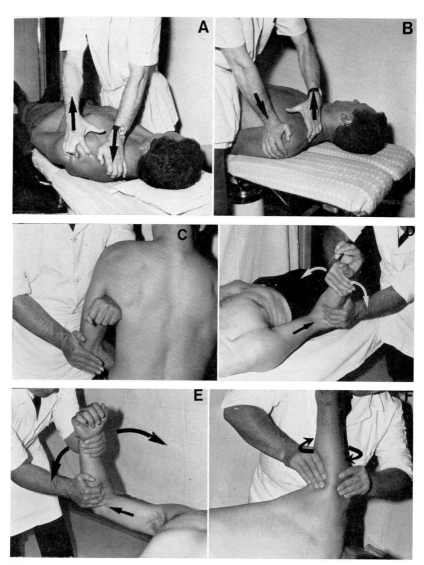

Figure 151. Mobilization. *Top,* Patient supine: the physician mobilizes the head of the humerus forward *A,* then backwards *B,* while the clavicle is stabilized. *C,* Separation of the humeral head from the glenoid fossa. Physician's knee stabilizes the lateral aspect of the arm while he pulls toward him the humeral head. *D,* Mobilization in rotation—one technique; *E,* Mobilization under continuous traction; the physician rotates the shoulder inwards and outwards, by applying slow developing effort. *F,* "Pilon" mobilization. The physician mobilizes the humerus as if it were a pilon in relation to the glenoid fossa.

DIFFERENT TYPES OF PAINFUL SHOULDERS

Painful shoulder is seen with one of the following four clinical pictures:

1. Acute hyperalgic shoulder.
2. Painful shoulder with free movements.
3. Chronic shoulder with completely blocked movements (pain-free at the steady period).
4. Limited and painful shoulder movements (see also Chapuis-Phankim, 1957).

Hyperalgic Shoulder

Pain is acute with complete functional inability to move the shoulder. It is usually due to acute bursitis with acute hyperinflammatory calcifying tendinitis (Codman, 1934). It may be the beginning of a chronically frozen shoulder. No manipulation should be considered in such cases. The shoulder should be placed at rest with ice, anti-inflammatory medication, and, possibly, infiltration of the stellate ganglion. As soon as the patient is relieved, one may ask him to start pendular exercises of small amplitude. Welfling *et al.* (1963) described a "syndrome of bursal migration." In these instances calcified tissue of the tendon of the supraspinatus erupts into the subdeltoid bursa. This is associated with acute pain. Radiologic examination shows calcified matter outside of the trochanter. Spontaneous recovery is the rule.

Chronic Painful Shoulder with No Limitation of Movements (Simple Painful Shoulder)

This is generally the case of pain originating in the tendons. Analysis of movements is done by manual resistance, while the other hand of the physician palpates the tendons or the insertion of the exercised muscles. In most cases one will find a tender tendon of the long head of the biceps, or that of the supraspinatus, more rarely that of the subscapularis or infraspinatus. The usual treatment is to inject cortisone locally, occasionally intraarticularly. It is well known that results are usually satisfactory, although some cases are very resistant to this treatment. Examination of the cervical spine should be done systematically in an effort to reveal a tender segment at the level of the lower central spine. The signs of minor intervertebral derangement will be looked for (see p. 52) . After a radiological checkup, manipulative trial may be attempted. Very often the patients improve after the very first maneuver. The improvement will not always persist although it does constitute a good prognostic sign. Indeed after three or four sessions the cervical spine becomes flexible again and the shoulder pain subsides, so that cortisone injection may no longer be required unless the therapeutic results are nil or incomplete.

Chronic Shoulder with Completely Blocked Movements

Frozen Shoulder—Adhesive Capsulitis

When a shoulder shows completely blocked movements in all directions with no motion between the humerus and the scapula, one deals with an adhesive capsulitis (de Sèze, 1961, 1962; de Sèze *et al.*, 1959) . The articular capsule is thickened and retracted, as is seen very clearly by arthrography. Spontaneous course is very long, one to two years. However, treatment consisting of intra-articular injections of cortisone and active-assistive mobilizations did permit de Sèze (1961) to shorten this course to only three months. In cases of adhesive capsulitis, some authors advise forced mobilizations under anesthesia. Although some spectacular results have been achieved at times, the occurrence of grave setbacks in other cases make this treatment ill-advised. It acts by breaking the lower part of the capsule, as determined by arthrographies made before and after the treatment. However, Bloch and Fischer (1958) claim to have treated 2,000 cases with no complications, actively mobilizing the shoulder the day following manipulation. We do not have sufficient knowledge of this technique to evaluate it. We believe that in any manipulative treatment, experience and skill play the dominant role. When one forces movement under anesthesia, one should feel when to stop and how to grade the maneuver. This is practically never done, as an articular mobilization under anesthesia appear to be so easy and simple. Unfortunately disenchantment comes the day after or when the patient wakes up.

We do not believe that cervical manipulations are indicated in the frozen shoulder. However, occasionally we feel that the reeducation of the frozen shoulder might be accelerated by cervical manipulation added to the program of passive and active exercises.

Blocked Shoulders Without Adhesive Capsulitis

While adhesive capsulitis always results in a blocked shoulder, Waghemacker, Cecil, and Buise (1963) found some cases of blocked shoulder without any adhesive capsulitis. They found the presence of capsular tears or lesions of the tendon of long head of biceps.

Blocked Shoulders of Psychosomatic Origin

One should always think of this possibility (Waghemacker *et al.*, 1955). The following case of Waghemacker seems to be particularly revealing: Mrs. X was a victim of a contusion of the shoulder during a fall. A severe completely blocked shoulder was observed afterwards. Three weeks of treatment by exercises and different modalities were ineffective. Arthrography was done which showed no abnormality. The patient was cured by narcoanalysis.

Painful Shoulders with Limited Motion

These chronic shoulders are commonly observed. Movements are limited, but there is a motion between the humerus and the scapula. Abduction and extenal and internal rotations are not completely blocked. The patient has difficulty placing his hands over his head, and touching his neck. Abduction is limited to 60 to 80 degrees. All attempts to passively force these movements are painful. In such cases cervical manipulations permit one to obtain satisfactory results at times which occasionally are surpising. At times, one may free the movements of a shoulder which has been stiff for many months.

It is of great interest to find that it is possible from the very first session to predict the outcome. In a favorable case, improvement has to be immediate. The latter may be slight and transitory, but if it is manifested, the prognosis is favorable if the treatments are continued. The improvement usually first concerns the placement of the hand behind the head. A patient who could scarcely touch his ear, may now be able to place his hand above his head. Following sessions will complete the results. Placement of the hand behind the back (internal rotation and abduction) takes the longest to recover. Three or four sessions with five-day intervals between are sufficient in favorable cases; five or six sessions are usually necessary in other cases. Exercise therapy should complete the treatments.

Cervical manipulations used in these cases are the same as those described for the cervicodorsal junction or for the lower cervical spine. One carries them out according to the rules which have been discussed. However in a case of scapulohumeral periarthritis, and in contradistinction to what is done for cervicobrachial neuralgia, for example, manipulation should be brief and forced, although it should remain elective and pain-free. It is always the case when reflex action is demanded. How can one explain this often instantaneous action of manipulation of the lower cervical spine upon a partially blocked shoulder if it is not by a reestablishment of a normal synergy of different muscle groups of the shoulder? Indeed, it is known that the abduction of the arm is due to perfect coordination of the abductors (deltoid and supraspinatus) on one hand, and of the muscles which lower the humeral head on the other, permitting, in this fashion, a free play of the tendon of the supraspinatus between the acromion and the head of the humerus. The disruption of this synergy makes it impossible to abduct the shoulder more than 70 degrees as the tendon of the supraspinatus is then pinched between the humeral head and the acromion, thus eliciting a sharp pain, particularly if there is tendinitis at the same time. In order to free this movement, one has to make the antagonistic muscles and their tendon pain-free and capable of elastically supporting the traction imposed upon them. There is frequently tenderness and muscular pain in these radicular neuralgias, just as the presence of a painful tendon of the biceps femoris, which often is marked in S1 sciatica and which is improved by a successful lumbar manipulation. It is probable that some tendinous pain of the shoulder muscles is of the same nature since cervical manipulation may relieve it also.

Massage (Fig. 152)

One should consider the muscular pain proper, which may prolong the suffering of the patient. Palpation of muscles (supraspinatus, infraspinatus, pectoralis major, biceps, deltoid, etc.) will reveal the presence of some contracted fasciculi, with painful induration and even some trigger points, the presence of which induces a referred pain (see p. 48). Such palpation may be carried out in relaxed muscles, but it is good to complete it by palpating contracted muscles (against resistance). Thus one will be able to reveal supraspinatus pain, which may be decreased by combined

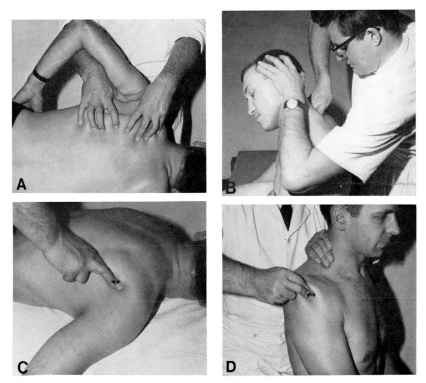

Figure 152. Maneuver of Petrissage. *A,* Petrissage of periscapular muscles; *B* and *C,* deep friction; *D,* friction at the insertion of the supraspinatus (Cyriax massage).

massage and local injections (see a few maneuvers of manipulation, Fig. 153) (see also Kohlrausch, 1961; Michelsen and Mixter, 1944).

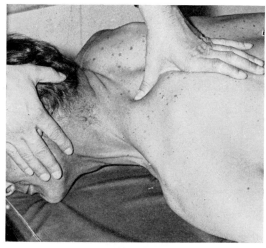

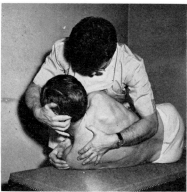

Figure 153. Two examples of useful cervicodorsal manipulations in the treatment of shoulder pain.

Other Painful Shoulders

Periarthritis following a fracture or dislocation of the shoulder is less amenable to manipulative treatments than so-called rheumatic periarthritis. The presence of multiple osteoligamental, capsular, and tendon lesions seems to be the explanation for these differences. Arthrography permits one to individualize cases and to prescribe appropriate treatments. One should remember that we frequently find an atrophy of the deltoid, usually reflex atrophy, but sometimes neurogenic ones as shown by systematically conducted EMG tests.

Extensive Traumatic Tears of the Rotator Cuff

A certain number of chronic painful and blocked shoulders are due to extensive tears of the rotator cuff. These resist all therapeutic efforts. Arthrography of the shoulder alone may reveal the explanation of some of these findings. (Lindblom and Palmer, 1939; Coste *et al.*, 1957; Kessel, 1950; Broscal and Claessens, 1957, de Sèze *et al.*, 1959). Waghemacker *et al.*, (1963) stress the importance of taking lateral pictures in addition to the AP views. Such pictures will show the lesion of the rotator cuff, those of the capsules, those of the tendon of the long head of biceps for which surgery is indicated. One may see them without any violent trauma to the shoulder. This is the case with elderly people in whom deterioration of the cuff is very frequent and often well tolerated. They may result, however, in intractable pain due to rubbing of two bones (acromion and great tuberosity). If such pain remains intractable and does not respond to medical treatment (hydrocortisone), surgery may be successful (Debeyre, 1962). It consists in displacement of the supraspinatus, the mass of which becomes interposed between the great tuberosity and the acromion.

Dislocation of the Bicipital Tendon

This is not rare. The tendon leaves the intertuberosity groove and slides medially. It usually results from sudden movement of abduction and external rotation. The palpation of the tendon is done medially to is usual location. The differential diagnosis with its rupture may be difficult (Claessens and Anciaux-Ruysen, 1956). In such cases arthrography permits one to make the diagnosis (Claessens and Anciaux-Ruysen, 1956). Manipulation consists of hooking the tendon by its medial aspects and pulling it laterally, while one internally rotates the arm (see also Denis, 1952).

Acromioclavicular Joint

One should not omit examination of the acromioclavicular joint even though one might find signs of tendinitis of the supraspinatus or long head of the biceps, to name only the most frequently observed conditions. This articulation has a small meniscus which may be torn or be dislocated during rapid and violent movements or even during a false shoulder movement. Besides such an acute block, there is chronic involvement of this structure which is said to deteriorate nine times out of ten above 50 years of age.

It is advisable not to forget this joint, as a pressure over its articular line with a tip of the index finger reveals acute pain when it is responsible for the shoulder pain. If the latter resembles the habitual pain, the diagnosis is made. A local injection of hydrocortisone is an excellent treatment. However, manual therapy may also be useful. One should push the lateral end of the clavicle backward, then forward, in order to determine whether or not these movements are painful. A few mobilizations directed in the opposite sense, helped by synchronous movements of the shoulder may be sufficient to help the patient. The radiological examination may at times show a pinching of the interarticular space, with condensation of the edges, osteophytes, and even in certain cases, deformities of the bony structures. At the beginning one may note only widening of the interarticular space. However, at times the latter remains normal despite an elective tender point.

The difficulty results from an association of the acromioclavicular involvement and a typical periarthritis. It is important, however, to consider it in order to help the patient.

One should not neglect the examination of the sternoclavicular joint. Although its involvement, particularly an osteoarthrosis, elicits a local pain, the patient may at times complain of shoulder pain (De Palma, 1957).

CELLULALGIA

When one deals with a simple painful shoulder and when the treatment of tendon pain or cervical manipulation is not successful, one should always check local skin and subcutaneous tissues, particularly if the movements remain free.

Painful infiltration by cellulitis is common at the level of the supraspinal fossa and of the humeral insertion of the deltoid. Using the maneuver of skin rolling, one should try to detect tender nodules, attempting to elicit habitual pain. If one does, a few sessions of massage with superficial petrissage with possible adjunction of Novocain injections into the tender points may help the patient considerably. One should keep in mind that it is not rare to find cellulitis in such cases.

Chapter 22

Paresthesias of the Hand

PARESTHESIAS OF THE HAND are expressed by the sensation of "pins and needles" or numbness which may be located at any part of the hand. They may be either unilateral or bilateral (Bonduelle, 1948; Dreyfus and Phankim-Koupernik, 1964). According to their topography and their character, they are distinguished as follows:

1. Global paresthesia (involving the whole hand) occurring mostly at night (Fig. 154D).
2. Radicular paresthesia (Fig. 154, A, B, C.)
3. Peripheral paresthesia (Fig. 154, E, F)—Involving the territory of the median nerve (carpal tunnel syndrome (E) or less frequently the territory of the ulnar nerve, "syndrome of the canal of Guyon" (F).
4. Finally, different symptomatic paresthesias of neurological origin (For example, in syringomyelia).

GLOBAL PARESTHESIA

This form of paresthesia is more frequent in female patients, particularly at the time of menopause. The trouble usually starts between 2:00 and 4:00 A.M., waking the patient who complains of the impression of having a "dead" hand.

Improvement by cervical manipulation is common, proving the cervical etiology of this complaint.

RADICULAR PARESTHESIA

This is a form of cervicobrachial neuralgia (Bonduelle, 1948), indeed, by irritation of a root: C6 in case of the involvement of the thumb; C7 in case of the involvement of the medius and C8 if the little finger is involved. A search for the anterior doorbell pushbutton sign is always positive (see Fig. 129, p. 83), the pressure over it reproducing the paresthesia in the habitual area.

Cervical manipulation well localized and correctly directed is an effective treatment.

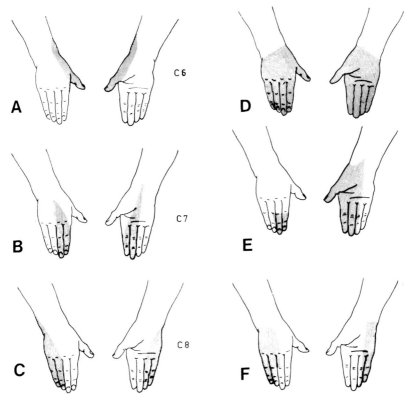

Figure 154. *A, B,* and *C,* radicular involvement; *D,* global involvement; *E,* peripheral involvement, median nerve; *F,* peripheral involvement, ulnar nerve. In all figures: *Left,* dorsum of the hand; *Right,* palmar region.

PERIPHERAL (TRUNCULAR) PARESTHESIA
Carpal Tunnel Syndrome

A compression of the median nerve in the carpal tunnel and much less often, a compression of the ulnar nerve in the canal of Guyon (Brain *et al.,* 1952) is the common origin of the paresthesias of the hand (Dreyfus, and Phankim-Koupernik, 1964) (Figs. 155, 156 and 157). These paresthesias are exacerbated at night, but are also distressing during the daytime, occurring by

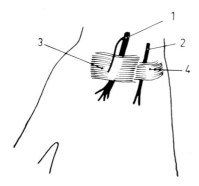

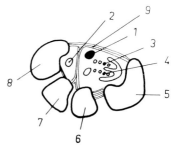

Figure 155. Anterior aspect of the median nerve in the carpal tunnel and of the ulnar nerve in the canal of Guyon. (1) Median nerve; (2) ulnar nerve; (3) transverse carpal ligament; (4) expansion of the ligament of the flexor carpi ulnaris.

Figure 156. Cross section of the carpal tunnel at the level of the second row of carpal bones. (1) Median nerve; (2) tendon of the palmaris longus (3) flexor digitorum sublimus; (4) flexor digitorum profundus; (5) hamate; (6) capitate; (7) lesser multangular; (8) greater multangular; (9) transverse carpal ligament.

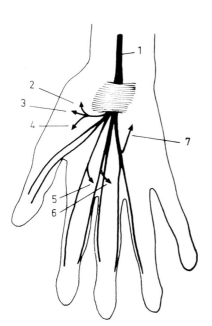

Figure 157. Median nerve.
1. Median nerve.
2. Nerve of the abductor pollicis brevis.
3. Nerve of the opponent.
4. Nerve of the flexor pollicis brevis.
5. Nerve of the 1st lumbrical.
6. Nerve of the 2nd lumbrical.
7. Anastomosis with the ulnar nerve.

brief episodes, or, in certain extremely severe cases, persisting all day long. Carpal tunnel syndrome should be suspected if the following are present:

1. The topography corresponds to the median nerve first three fingers and half of the fourth one; however, often only two fingers are involved.

2. Pressure of the tunnel for one minute reproduces the patient's complaints.

3. Hypoesthesia and, occasionally, atrophy of the muscles of the thenar eminence are present, as well as a decrease of muscle strength of the abductor pollicis brevis and opponent.

4. Increase of the terminal latency following stimulation of the median nerve at wrist.

5. A therapeutic test: injection of hydrocortisone in the tunnel or surgical section of the ligament brings about an improvement or cure.

Syndrome of the Canal of Guyon

There is the same clinical picture as in the carpal tunnel syndrome, but involving the ulnar nerve (last two fingers) (Figs. 158 159).

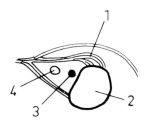

Figure 158. Cross section of the Canal of Guyon.
1. The tendon of the flexor carpi ulnaris and its expansion.
2. Pisiform.
3. Ulnar nerve.
4. Ulnar artery.

MANIPULATIONS AND PARESTHESIAS OF THE HAND—PRACTICAL CONSIDERATIONS

As discussed earlier, cervical manipulations may be useful in cases of paresthesias of the hand. They are obviously legitimate in parasthesias of spinal origin, if the involvement of the root is purely mechanical. However, they do not seem to be justified in cases of the carpal syndrome tunnel or of that of canal of Guyon.

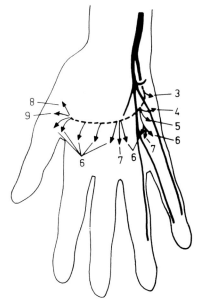

Figure 159. Ulnar nerve.
3. Nerve of the opponent digiti quinti.
4. Nerve of the abductor digiti quinti.
5. Nerve of the flexor digiti quinti.
6. Nerve for the dorsal and palmar interossei.
7. Nerve for the 3rd and 4th lumbricals.
8. Nerve of the deep portion of the flexor pollicis brevis.
9. Nerve of the abductor pollicis.

Yet in a certain number of cases where diagnosis of the carpal tunnel is revealed (1) by the topography of the complaints, (2) by their reproduction following carpal compression and even (3) by temporary improvement due to a local cortisone injection, one can obtain remarkable improvement by a cervical manipulation. In some cases sensory disturbances alone are seen without any motor deficit of the opponent or abductor brevis and in which traumatic or microtraumatic involvement of the wrist was absent. Originally, we were led to try a manipulation in such a patient because of the presence of the anterior doorbell pushbutton sign. The presence of this point would bring about the habitual complaints (p. 83).

In a number of cases the duration of improvement by cervical manipulation was about the same as the duration of the improvement by local cortisone injections. Combined treatments by these two methods gave better results than those obtained by the application of only one of the theraeputic methods under consideration. It seems, therefore, that in cases which respond to such a combined treatment, irritation of a cervical root could be responsible for the edema at the level of the carpal tunnel. We would like to mention that in cases where surgery was performed, the source of the compression of the nerve was not always found, the nerve and other structures appearing quite normal.

Moreover we have observed a few cases of carpal tunnel syndrome following typical radicular cervicobrachial neuralgia in which the original involvement of the tunnel could be excluded. In one such case, a young woman, following an acute torticollis, complained of a pain with a typical segmental topography corresponding to C6, with the sensory disturbances localized to the thumb. An anterior doorbell pushbutton pressure increased referred pain. Anti-inflammatory treatment decreased the patient's complaints with only slight residual pain. Fifteen days later she came complaining of paraesthesia of the first three fingers increased by dorsiflexion and percussion of the wrist. She was improved for three weeks following cortisone injection in the carpal tunnel. Following this period, she had a relapse, showing the same symptomatology, but this time she showed a positive anterior doorbell pushbutton sign. The presence of this tender point reproduced the entire picture of the numbness of the first three fingers. A cervical manipulation resulted in persistent improvement. It is obvious that in the absence of cervical signs, cervical manipulations should not be performed. Also, in a certain number of cases, carpal mobilizations as well as mobilizations of the wrist were followed by improvement of the parasthesias.

There is a simple test which seems to predict whether or not such a patient is going to be improved by manipulations. One asks the patient to maintain elevated upper extremities for a certain time. In most cases, but not in all, habitual numbness appears after 20 to 30 seconds. This offers the possibility of checking the topography of the patient's complaints, which may be somewhat vague in certain cases. One notes exactly the number of seconds elapsed before the appearance of the symptoms. Then one repeats this test after a cervical manipulation. In all cases which were improved by a series of manipulations, this period of time increased, and no symptoms appear during the *second* trial (see also Rageot, Maigne, and Nataf, 1968; Serre, Simon, and Claustre, 1965; Wattebled, 1964).

Chapter 23

Tennis Elbow (Epicondylitis)

INTRODUCTION

Tennis elbow characterized by pain localized to epicondyle has been classically attributed to tendinitis of the muscle originating from this anatomical structure (Fig. 160). As a result of this pain, patients have difficulty making a fist, filling a cup, etc., or may be incapable of performing these movements. This condition is often observed in the individual who plays tennis; hence, the name of "tennis elbow." However, one may find this same clinical picture in some manual workers and it may be seen in patients who are not engaged in either sports or manual labors.

Before deciding as to the origin of pain arising from the epicondyle, it is good practice to examine the wrist. We have observed in almost 25 percent of cases with complaints centered around the epicondyle that there is a decrease of passive mobility of the lower radio-ulnar joint, associated with a decrease of the lateral mobility of the elbow. The technique of the examination is as follows (Fig. 161) : one grasps the lower end of the radius between the thumb

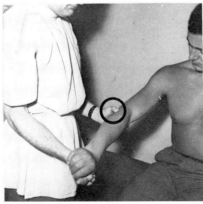 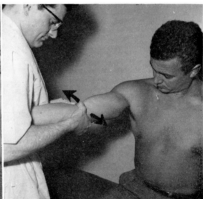

Figure 160. Epicondylian point.   Figure 161. Lateral mobilization of the elbow and testing of the lateral mobility.

and index finger of one hand and that of the ulna between the thumb and the index finger of the other hand, and one elicits reciprocal movements (backwards and forwards) of these two bones. One finds in such cases that the mobility is decreased and tenderness is increased in comparison with the other side. It is sufficient to repeat this maneuver several times, using slightly forced movements, in order to reduce the joint block.

DIAGNOSIS

The diagnosis is established, essentially, on the basis of the patient's complaints of pain centering around the tip of epicondyle or its anterior aspect, at times over its entire surface. One always finds local tenderness while palpating muscles originating from the epicondyle, as well as small cordlike formations within these muscles. In more chronic cases one finds tenderness of the skin while attempting a skin-rolling maneuver. Skin tenderness may spread upwards over the external aspect of the arm and downwards over the lower half of the lateral aspect of the forearm.

It is helpful to complete the examination by the following procedures which may indicate effectiveness of some therapeutic maneuvers. Thus the pain may be affected by resisted dorsiflexion of the hand, the arm of the patient being stretched out, and handshake, also with outstretched arm. These simple tests should be carried out (1) in neutral position, (2) in resisted supination and (3) in resisted pronation.

It is advisable to repeat these procedures before and after each therapeutic maneuver in order to evaluate their efficacy.

DIFFERENT ETIOLOGIES OF EPICONDYLITIS

Pain originating from the tendons originated from epicondyle and may be due to several causes.

1. It may be of *cervical* origin. It is remarkable to find that certain patients presenting a clinical picture of "tennis elbow" may be substantially relieved from their pain or even cured after a single session of cervical manipulation.

2. It may be of *local* origin. Different disturbances may be found at the level of epicondyle, such as (a) periarthritis of the

elbow which may be manifested solely by pain at the level of the epicondyle, or (b) a simple mechanical derangement of the humeroradial joint.

3. *Mixed* etiology is characterized by the presence of a cervical element in a patient suffering from a periarthritis of the elbow.

4. In rare cases no pathology exists at the level of the cervical spine nor at the level of the elbow. One may be confronted with (a) a case of a peritendinitis of a muscle of the area or with (b) a painful muscle itself.

5. Finally, particularly in chronic cases resistant to all therapy, a specific metabolic background such as hyperuricemia, for example, should be considered and the patient treated in accordance with the clinical findings.

Epicondylitis of Cervical Origin

Certain cases presenting themselves from the clinical point of view as epicondylitis may be helped by cervical manipulation. Sometimes four to five sessions may be necessary in order to bring about a definitive therapeutic result without using concomitantly any other treatment, although the patient's pain resisted all other treatments prior to the beginning of cervical manipulation sessions.

In such cases one always finds the signs of an involvement of C5-C6 segment, or less often those of C6-C7 segment. These signs will be looked for, according to the previously described procedure. The most constant sign is the tenderness to the pressure exerted over the posterior joint at C5-C6 or C6-C7 levels on the side of the epicondylitis, the pressure exerted on the opposite side being painless. The patient may have complained spontaneously of cervical pain or of brachial pain suggesting cervical radiculitis. However, in many cases no cervical or radicular complaints are elicited. X-ray films may show some minor abnormalities or remain normal. Positive therapeutic results obtained by manipulations confirm the etiological hypothesis based on the signs elicited from the examination of the cervical spine. This examination should be repeated after each session, as well as the search for the local diagnostic signs—handshake and its dorsiflexion with resisted pronation and supination. Often these local signs disappear immediately after cervical manipulation, as well as the patient's complaints. They may return some time after the first session, but the patient is usually either cured or considerably improved following a series of treatments.

In cases of long-standing complaints it may be particularly helpful to look for the skin-rolling tenderness at the lateral aspect of the arm and forearm, and if it persists following manipulative sessions, a few treatments of skin-rolling massage may be helpful. Also we should not omit searching for small stringlike formations in the muscles originating from the epicondyle. These intramuscular indurations may be quite tender. They too usually disappear following cervical treatment although some of them may resist manipulations. In such a case Novocain injections or stretching of the muscle may be indicated.

According to our present statistics there are about 60 percent of cases with clinical epicondylitis having a "minor intervertebral derangement" at the C5-C6 or C6-C7 levels on the side of the "tennis elbow." About one half of these cases are associated with some degree of a periarthritis of the elbow (see below), thus to be considered as "mixed forms."

Cervical treatment alone may be helpful in about one third of cases of epicondylitis. In both clinical conditions, either purely cervical or mixed, one to five manipulations are generally sufficient. Cervical traction may also be helpful at times.

Epicondylitis Originating from the Elbow

Once the cervical region has been examined, one should proceed with the examination of the elbow and firstly with the investigation of its passive lateral movements (Fig. 162). These nonvoluntary movements, minimal in tense individuals, may be quite noticeable in a relaxed subject. The elbow of the patient placed in almost complete extension and in supination is grasped by the operator who faces the patient. The thumbs of the physician touch each other in the fold of the elbow while he immobilizes the wrist in supination under his arm. He then induces movements of laterality of the elbow from right to left and clearly perceives the play of the joint. The skill necessary to carry out this test may be easily acquired after some practice. One may find that (1) these movements are free and painless, or (2) they are limited and painful. If so, one may deal with one of two cases: a periarthritis of the elbow or an acute frozen humero radial joint.

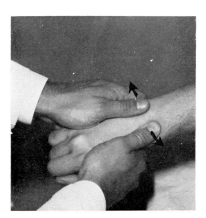

Figure 162. Lower radiocarpian mobility.

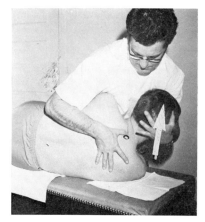

Figure 163. One of the cervical manipulations useful for treatment of tennis elbow of cervical origin.

Periarthritis of the Elbow

In such a case lateral mobility is suppressed when compared with the normal side. The procedure necessary to elicit such movements is painful or at least disagreeable, while the patient does not complain when the other side is examined. This maneuver may have a therapeutic value if repeated several times, or slightly forced. Sometimes this is all that is needed to relieve the pain from the tennis elbow.

Just as in the case of periarthritis of the shoulder one may find dissociated forms of the periarthritis of the elbow, by palpation of the muscles or tendons during resisted contractions. Thus, some of the muscles or tendons may be more involved than the others.

The above described signs may be found in about one half of cases of epicondylitis. In 50 percent of them one also finds the signs of the involvement of the C5-C6 or C6-C7 segments. These are the mixed forms. In the remaining 50 percent there is no evidence of cervical involvement, and therefore, one deals with purely local pathology.

Treatment consists in lateral mobilization of the elbow, repeated about twenty times per session in the same fashion as described for the examination. One may add mobilization in supination and at times *intra*articular injections of cortisone, much more effective than periarticular infiltrations.

Epicondylitis Due to Intraarticular Humeral Radial Derangement

This is a form which we described in 1960 as it involves a particular mechanism. It responds to a specific treatment, as the alleviation of this form may be obtained immediately following the appropriate manipulation of the elbow. Several arguments, both clinical and therapeutic, led us to conclude that this form of epicondylitis is due to a mechanical intraarticular humeral radial derangement in about 8 per 100 of cases, according to our statistics:

1. This form of epicondylitis starts suddenly during an effort or false movement.

2. During the examination, signs of the involvement of the radial humeral joint are obvious; thus, there may be a limitation of the hyperextension of the elbow or a limitation of the supination or of the pronation. This can be demonstrated in the following way: The patient faces the physician with his arms outstretched, elbows pressed against the body. The physician holds the lower part of the forearms and imparts to the patient the movements of pronation-supination. There is an evident limitation of supination of the involved side. Any attempt to force this movement is painful.

Exploration of the lateral play of the elbow does not show global restriction found in periarthritis, but elicits acute pain in adduction and abduction. Palpation of the humeroradial articular line is very tender and sometimes one may perceive a slight proturbance at the level of the articular line, very sensitive even to superficial palpation. In this particular form, when manipulation is possible and successful, one may observe instantaneous improvement of pain with disappearance of all of the described signs, analogous to the case of a knee with a locked meniscus, when an appropriate maneuver is successful.

How can one explain the pathogenesis of this intraarticular derangement? In the humeroradial joint there is a local thickening of the capsule which resembles a small meniscus. This was described under the name of humeroradial fold by Testut (1929) or falsiform folding of Poirier (Testut and Latarjet, 1931). It is undoubtedly a small fragment of this small meniscus which one perceives in certain cases over the interarticular line. In some cases where manipulative treatment was not successful and where surgery was performed by our friend Benassy, orthopedic surgeon, a small torn meniscus was found in effect. Its removal completely relieved the patients. However, it is possible that in other cases, the pathogenesis of the humeroradial joint derangement is different: there may be, for example, a pinching of the synovial fringe. May we recall on this occasion that a number of authors consider the lesions of the humeroradial joint in the pathogenesis of the tennis elbow. Thus, epicondylitis was attributed to radio humeral bursitis (Osgood, 1922; Carp, 1932; Dittrich, 1929). However, Stack and Hunt (1946) found the presence of such bursae in only 10 percent of the cadavers which they examined.

Belin du Coteau (1935) noticed that often pain which is electively located at the level of the interarticular humero radial line may be attributed to "chondritis of the condylar articular cartilage" and to "synovitis by inflammation of the falsiform folding of the fatty fringes." Stack and Hunt (1946) proposed the hypothesis of pinching of a synovial fringe. According to Moure (1952), there is a fringe originating from the lateral synovial membrane of the elbow, located between the humerus and the radius and which may be pinched during hyperextension of the elbow, this pinching being increased by forced supination. Repetitions of such trauma elicits a congestion and a thickening of the synovial membrane which thus becomes increasingly painful and fragile. Be that as it may, there are cases of epicondylitis due to mechanical derangement of the humeroradial joint and which may be greatly improved by manipulations.

When these forms are chronic, they may become complicated by periarthritis of the elbow and their treatment becomes more difficult.

Manipulations To Be Used

Manipulations to be used will be variable according to different cases. At times, one should manipulate in hyperextension, at times in adduction, at times in abduction, at times in rotation with simultaneous traction. It is the application of the rule of no pain which will determine the choice (Figs. 164 and 165) (see also Mills, 1937).

Manipulation in Adduction

The physician grasps the elbow of the patient with his fingers against its medial aspect and with the other hand, holds the wrist. The manipulation consists of a brisk movement which forces the elbow in adduction.

Manipulation in Hyperextension

This procedure may be used in a case of epicondylitis. The right hand of the physician holds the right wrist of the patient. The left thumb is placed just behind the head of the radius. The forearm is set in supination and hyperextension by the right hand while the thumb exerts firm pressure over the head of the radius. Finally, the right hand increases the extension of the forearm by a small sudden thrust. One can hear a cracking sound. The improvement is usually immediate, but sometimes manipulation should be repeated three or four times with a few days interval between each session.

Manipulation in Abduction

The same principle as that used in manipulation in adduction is applied in this case except that the way the elbow is grasped and the direction of the maneuver are reversed.

Manipulation with Traction

The patient is in a sitting position holding his arm against his body with his forearm flexed at a right angle. An aide, standing behind him, grasps the lower part of the patient's arm while a second aide standing in front of the patient grasps his wrists. Both aides exert a firm sustained traction while the physician manipulates the head of the radius; at the same time the second aide exerts a slow movement of pronation and supination.

Mixed Epicondylitis

In such patients there are signs of involvement of the C5-C6 segment or C6-C7 on the side of the epicondylitis as well as disappearance of the lateral joint play of the elbow. One therefore deals with patients having epicondylitis with both cervical involvement and periarthritis of the elbow. In most cases there is a long history of the disorder and it seems that the periarthritis constitutes a complication secondary to "cervical epicondylitis." The role of the cervical spine in the pathogenesis of periarthritis of the elbow appears to be analogous to that which is habitual in periarthritis of the shoulder. At times cervical treatment (Fig. 163) alone alleviates both epicondylitis and periarthritis, but in general, we apply a mixed treatment which aims at both the cervical spine and the elbow, the latter being treated by progressive mobilizations as described above.

Epicondylitis Due To a Pure Tendinitis

In certain cases, one may fail to find either cervical etiologies or local pathology of the elbow or wrist. Systematic palpation may reveal exquisite tenderness of a muscular fascicle attached to the epicondyle. At times, one finds within the epicondylian tendon, a small nodule the size of a glass pin head. Extremely sensitive to pressure, it is located near the epicondyle. Local injection of cortisone and Novocain into the tender muscular fascicle or into the small nodule is the treatment of choice, but it is difficult at times to reach it with the needle. Certain kinds of massage with deep friction or transverse massage according to the technique of deep massage by Cyriax (1960) may be effective.

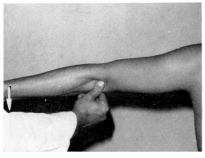

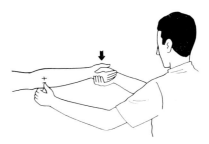

Figure 164. Manipulation in hyperextension, pushing the humeral head forward.

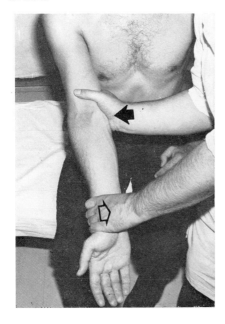

Figure 165.
Lateral manipulation: the supinated wrist being well immobilized, the physician forcibly adducts the elbow with his right hand.

Epicondylitis of Muscular Origin

There are cases of epicondylian pain of strictly muscle origin. This pain tends to disappear spontaneously if the elbow and spine are normal and if one mobilizes the arm. This form of epicondylitis, if observed in tennis players, is due to poor training or to the use of either a too heavy racket, or one that is poorly balanced.

Epicondylitis and Hyperuricemia

Some cases of chronic epicondylitis which are resistive to treatment are due to hyperuricemia. These patients usually have never had an attack of gout, and most authorities agree that specific medication should not be administered to the patient who has hyperuricemia unless they have an attack of gout. Yet, the use of anti-gout agents often have a very favorable effect in cases of persistent epicondylitis.

Chapter 24

Chronic Dorsal Pain of Cervical Origin

Obviously, we are going to consider here only the benign (functional) cases of chronic back pain. We therefore will omit the discussion of back pain of tumoral, infectious, inflammatory, or metabolic origin as well as back pain due to visceral diseases.

The difficult problems related to common cases of back pain are well known. The description by the patients of their pain, lacking in precision but full of images, the frequent absence of any radiologic sign, the meagerness of clinical manifestations, and the deceptive results of habitual therapy cause the physician to consider these conditions functional. It is generally accepted that a neurotic background, combined with poorly developed muscles constitutes the essential cause of this painful syndrome. If it is true that these factors are frequently found, it is difficult to consider them as the immediate cause of the dorsal pain even though they may favor, increase or maintain it.

We do not agree with this opinion. It is our conviction that most cases of back pain are due to a simple vertebral origin which is easy to identify and treat. However, most often one should not look for the origin of this pain at the level of the thoracic spine but at the level of the cervical spine.

This is why we believe that one should consider two classes of upper back pain: (1) those of cervical origin and (2) those of dorsal origin. It is also important to mention the role of the spasmophilic diathesis which is very often found in these patients.

"INTERSCAPULOVERTEBRAL PAIN"

We could show that 70 percent of the common dorsal pain is of lower cervical origin and is predominant in the interscapular region. These represent almost entirely the postural dorsal pain, such as manifested by typists and secretaries. It is, therefore, this form which we will study first; we call it "interscapulovertebral pain, or ISP."

Dorsal pain of cervical origin (ISP) is particularly frequent in women and our statistics concerning benign dorsal pain confirm it: one man to six women (200 cases).

By definition, it is localized between the scapula and the spine. It is almost always unilateral. It radiates very little, at times to the latter border of the scapula, at times, upwards. It may give the patient the impression of being deep seated, intrathoracic. This pain is, at times, described precisely as a nail or an abscess. In other cases, it is more diffuse giving the impression of a weight, a burn, or a painful tension between the scapula. It is in the latter case that the search of an interscapular point may reproduce the pain of which the patient usually complains.

Occupational factors are obvious and the most important point to be noted is presence of postural factors in this dorsal pain. It is most frequently found in occupations during which the hands are used at the level of the chest and where the elbows are not supported. For example, a farm girl did not suffer when strenuously working in the fields but when she started knitting, she developed acute interscapular pain.

Therefore, this pain will not be present unless the habitual occupation requires unfavorable posture. The pain will be absent during other activities unless we are dealing with a particularly severe case. Domestic activities (ironing, housework, sewing) elicit this pain frequently. Also carrying heavy packages may cause it. It does not seem to be paradoxical to assume that if men were engaged habitually in typing or sewing, the frequency of the occurrence among men would be increased considerably. In some cases, the pain occurs at night (6%) depending on the position of the head on the pillow, the height of the pillow, and the side on which the patient lies.

In other cases, the dorsal pain occurs in the morning, particularly on awakening. It disappears after the patient begins daily activity, but may reappear later in the day depending on the type of work that is being performed.

In some cases, the dorsal pain may have a particular character.

For example, we often find what we call an "overcoat sign," thus meaning a heavy overcoat, particularly during prolonged standing which elicits the pain very rapidly. This sign may be found, not only in women, but also in men, even those with well developed musculature.

Finally, we should underscore the fact that this sharp pain may occur three to four hours after working at a sewing machine for example. On the other hand, it may occur a few minutes after the patient begins work, causing these patients to claim they have to stop working. In other cases, pain is episodic, elicited by a faulty movement (almost always of the same type, *e.g.* reaching back behind the car seat) and may last several days, then disappear until another faulty movement brings it back again. It is almost always a movement of extreme rotation of the neck toward the painful side, or a stretching an aducted arm backwards.

The medical examination is reassuring if the benign nature of the complaint may be ascertained. However, the absence of effective treatment and a repetition of the x-ray examination in order to rule out any major organic disease inevitably increases the patient's anxiety which is so often associated with the back pain.

INTERSCAPULOVERTEBRAL POINT OR "CERVICAL POINT" OF THE BACK

What the clinical examination reveals in this syndrome is the *absolutely constant* presence of a tender point which we will call interscapular point of ISP. This point is very easily revealed by examination (Fig. 166). It is (1) constant, (2) remarkably fixed as to its position, being located 2 cm from the line of the spinal processes at the level of D5 or D6 (see diagram), and (3) very tender. The pressure of the finger, on this point *only,* reproduces exactly the dorsal pain of the patient. This is the epicenter of the pain.

This point should be investigated with the patient in sitting position with head flexed, hands over the knees, and as relaxed as possible. The finger of the physician slowly glides parallel to the line of the spinal processes at a finger's width from this line. It is

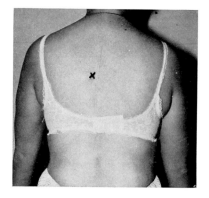 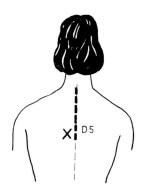

Figure 166. Interscapulovertebral point (ISP).

particularly helpful to use the index for the left side and the middle finger for the right side, both fingers forming a fork, with both fingers slowly gliding over the skin. Every half centimeter the physician exerts a slight pressure (the same at each level and on both sides). He may find points which are more or less tender, but none of them will be associated with this acute pain which is so characteristic. The skin-rolling maneuver applied to the skin is often very painful at this level. However, superficial anesthesia does not suppress the tender point. If one produces a deeper anesthesia, plane by plane, the pain is only partially suppressed, or only for a short time.

We have used the method of Kellgren (1939) consisting of injecting one milliliter of a hypertonic saline solution (following superficial anesthesia of this interscapular point). This injection elicits for a few minutes the sharp habitual dorsal pain which the patient complains of.

If the injection is made in a nontender symmetrical point, or in an analogous point in a normal individual, it will produce a sharp dorsal pain which is located two or three segments below the injected point and will vaguely radiate towards the intercostal space, but will have no character of the interscapular pain under discussion.

The measure of the local skin temperature does not provide any additional information of clinical significance.

ANTERIOR CERVICAL DOORBELL PUSHBUTTON SIGN

The search for this sign is important as, if positive, it confirms the cervical origin of this dorsal pain (Fig. 167).

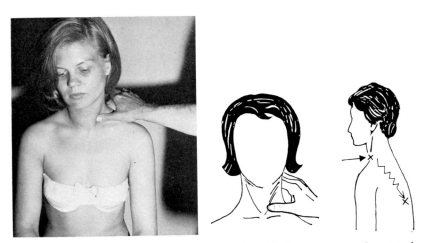

Figure 167. Anterior doorbell push button sign. Moderate pressure is exerted, at one level after another, in the anterolateral aspect of the lower cervical spine. At one point, it elicits an habitual dorsal pain of the patient.

In order to reveal this sign, the physician should stand facing the seated patient and exert moderate pressure with his thumb maintained horizontally (right thumb for the left side and left thumb for the right side) thus exploring segment by segment the anterolateral aspect of the lower cervical spine at the level of the emergence of the cervical roots. The doorbell sign exists only on the side of the interscapular pain. A moderate pressure maintained for only *two or three* seconds *reproduces immediately the dorsal pain of the patient which he recognizes as his usual complaint.*

If such pressure is applied to other segments or to any segment in a normal individual, a disagreeable sensation is produced or even a feeling of numbness in the corresponding dermatome. However, such pressure never *elicits* dorsal pain. It is in this fashion that one may, in the case of cervicobrachial neuralgia with poor localization, reactivate pain by pressure of the involved emergent root. This cannot be found either above or below the critical point nor on the opposite side. In some cases this sign may not be easily found. Occasionally, it may be present at the level of two segments. *The most important finding is the propensity of such pressure on the cervical spine to reproduce exactly the kind of dorsal pain which constitutes the patient's complaint and which, therefore, expresses a projected pain, not a local one.*

Thus, one may reproduce a dorsal pain by a purely cervical maneuver, and it is by this cervical manipulation that one is able to relieve the pain. Such manipulation will suppress the doorbell pushbutton sign as well as the interscapular point and this may occur immediately after the manipulation.

Let us add that this interscapular pain may be elicited, however, by a poorly conducted cervical manipulation. Also, the ISP may be found in patients who have had recent cervical trauma.

We recently observed a case of herniation of the C6-C7 disc which had manifested itself for six months by isolated interscapular pain, within the interscapular point at the level of D6 and with a particularly manifest doorbell pushbutton sign. Six months later the shoulder pain appeared to be radiating to the axillar region. A myelography and subsequent surgery confirmed the diagnosis of the discal herniation.

Whatever the situation and whatever hypotheses are formulated, the fact remains: there is a minor cervical intervertebral disturbance which may be attacked therapeutically.

TREATMENT

While in most cases, x-rays of the dorsal spine are negative, sometimes some changes are found. Then a frequent error consists of relating the dorsal pain of the patient to the lesion of the spine—in minimal scoliosis, a sequal of Scheuermann's disease, or dorsal arthrosis, which are observed so frequently without any clinical signs. In other cases, the association of dorsal pain with a local dorsal region may appear justifiable as in the following case:

Mrs. X, age 47. Her history included a fall from a horse with fracture of the 6th dorsal vertebrae. For several years following the fracture, she complained of a very tender paravertebral point at that level. All treatment was unsuccessful and the pain continually increased and was aggravated by fatigue. Intensive exercise, which she scrupulously followed, brought no success. However, in this patient the finding of the anterior cervical doorbell pushbutton sign at the level of C7 with the reproduction of the same dorsal pain permitted us to make a diagnosis of interscapular pain. We therefore had to conclude that there was at the same time a dorsal fracture and a cervical strain and that it was the cervical minor intervertebral persistent disturbance which caused the dorsal pain. Two cervical manipulations were sufficient to completely suppress this pain which had persisted for all those years.

In summary, a persistent dorsal pain in a woman who suffered a fracture of D6 years before, was suppressed by cervical manipulation and therefore should be classified as interscapular pain of cervical origin.

The radiological examination of the cervical spine is negative in most cases, although in some cases an isolated lesion of C5-C6 or C6-C7, or C7-D1, suggests a discogenic disease. In other cases, marked intervertebral pinching of the intervertebral space may be found in a young individual with persistent dorsal pain due to an old and forgotten trauma.

Clinical examination of the neck should be concerned mostly with the segment where the anterior doorbell pushbutton sign is present. The pain will be elicited at the same segment in the posterior paravertebral groove by the pressure of the corresponding posterior intervertebral joints and at times by the lateral pressure of the spinal process of C6 or C7. These signs confirm the presence of a segmental, cervical, intervertebral disturbance.

A careful examination of the movement involving this segment will be made in all directions with a tautening of the corresponding joints. According to the results of this examination, the manipulation which constitutes the principal treatment of this type of dorsal pain should be applied according to an appropriate technique. Long experience is necessary to conduct these maneuvers precisely and effectively. In certain difficult cases, as in cases where manipulation is contraindicated, the prescribing of a collar to be worn for 15 to 20 days has resulted in excellent improvement. Stellate ganglion infiltration may be particularly helpful in acute cases. In some cases physical therapy modalities and radiotherapy may be indicated. The ganglioplegic drugs and particularly the sedatives of the sympathetic nervous system may be of value. Finally, neck muscle reeducation is important. It should involve first the flexor (anterior) muscles of the neck and then the extensor muscles.

In summary, this dorsal pain of cervical origin is most frequent among cases with back pain. It can be diagnosed easily by the following:

1. Constant presence of a manifest fixed tender point very sensitive to pressure located at 2 cm from the midline at the level of D5 or D6 (interscapular point).

2. The possibility of reproducing the dorsal pain of the patient by pressure maintained for a few seconds and exerted at the level of the corresponding segment against the anterolateral aspect of the spine (anterior cervical doorbell pushbutton sign).

3. The efficacy of cervical treatment (manipulation, collar, and physiotherapy).

4. Whenever recurrent interscapular pain is observed, one should keep in mind that spasmophilic contributions may be involved, as we pointed out previously (Chapter 4).

THE NATURE OF THE INTERSCAPULAR POINT

The following two questions arise:

1. What is the significance of an interscapular tender point which is so constant and so consistently found?

2. What is the relationship between this point and the cervical spine?

Let us review once more, the work of Cloward (1960), an American neurosurgeon. In his papers devoted to discongenic cervical pain, he repeated some experiments of Frykholm (1947, 1951) and found that mechanical or electrical excitation of the anterolateral portion of the annulus of the lower cervical discs elicits scapular pain which may also be elicited by directly stimulating the ventral root of the lower cervical segments.

Cloward (1960) tried, in this work, to explain the interscapular spread of pain in the cervical discal herniations. He found on the basis of EMG recordings that such excitation elicits abnormal potentials in the muscles stabilizing the scapula. He concluded, therefore, that the muscular pain originating in the angular or rhomboid muscles explains the interscapular pain commonly observed in these patients. He thinks that there is irritation of the sinu-vertebral nerve which elicits a segmental reflex in the spinal cord resulting in the transmission of potentials along the ventral root of the same or adjacent segment. Thus, he considers again the opinion of Frykholm (1951) according to whom, a part of the neuralgic pain of mechanical vertebral origin is due to irritation of the ventral root.

While this work shows the possibility of eliciting dorsal pain from a cervical disc, the fact that seems of basic importance to us is not explained. This fact is the consistency of the localization of the interscapular tender point in all cases, whatever the cervical level involved. This is particularly obvious when we deal with interscapular pain associated with cervicobrachial neuralgia where the interscapular tender point is always adjacent to D5 or D6 whether the original cervical disturbance is at C6, C7 or C8 levels.

We do not believe that this point originates in the rhomboid or the trapezius muscles inasmuch as a resisted isometric contraction of these muscles does not always increase either back pain or tenderness of the interscapular point. The same can be stated about the muscle complexus or the splenius cervici. When one carefully studies the anatomy of the region one finds that this tender point corresponds exactly to the emergence of the posterior branch of the second dorsal spinal nerve. The posterior branch of the second spinal dorsal nerve is described by Hovelacque (1927) as the most important of all the dorsal nerves because it distributes itself over a very large skin area which extends from the middle part of the back to the lateral borders and up to the acromion (Figs. 168 and 169).

This nerve originates between D2 and D3, curves around the bony structures carrying posterior joints' articular surfaces to which it becomes intimately related and passes through a narrow osteofibrous canal. This canal consists of posterior intervertebral ligament of Cruveilhier limited above by the transverse processes

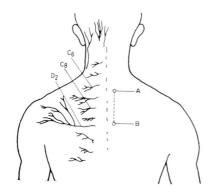

Figure 168.
Superficial nerves of the dorsal plane (after Hovelacque).

of D1, below by the neck of the adjacent rib, and laterally by the superior costotransverse ligament. It then descends vertically into the depths of the paravertebral groove. It branches out into two rami; one lateral which is purely motor and which innervates the muscle dorsalis longisimus and the other medial of larger diameter which is musculocutaneous and which innervates transverse and interspinal muscles. The medial ramus becomes superficial between D5 and D6 at 3 cm lateral to the midline; in other words exactly where the interscapular vertebral point is located. From there it fans out horizontally, supplying a large skin area,

Figure 169.

Posterior branch of the second spinal nerve (after Hovelacque). It is originated from D2-D3; it becomes superficial after perforating paravertebral muscles innervated by the cervical spine. It emerges at the level of ISP. Its territory corresponds to the area of hyperesthesia and of cellulalgia which are often found in this type of dorsal pain. Anesthesia of this nerve at its origin (between D2 and D3) relieves pain and makes ISP disappear. It is, therefore, probable that this branch plays a role in the genesis of interscapular dorsal pain.

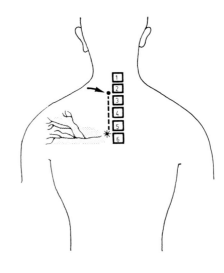

larger than any one corresponding to other dorsal nerves reaching the acromion above. This area corresponds to the skin hyperesthesia often observed and involved in local cellulitis.

During its course, the medical branch may give a twig to the rhomboid or the trapezius (Hovelacque, 1927). This explains why occasionally there is tenderness of some fascicles of these muscles which may be detected by palpation simultaneously with this resisted isometric contraction. In order to check this hypothesis, we anesthetized this posterior branch of D2 at the point of its emergence between D2 and D3 in more than forty patients suffering from interscapular pain, or in those with chronic interscapular pain such as observed in seamstresses. During the examination, these patients showed an obvious intrascapulovertebral tender point, adjacent to D5, the center of the area of the back pain. In all these cases, particularly in those with acute back pain, we could immediately suppress spontaneous pain and eliminate the tender point. The band of "cellulitis" then becomes painless during the skin-rolling maneuver and the skin hyperesthesia disappears.

RELATIONSHIP BETWEEN THE SECOND DORSAL NERVE AND THE CERVICAL SPINE

The fact that the posterior branch of the second spinal nerve may be responsible for back pain does not explain the mechanism of the cervical doorbell pushbutton point or the cervical origin of the back pain. At the present time, we found, on the basis of personal anatomical research, that there are anastomoses between the posterior branches of the lower cervical and of the upper dorsal nerves, particularly the second dorsal nerve which Hovelacque (1927) showed to be largest of these nerves, and which seems to us as resulting from the merging of the above nerve branches (particularly those supplying the skin.) One should also note that the D2 segment is an important one as far as the cervical sympathetic nerve is concerned. As already mentioned, infiltration of the stellate ganglion may often suspend dorsal pain, particularly in acute cases; then the pressure over the cervical doorbell pushbutton point does not elicit dorsal pain any more.

As to the sinu-vertebral nerve, it does play a definite role as it innervates the superficial fibers of the intervertebral disc. It certainly constitutes the first segment of the sensory pathway of the dorsal pain. However, it appears to us that one should correct the concept of Cloward (1960) so that instead of considering potentials which are transmitted through the spine and reach a spinal nerve, one considers those transmitted through the posterior branch of the second dorsal nerve supplying the involved muscles (see also Maigne, 1962, 1964, 1967).

Chapter 25

Other Causes of Chronic Benign Dorsal Pain

DORSAL PAIN OF DORSAL ORIGIN

Postural Pain

T HERE ARE cases of postural dorsal pain which offer a clinical picture resembling the one which we described for the intra-scapular pain but which is of dorsal and not cervical origin. In such cases, however, the pain is not always localized in the D5 and D6 segments.

In this case, clinical examination reveals the presence of a minor intervertebral disturbance of a thoracic segment with the following:

1. Pain following lateral pressure on one side of the spinal process (Fig. 170, left).

2. Elective pain elicited by "resisted" pressure of the spinal processes in one direction (Fig. 170, right).

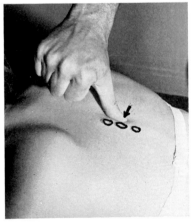 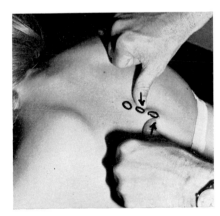

Figure 170. Pressure over spinal processes of the dorsal spine. *Left,* lateral pressure; *Right,* opposed lateral pressure.

3. Tenderness of the corresponding supraspinous ligament (Fig. 171).

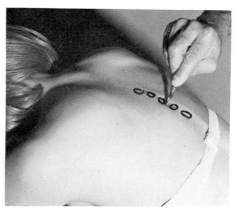

Figure 171. Key sign.

4. Frequent presence of a tender infiltrating cellulitis tested by the skin-rolling maneuver of the neighboring skin (Fig. 172).

Treatment

In this case, one may use a direct manipulation or an indirect manipulation. Direct manipulation is rarely indicated, but if effective in this case, should also be carried out according to the rule of no pain. One should, therefore, find a nonpainful direction

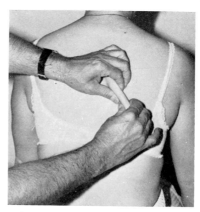

Figure 172. Skin rolling maneuver.

for the maneuver of resisted pressure of the spinal processes (Fig. 170). Once this direction is found, the manipulation will be effected by applying pressure on the right transverse process (as in the example in the figure) of the upper vertebrae and the left transverse process of the lower vertebrae so that a rotation in the nonpainful direction is produced at the level of the corresponding intervertebral joint. One may also apply pressure only on the right transverse process of the upper vertebrae.

In a case where the pain of the interspinal ligament persists its infiltration with Novocain and cortizone and in very rare cases, an infiltration of sclerogenic solutions (Hackett, 1956) may be very helpful when there is an unstable joint.

One should not forget to prescribe a few sessions of skin-rolling massage (Fig. 172) involving the tender skin if its tenderness persists after the correction of the intervertebral disturbance.

Finally, muscle reeducation and postural exercises should be prescribed as well as correction of static deficiencies (e.g. in the case of one leg being shorter than the other) (see also Fig. 173).

Dorsal Pain in Scoliosis

This is a case of a spine presenting dorsal scoliosis. It is common that the vertebrae placed at the summit of the dorsal curve becomes painful after fatigue. Manipulations usually improve this pain for a sufficient length of time so that if they are repeated two to three times a year the patient will be relieved and the effect of the muscle reeducation will be increased.

Tenderness of the Spinal Processes

Tenderness of the spinal processes to touch or pressure is frequent in some instances.

When it is associated with minor intervertebral disturbance, one should treat this disturbance.

It may be an isolated apophysitis. In some cases, it is provoked by a direct shock or a trivial contact (with the back of a chair) and constitutes a case of intractable dorsal pain. The treatment consists of local injections of cortizone and Novocain.

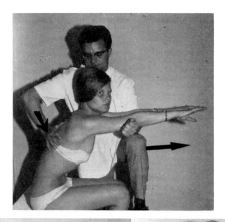

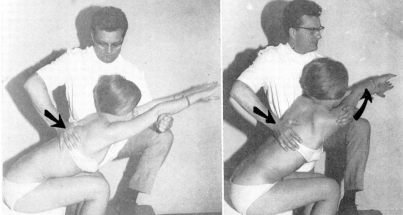

Figure 173. An example of gentle progressive mobilization of a stiff back.

However, occasionally, several processes may be tender together with other multiple tender points in the muscles and in
the skin. In this case, we usually deal with neurotic patients with
whom local treatment is usually ineffective.

Arthrosis and Dorsal Pain

Before considering thoracic arthrosis as responsible for benign
dorsal pain (obviously after having ruled out the possibility of a
projected pain due to a visceral disease, etc.), *one should be absolutely sure that one does not deal with interscapular pain of*

cervical origin, suspected by the presence of interscapular point at the level of D5 or D6 (p. 225), and confirmed by the presence of the anterior cervical doorbell pushbutton sign. In such cases a more complete examination of the cervical region should be done and the treatment should consist of manipulation, wearing a collar, cervical radiotherapy or stellate infiltration (see above).

One should also rule out the presence of an arthritic inflammatory episode; thoracic arthrosis may cause pain during such an episode. If this were the case, no manipulation or immobilization should be done. Instead, rest and anti-inflammatory therapy, possibly associated with radiotherapy, should be prescribed. Indeed, in these cases, manipulation may aggravate the pain.

Finally, one may deal with a case of dorsal pain due to rigidity produced by arthrosis, and then careful mobilization in extension and rotation may be very helpful. Manipulations are rarely advisable in such cases.

Dorsal pain in Scheuermann's disease should not, as a rule, be treated by manipulation. Such treatment should never be applied during an acute period in a young subject. Manipulation may at times be helpful at a later date if the spine is not too difficult to manipulate; it is much better to use progressive mobilization in extension.

PSYCHIC CAUSES

Although this subject is clearly beyond the limits of this monograph, we would like to say a few words in this regard. These causes should never be neglected inasmuch as their common occurrence is well known. The common French expression of having a "full load on one's back" is quite appropriate. This pain may be purely psychological and then it does not appear as a systematic condition. By its character and with the results of a skillful interview, a diagnosis of the psychological nature of the pain is much easier than its treatment. However, one should not forget that the most frequent cases are those of organic pain amplified by emotional tension. While one should recognize the cause of the amplification, it is just as important to detect the organic cause (after appearing as an interscapular pain). When one suppresses the latter; the additional use of some sedative drugs is generally effective unless the psychological factors play a dominant role (see, however, Bret and Bardiau, 1951; Toussaint, 1951; Arlet, 1952-54).

Chapter 26

Acute Dorsal Pain

A CUTE DORSAL pain may be seen under different circumstances.

"DORSALGO"

Dorsal pain may occur acutely just as it does during torticolis or lumbago. de Sèze (1951) called such a syndrome "dorsalgo."

There is a marked local contracture, a vertebral tenderness to pressure and signs of an acute intervertebral disturbance, probably of discogenic nature (see also Dreyfus and Levernieux, 1966).

Manipulations should be performed according to the principle of no pain using a technique which will depend on the circumstance. The results are good, with at times, total and instantaneous improvement.

INTERSCAPULAR PAIN

In some cases one deals with an acute interscapular pain which we feel is more frequent than dorsalgo. We have described its signs such as tender point near D5 or D6 vertebrae, and particularly, the possibility of reproducing this pain by pressure at the level of the lower cervical spine (anterior doorbell pushbutton sign, p. 259).

It is not rare that this acute interscapular pain precedes severe cervicobrachial neuralgia which manifests itself a few days later. Cervical manipulation and stellate ganglion infiltration may relieve the pain. The use of a cervical collar, particularly at night, may be very helpful.

REPETITIVE DORSAL PAIN OCCURRING "IN A FLASH"

This is a type of acute dorsal pain the description of which is not in the literature, but which we observed in a number of cases. The following clinical history gives a pertinent example of such cases:

Mr. C, age 44, prior to the first visit, while putting his arm through the sleeve of his vest, suddenly felt a severe pinching in his back. This lasted for a few minutes, then decreased while the patient immobilized his thorax by breathing as shallowly as possible. An attempt to take a deep breath again elicited a severe flashing pain. Following this episode, a certain tenderness of the back persisted but each time the patient felt himself relieved and would make another movement, the pain would recur. The periods of relief and the very acute episodes immobilizing him for a few seconds or minutes occurred alternately up until the time he sought treatment.

The examination showed a flexible spine. There was no limitation of movement and no consistently painful movement. However, during the examination, certain movements by either the physician or the patient did elicit an extremely severe episode. In trying to find a movement to initiate an episode, it was felt that the deep inspiration was the most successful. However, a radiological examination carried out the same day did not show any abnormality.

Different maneuvers of mobilizations carried out for diagnostic as well as therapeutic purposes had no influence whatsoever on the episodes. However, a definite improvement lasting for several minutes was obtained by slow intravenous injection of thiocolchicoside.

This patient experienced three identical episodes in four years with no clinical or radiological signs. In view of the therapeutic results during the first episode, two others were treated by the same drug as early as possible.

We now have about thirty cases of this kind. They are all identical. We have no pathogenic hypothesis to suggest but we advise treatment by intravenous injection of thiocolchicoside which appeared to be the best therapeutic agent in these cases, while the same drug had little effect in cases of lumbago or acute torticollis.

Chapter 27

Costal Sprain

Figure 174 shows costovertebral and costotransverse joints.

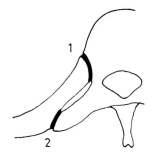

Figure 174.
1. Costo-vertebral joints.
2. Costo-transverse joints.

Costal sprain is often neglected. Yet, it is very frequent and we have described its clinical signs. The costal sprain is expressed by a thoracic or an upper lumbar pain. It follows either a contusion, an effort, or a faulty movement. It shows either a manifest costal localization or it offers a vague clinical picture, particularly when the false ribs are involved with pain radiating at times toward the lumbar region or the inguinal region. Clinical examination does not reveal any tender point of the spine, but pain is produced by pressure on one rib only, with pressure exerted over the neighboring or symmetric ribs remaining painless. Such pressure increases the spontaneous pain.

Without manipulation, which is immediately successful, the course of this sprain is favorable and the cure is usually apparent within a few days. However, there are cases of costal sprain that become chronic originating thoracic or lumbar pain and responsible for diagnostic errors, particularly when the false ribs are involved.

The diagnosis may be asserted by presence of only one sign which is necessary and significant for the diagnosis. This diagnosis is interesting because a simple single manipulation brings about immediate relief and particularly because in undiagnosed chronic cases, unnecessary examinations, such as kidney examinations, are usually carried out. The following case histories illustrate the clinical picture:

Case 1: Mrs. L, age 42, felt a knife-like pain on her right side as she flipped a bedspread on the bed. The maximum pain was localized at the level of the false ribs and radiated in the crotch and even toward the internal aspect of the thigh. She was suffering a lot and had to go to bed. Little by little, the pain decreased as long as she did not move. After three days of bed rest, she improved somewhat and then came for treatment.

Trunk movements, as well as deep respiration, elicited pain. There was no anthalgic attitude. Flexion of the spine was free, while its extension as well as right rotation and lateral flexion of the trunk were painful. There was no tender point at the level of the spinal processes. There was a definite tender point two fingerwidths to the right of D12. Pressure was painful all along the last rib and completely painless above it and on the other side.

The previous year she had had an identical episode. She was sent to the GU Service where several renal and radiological examinations were made with negative findings. The pain slowly disappeared in the next five to six months. She was very uncomfortable during the first month.

Case 2: Mr. B, age 30, during a judo exercise, while being held by his opponent in a scissors hold (the base of the thorax being squeezed between the legs of his opponent), experienced an extremely severe pain which caused him to stop the fight. He was bent double, clutching his left side at the level of the false ribs. His breathing was difficult since each movement seemed to produce pain in the spine, although the maximum pain was found to be all along the left rib, but particularly at the tip. Manipulation brought about instantaneous relief.

Both of these patients were immediately relieved by a single maneuver aimed at the painful rib.

If not treated, in most cases, the pain will stop after a few days. However, at times, it may recur with a slight movement of the trunk in rotation or lateral flexion or during a spell of coughing. Occasionally, the disturbance is more prolonged and marked as illustrated by the following case:

Case 3: Mrs. D came for treatment after suffering pain in the left upper lumbar region for a year. Onset was brutal during the lifting of a heavy pot. In the following days the pain was so severe that her family physician thought she was suffering from kidney stones. She was hospitalized for examination and tests, but all the findings were negative including radiological examination of the spine. She remained uncomfortable and whenever she lifted even the slightest weight she had to go to bed. At times the pain would again become sharp, particularly after exertion, housework or the assuming of a faulty position. Clinical examination revealed a mild dorsal lumbar scoliosis. The spine was flexible, although left lateral flexion of the trunk remained difficult and painful. The pain was localized at the level of the left false ribs, the last one being the most tender.

Manipulation was difficult since the patient was obese. It was, however, successful, as immediately afterwards the rib was no longer tender. The patient was seen five months later and did not report any reoccurrence of pain.

We have seen many patients who have undergone kidney examinations because the correct diagnosis of costal vertebral sprain was not made in time. Two of them even had surgery performed which did not help.

There are also cases of anterior costal sprain which are located at the chondrocostal juncture as illustrated by the following case:

Case 4: Miss P, age 38, fell over a large stone and struck the anterior aspect of the thorax under her left breast. The pain was very sharp and she fainted. A surgeon made a diagnosis of rib fracture. A supporting bandage was applied but brought little relief. The pain persisted, being aggravated by movements and coughing. The mere touch of the traumatized region elicited a syncopal pain at the level of an area located under and lateral to the left breast. Then the pain became less severe although still present and two months later the surgeon decided to repeat a complete radiological examination of the area. The pain continued to decrease during the ensuing months but manual efforts were impossible to carry out and the point under her breast remained tender. The patient had to be constantly sure that this area was protected and was unable to wear a bra.

The patient had, therefore, suffered for a year prior to the examination during which pain was elicited by touch all along one rib while pressure on the other ribs was painless. The patient complained of pain during deep inspiration.

The diagnosis of anterior costal sprain was made and manipulation instantly relieved the pain.

Once the existence of this sprain is known, it is easy to make the diagnosis in a patient who, following a faulty movement or effort, has a sharp thoracic pain. However, one should think about such a diagnosis in an intercostal pain of long-standing, imitating a precordial pain or "pleurisy pain" or intercostal neuralgia. It is not rare to find that the trauma which produces a real fracture of a rib is also responsible for an articular sprain of long duration involving the same rib. It is however, at the level of the lumbar region that the costal sprain is responsible for the greatest number of diagnostic errors: *it is, indeed, at the level of the false ribs that the costovertebral sprain is most frequent.*

Patients complain of a continuous soreness at the costovertebral angle aggravated by certain movements or positions, which goes from a simple uncomfortable feeling to a pronounced chronic lumbar pain. At times, painful episodes occur following false movement or exertion. However, the patient is not always aware of the cause of the pain and in view of the normality of the spine from the clinical and radiological standpoints the examinations are mostly oriented toward the evaluation of the renal function.

CAUSES

Direct Trauma

In a case of thoracic contusion or a fall, one deals mostly with the anterior chondrocostal sprain.

Costal sprain may be associated with a rib or vertebral fracture. A certain number of patients with persistent thoracic pain following a rib fracture may in fact suffer from the residual vertebral or costal sprain and be relieved by manipulation.

During judo exercises, costal sprain is frequent, particularly at the level of the false ribs; the hold which is commonly used consists of squeezing the base of the thorax of the opponent between the knees and to force him to give up by continually increasing the pressure. The fighter who is being held in this way resists by blocking his respiration and contracting his diaphragm as well as his abdominal and lumbar muscles. However, it may happen that if he relaxes his muscles while his opponent maintains his hold, he experiences an extremely sharp pain in the lumbar region. This pain, due to the costal sprain, generally decreases in the following days, but may reappear following certain movements or positions. At any rate, from this point on, the fighter is not able to endure this hold since the involved rib remains tender to pressure unless treated by manipulation.

False Movements and Exertion

In our experience these are generally false movements in rotation: at times minimal movement, such as shaking a bedspread or reaching back to roll up the back window in a car, etc. At times a brisk muscle exertion is responsible, such as lifting a weight or even sneezing.

Is It a Costal "Sprain"?

We are aware that the term "sprain" is undoubtedly not entirely correct. However, it seems to us less advisable to call it subluxation or dislocation inasmuch as we could never secure radiological proof of this. We could call it a block in a faulty position, but it appears to us more simple to call it costovertebral or chondrocostal sprain.

What is the Mechanism of the Sprain?

In the case of a false rib the mechanism is not in doubt inasmuch as there is no costotransversal joint; but what about the other ribs? Theoretically, one may consider two types of sprain: one having for its site the costovertebral joint and the other involving the costotransversal joint. In both cases, the other joint is not involved. Anatomically, the involvement of the costotransversal joint with the costal vertebral joint remaining uninvolved seems to be the most likely mechanism.

DIAGNOSIS

In case one suspects a costal sprain, the search for the following sign is essential ("rib maneuver") (Figs. 175 and 176) :

1. The patient is in sitting position with the physician standing behind him.

2. The patient's trunk is moved in lateral flexion to the side opposite the painful one with his arm on the painful side being raised over his head.

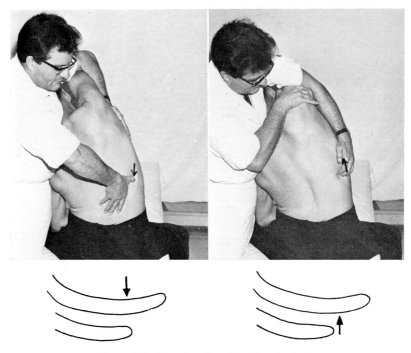

Figure 175. Examination of a "floating" rib.

3. With the tips of the fingers, one hooks the upper border of the painful rib and pulls downward. Then the same maneuver

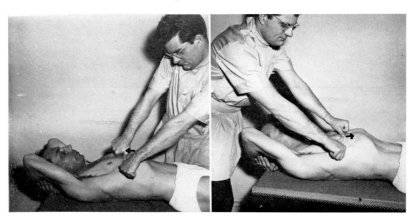

Figure 176. Examination of an anterior "floating" rib.

is applied by hooking the lower border of the rib and pulling upward. *If it is a costal sprain, one of these two maneuvers will increase the pain while the other is painless.* This sign exists only in cases of costal sprain. Indeed, in the case of *rib fracture* both maneuvers are equally painful. *If there is intercostal pain of radicular origin,* due to a vertebral sprain or vertebral discal disturbance or to any other inflammatory or tumoral cause, this maneuver does not change the character of the pain. Also, if the *pain is muscular,* it is not influenced by the rib maneuver. Nor is it influenced by this maneuver if it is a projected pain, as in the case of certain patients with liver or kidney diseases.

The anterior costal or chondrocostal sprain is frequently confused with the Tietze syndrome which is characterized by a progressive swelling of the rib cartilage which becomes spontaneously painful and tender to pressure and which is best treated by local hydrocortizone injection.

The examination is sometimes difficult in an obese patient. It is not easy in such a case to hook the rib. It is important in such cases to exaggerate to maximum the lateral flexion of the trunk to the side opposite the painful rib in order to facilitate the test.

MANIPULATIONS

All useful techniques are described in Part IV in the chapter, "Articulations of the Ribs." Manipulation is performed by pulling in the nonpainful direction (Maigne, 1957; LeCorre and Maigne, 1966).

Chapter 28

Acute Lumbagos

MORE THAN any other painful condition, acute lumbago has contributed to the reputation of manipulation and manipulators. It is, indeed, quite spectacular to see a patient, bent over as a result of acute pain, instantaneously recover following a maneuver which would appear to be too simple if it were not associated with the famous cracking sound. It is even often considered that a lumbago occurring in a young subject is the most typical indication of manipulation. Let us state at once that although acute lumbagos do constitute a good indication for manipulation, traumatic cervical pain, as well as traumatic involvement of the coccyx, offer still better therapeutic opportunities for manipulation.

The results of manipulation in acute lumbagos often are excellent and instantaneous indeed. However, inasmuch as acute lumbago in most cases recovers spontaneously by simple bed rest of relatively short duration, treatment by manipulation is of lesser importance than when it relieves a patient suffering from a headache, persistent for years, with no tendency toward spontaneous remission. It is certainly less convincing than in a patient remaining uncomfortable because of tender coccyx, or because of costal sprain for which manipulation is practically the sole efficacious treatment. Acute lumbagos are seen in different clinical conditions which react differently to manipulation. A great number of lumbagos seen in our clinic permitted us to establish the following statistics: 75 percent of the cases are associated with *antalgic* attitude. In 40 percent, the resulting deviation is *crossed* (often associated with some kyphosis). (Fig. 177, left). In other words, the patient is bent toward the side opposite to pain and is unable to assume a position of lateral flexion in the direction of the painful side. The pain is usually strictly lumbar. In 25 percent of the cases, *antalgic* posture is direct (the patient being bent in the direction of his pain) (Fig. 177, center). The pain then usually predominates in the sacro-iliac region. In 10 percent of the cases, the patient exhibits a pure kyphosis, the pain is in the midline over the lumbosacral juncture (Fig. 177, right) .

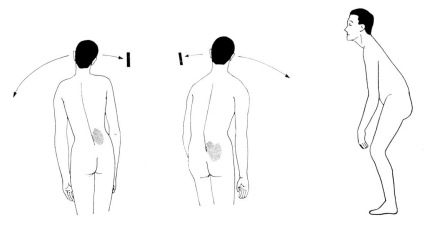

Figure 177. Antalgic attitudes. *Left,* crossed; *Center,* direct; *Right,* kyphosis.

In the remaining 25 percent of cases, the patient's posture remains erect; he exhibits only a vertebral rigidity, limiting most often his ability to bend forward, sometimes backwards.

In 20 percent of the total number of cases, the patient is not able to bend over forward and suffers from a pain across the lower back. In 5 percent of the total cases, pain is located very low on the midline of the sacrum. The onset of lumbago is usually very abrupt; in a few hours the patient is "nailed" in a rigid posture, incapable of either flexion or extension of the back which remains stiff but not bent laterally, although the patient may be slightly bent forward. There is no kyphosis. In contradistinction to the usual cases, there are no tender points over the spinal or transverse processes, nor for that matter over the muscles in the lumbar or gluteal regions.

TREATMENT

As always, the rule of no pain and free movement permits one to make a proper choice of the treatment in each individual case.

Case 1

When the patient shows a crossed antalgic attitude and a slight kyphosis, the maneuvers illustrated in Figure 178 are considered: the patient is placed astraddle a table, the physician imparting to the lumbar spine in slight flexion and lateral bending, a rotation toward the side opposite to the painful region. In other cases, the patient may be lying on his painful side and the maneuver shown in Fig. 179 is carried out.

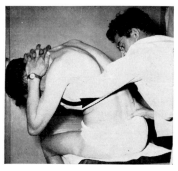
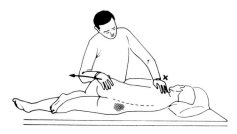

Figure 178.   Figure 179.

Case 2

In a patient having a *direct antalgic position,* the maneuver represented in Fig. 180 will be conducted, namely, lateral bending toward the side of pain and rotation to the opposite side. In some cases both maneuvers (lateral flexion and rotation) will be directed toward the side of pain. One could even select the maneuver described on p. 382, with the patient lying on the side opposite to pain, or the technique using the belt, as shown on Fig. 327.

Case 3

When the antalgic attitude is in marked kyphosis, treatment is particularly subtle. The manipulation in kyphosis shown in Fig. 182 with the patient in a side-lying position is certainly the preferred maneuver, the degree of rotation being slight at the beginning, then progressively increasing. It is mandatory to proceed

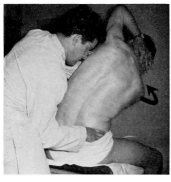

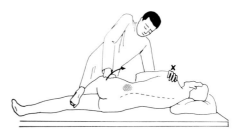

Figure 180. Figure 181.

with maneuvers of relaxation and mobilization in kyphosis prior to the manipulation.

In cases of lumbago with no antalgic bending, but where there is only a limitation of mobility most often in flexion, it is the knee maneuver which should be preferred as shown in Fig. 183.

Finally, in cases where pain is very low, in the mid-sacral region, in a patient without any history of trauma or a patient nailed by contraction of the psoas, manipulations usually are not successful. Epidural injection seems to be the most efficacious treatment.

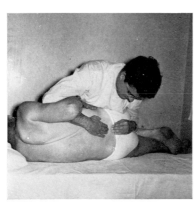

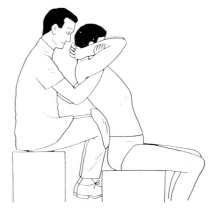

Figure 182. Figure 183.

The rapidity of therapeutic success is without doubt the most obvious characteristic of manipulations in these as in many other cases. In one half of the treated cases, the first manipulation brought about the cure, the other half being clearly improved. However, it is helpful to manipulate a second time, a few days later, in order to improve the flexibility of the spine. If one considers two manipulations in a patient having the first one done three days after the onset of pain, the results on the fifth day may be summarized as follows (patients cured) :

Crossed antalgic bending	80%
Direct antalgic bending	75%
Kyphosis	30%
No lateral bending, pain across the lumbar region	70%
No antalgic bending pain in the low sacrum	20%

It is obvious that after eight days of treatments, with three manipulations performed, the percentage of cure increases to 95 percent with the exception of the antalgic bending with kyphosis which is often followed by sciatica which, in turn, is surprisingly improved by manipulations.

Finally, the restoration of normal mobility of the lumbar spine after lumbago in subjects having had several lumbagos seems to be facilitated by appropriate therapeutic exercises.

Chapter 29

Chronic Lumbagos

W E WILL consider here only benign chronic lumbagos of vertebral origin. We will omit those due to infectious, inflammatory,
or tumoral involvement of the spine as well as those which are
due to visceral disease or those of psychic origin.

Radiological examination is of major importance for the
diagnosis. All lumbagos are suspect. Only by x-ray can one reveal
a spondylitis, beginning rheumatoid pelvispondylitis, or bone
lesions due to metastases or other causes. Only x-ray can reveal the
condition of the disc, the existence of a transitional anomaly, or
the extent of osteoarthrosis. However, it is well known that x-ray
in cases of true lumbago can be very deceptive. The spine may
be completely normal or may show an anomaly such as sacraliza-
tion, lumbarization, spondylolysis or even spondylolisthesis. The
x-ray may show various degrees of osteoarthrosis; an extensive or
a mild one. It may show a slight marked pinching of the intervertebral space. Finally, all of this is of only relative importance
for the treatment as it is well known that all of these particular
conditions are not the causes of lumbago inasmuch as there are
patients with the same radiological images who do not experience
pain and the patients who do will continue to show the same
radiological signs even after being relieved.

It is helpful to know the shape of the spinal processes, in
particular, whether or not there is a Baastrup syndrome (1933)
(kissing spines) . Most of all the radiological examination will aim
at measuring the comparative length of both legs as well as
establishing that the pelvis is level. These factors are not the immediate cause of lumbago, but they favor it and one should therefore keep them in mind for the prognosis. It is essentially the
clinical examination which will have to identify the pertinent
signs, thus leading to good treatment and individual care of
lumbago (see also Robert d'Eshougues *et al.,* 1960) .

THE CLINICAL EXAMINATION

Interview

The interview should be precise and very detailed. After taking the history, which is often extremely revealing, one should determine the rhythm of the pain, its topography (unilateral, bilateral or midline, high lumbar, low lumbar or sacral) and its radiations (in the lower leg, lateral, median, posterior or anterior aspect; at the inguinal or gluteal region) as well as the influence which may be either favorable or unfavorable for different positions (in bed, standing, sitting, arising). One should also ask whether coughing, sneezing, defecating or any other effort increases pain.

Study of Movements

Examination is aimed first at determining the flexibility of the spine and analytical differentiation of various movements of flexion, extension, lateral bending, and rotation. This examination is carried out on patients while they are standing and actively effecting these movements. The patient is then asked to straddle the end of the table with his back to the physician who will put him through the same movements passively. The directions of the free movements and painful or limited movements will be marked on the star diagram.

Identification of Minor Intervertebral Derangements

One will then examine the lumbar spine segment by segment. For this examination, the patient should lie prone with a cushion under his abdomen and also should be examined lying across the table (Fig. 184). One will effectuate the following:

1. Pressure over the spinal processes.
2. Pressure over the interspinal ligaments.
3. A search for paravertebral tender point (2 cm from the midline).
4. Lateral pressure over the spinal processes. (This examination is carried out on the patient lying across the table).

If one finds that this pressure is painful, one will exert pressure in the opposite direction over the spinal processes immediately adjacent to the first one, above and below it, so that a minor intervertebral derangement justifying manipulation may be properly identified.

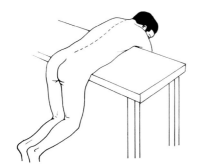

Figure 184.
Position of the patient for the palpation of the lumbosacral region. The examination of the gluteal region is mandatory.

The Muscles of the Gluteal Region

One should study the different gluteal muscles. It will often be found that one or several of the muscles will have hard, infiltrated fascicles which are at times cordlike. They may be very sensitive to pressure. In order to identify the tender muscle, one should make it contract against manual resistance; first the gluteus maximus, then medius, then minimus, the fascia lata, and the external rotators, while the other hand palpates the corresponding muscle. According to our experience the gluteal muscles pain is responsible for a considerable number of instances of lumbar pain. Deep massage (petrissage) gives excellent results in this type of chronic lumbago.

The Skin

This study would not be complete if one did not mention the importance of the skin and subcutaneous tissue of the lumbar, sacral, and gluteal regions. This examination is made by using the method of skin rolling (grasping a large fold between the thumb and index finger and rolling it like one rolls a cigarette). This maneuver, normally barely perceived by the patient, permits one to reveal areas where the fold becomes particularly large and contains tender nodules which are extremely sensitive to the least pressure.

The Ligaments

Careful attention during this examination should be given to the interspinal ligaments as well as to the iliac insertion of the iliolumbar ligament.

Static Disturbance

The difference between the lengths of the legs is of particular interest as is the postural study of the feet. We will return to this problem later.

TREATMENT

Manipulation with many different variations, determined by the individual case, constitutes basic treatment for most instances of low back pain. We rarely use direct manipulation. In such cases, the patient should be well stabilized lying on his abdomen or sometimes across the table. One exerts pressure over the transverse processes so as to elicit in the intervertebral joint, a movement in the reverse direction to that produced by the lateral pressure of the spinal process which was found before to be particularly sensitive. However, almost always we consider that the semi-indirect assisted maneuvers are the best and the most helpful. In such cases, the patient is lying on his side or sitting astraddle, if a knee technique is used. These maneuvers are preceded by the habitual relaxing procedures and by mobilizations. The direction of these maneuvers is determined by our rule of no pain.

If the movements are simply stiff, one will carry out a few sessions of mobilizations using the technique described in the last part of this monograph. During the last session, one may force the movement a little, so that a manipulation is done in all directions. There are cases where all movements are painful. It is evident in these cases that manipulation as well as mobilizations are contraindicated.

If there is muscular pain (and this is extremely frequent) revealed by the pressure of the gluteal muscles, such pain may subside following correction of intervertebral derangement. However, the pain may persist or exist independently of the derangement.

Most often it is sufficient to treat by deep petrissage using slow and tenacious movements.

Under the influence of such treatment which may be very disagreeable at the onset, the muscle may become flexible again and lose its abnormal sensitivity while the low back pain subsides. We would like to stress this point which is never mentioned. The gluteal muscles are the most important extremity muscles to be examined in low back pain. It is possible sometimes, that despite the treatment, there is a tender point in the treated muscle which will elicit pain radiating over the whole gluteal fossa or toward the thigh. This is a trigger point such as described by other authors, Travell (1955) for example. It should be treated by Novocain injection.

Some local infiltrating cellulitis revealed by the skin-rolling maneuver may elicit the patient's habitual pain. The latter may subside immediately following lumbar manipulation. If, however, it persists, which may be the case in low back pain of long duration, the treatment should consist of several sessions of massage (6 to 8) with superficial petrissage, using the same skin-rolling technique. This maneuver is extremely disagreeable at the beginning of the treatment but becomes pain-free at the end.

Tenderness of the supraspinous ligament is very often associated with intervertebral derangement, and decreases or disappears after manipulation, sometimes very slowly. However, if it persists unabated, one should treat it by injection of Novocain and cortisone, which is sufficient for most cases. Such injections, moreover, permit one to evaluate the role played by this ligament in low back pain. When the needle penetrates the ligament, the habitual low back pain is reproduced. When the ligament is anesthetized, the pain subsides.

In some cases where involvement of this ligament produces instability of the joint and when the tenderness remains quite acute, and so its role in low back pain is established, one may inject sclerosant agents according to Barbor's (1966) method. Finally, in some cases, it is at the iliac insertion of the iliolumbar ligament that one may discover extreme tenderness to pressure. If the pain induced in this fashion is the habitual one, injections of these insertions are advised. Very often this pain is associated with intervertebral derangement and disappears after its correction. It often radiates toward the inguinal region.

If one leg is shorter than the other, one should never prescribe a lift before the spine regains its flexibility. Then the correction should be made progressively without achieving complete correction except in very young individuals. One should learn how to respect those cases of leg differences which are well compensated for and well tolerated.

If there is a valgus deformity of the foot, one should place a supinator lift under the heel and if there is also a collapse of the arch, one should add a pronator lift under the ball of the foot. Prescribing of a corset should be avoided. A corset may sometimes be useful at the beginning of therapeutic exercises in order to retain the results obtained on low back pain by manipulative treatment or other therapy. However, as soon as muscle strength is restored, the corset should be discarded. In certain cases, however, it will remain indispensable, for example, in those cases when the patient complains of pain after a given period of standing and when the pain progressively increases.

Finally, one should give the patient the following advice:

1. *Bed:* It is of utmost importance for a patient suffering from low back pain to sleep on a firm mattress.

2. *Chairs:* Soft and low chairs are to be avoided.

3. *Posture:* One should teach the patient not to bend over, but to stoop; also, not to twist the body in turning but, rather change position of their feet. One should explain the effect of poor posture on the spine. Most of all one should prescribe lumbar abdominal exercises.

Muscle Reeducation by Lumbar Abdominal Exercises

The exercises illustrated in Figure 185, A through E, are so intimately integrated in our treatment of low back pain following manipulations in order to recover flexibility of the spine that it is essential to review the principal exercises prescribed for our patients. The rule of no pain should be respected here also and any movement which is painful should be avoided. In 90 percent of cases, the helpful movements are those in flexion, in 10 percent they are in extension.

These therapeutic exercises, which we like to call antalgic exercises, do not appear to be effective because of the increase of muscle strength but rather because of learning of better utilization of the muscles, their better coordination and the awakening of the regional proprioception.

These therapeutic exercises, only the first stage of a program, are, however, very often sufficient by themselves. Later on, more complex and complete exercises may be prescribed, based on quadrapedic exercises of Klapp (1955). Once the patient has learned these different movements, one asks him to perform two selected exercises each morning for two to three minutes.

1. All these exercises should be done with the pelvis positioned to correct lordosis. The first purpose of this reeducation is to make the patient aware of the tilt of his pelvis. The explanation of the pelvis tilt is made to the patient while he is in a supine position by asking him to retract his abdomen, to pinch his buttocks together, to press his lower back against the floor or table, and then relax and start all over again. One should demonstrate to him the mechanism of the tilt which places the lower back in kyphosis and which shortens the distance between the pubis and the sternum (see also Peillon, 1958; Weiser, 1966). At the beginning one may place a pillow under the neck.

2. This position of the pelvic tilt should be maintained for the duration of all the exercises.

3. The respiratory rhythm should be the pacemaker for the exercises. The patient should inhale prior to the effort and exhale just afterwards. The expiration should in principle, coincide with the shortening of the distance between the pubis and the sternum (Balland and Grozelier, 1952).

4. Progressive difficulty of the exercises will be determined by the initial position. In all these movements, the angle of the hip joint should be between 80 and 100 degrees. This avoids contraction of the psoas in this position which produces lordosis (Fig. 185D). The working angle is therefore 40 degrees. This exercise strengthens the abdominal muscles.

Figure 185A.

First Series

First initial position: Patient is supine, thighs semiflexed without elevating the buttocks.

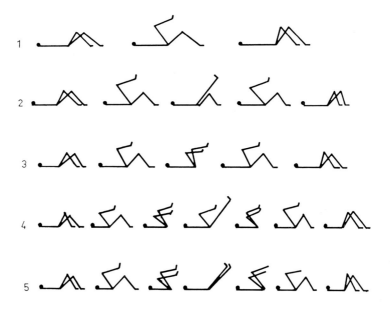

Figure 185B.

Second Series

Second initial position: Patient sits in a half-reclining position supported by his elbows. The hip angle remains the same.

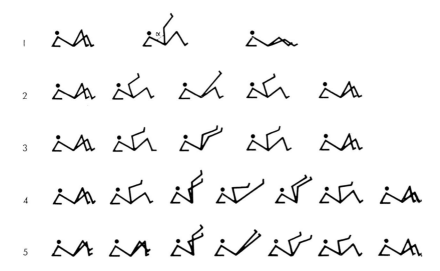

Exercise of the obliques: Starting with the same initial position, the patient raises his knees with legs flexed and makes a balancing movement with his thighs which are inclined to the left and to the right alternately.

Exercise of the transverse muscles: The patient is on all fours. The abdomen is retracted maximally and he exhales forceably and slowly through his almost closed mouth. Then he is asked to pretend he is blowing out a candle.

Figure 185C.

Third Series

Third initial position: Patient is in a sitting position on the floor, propped up by his hands extended behind him. Patient carries out same movements as in 1 and 2 with the angle of movement remaining the same.

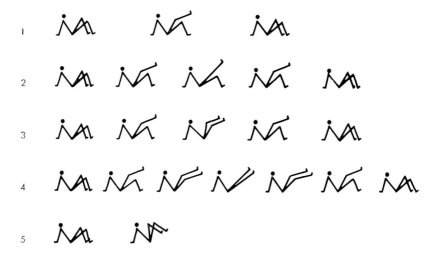

Figure 185D.

Fourth Series

Fourth initial position: Up to this point, it was the light body segments (lower extremities) which were mobile; the heavy segments (trunk and arms) being immobilized. Now it is the heavy segments which will be mobile while the feet are immobilized by a heavy weight.

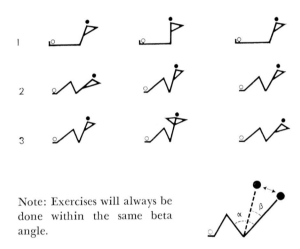

Note: Exercises will always be done within the same beta angle.

1. Progress is made by position of the arms: arms crossed on the chest; hands placed on shoulders; hands placed behind the neck; arms elevated.
2. Same position as 1.
3. Rotation of the trunk to right and then left. Progression is made by changing position of the hands: arms crossed on chest; hand placed on shoulders; hand behind the neck; arms horizontal.

Figure 185E.

Fifth Series

This is the end of the continuous progression which consists of very difficult exercises as both the light and heavy segments are mobile.

Initial position: Patient is sitting balanced on the buttocks, leaning backwards, knees half-flexed and hands placed on the shoulders.

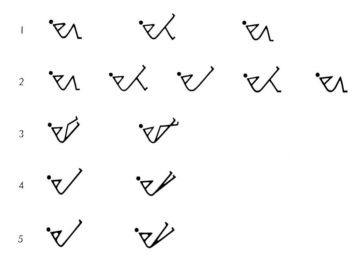

Pedaling: Kicking motion with the knees stiff; circling movements also with knees stiff.

Exercises of the obliques: Trunk and arms effect movement of rotation to the right while the legs lean to the left and then the process is reversed.

Chapter 30

Sciatica

Common sciatica is due to interference of the disc with the L4, L5, and S1 roots (Krayenbuhl and Klinger, 1949; Kuhlendahl, 1950). The frequency of this interference is explained by the local peculiarities. Indeed, it is only at these levels that the dural envelope of the root faces the disc and therefore, the root adherent to its envelope cannot escape the discal protrusion. Involvement of the L5 root is expressed by pain which travels from the buttocks along the posterolateral aspect of the thigh, the lateral aspect of the lower leg, and then turns and travels over the instep in order to reach the big toe. Involvement of the S1 root elicits pain which travels more posteriorly, namely along the posterior aspect of the thigh and the calf and passes under the heel in order to reach the little toe and the lateral border of the foot. The patient may complain of a crawling sensation or numbness, particularly in the distal parts of the extremity in which case they have the same localizing significance as above.

In some cases, there may be motor involvement. It is localized in the dorsal flexors of the foot in cases of L5 sciatica (except perhaps the tibialis anticus which may be supplied by L4). In these cases, the patient has a foot drop. In less-pronounced disabilities, the patient scuffs the floor with the toe of his shoe. In cases where motor involvement is even more discrete, one should elicit the involvement by opposing a forced voluntary movement of the big toe. When there is motor involvement of the S1 root, there is weakness of the calf muscles and the patient cannot stand on tiptoe. However, as Troisier (1962) showed, the systematic evaluation of strength of different muscles in sciatica reveals that motor involvement is much more frequent than expected. For example, the gluteus medius is involved in 33 percent of L5 sciaticas (Fig. 186).

There is absence or diminution of the ankle jerk in S1 sciatica. There is no reflex corresponding to L5 root.

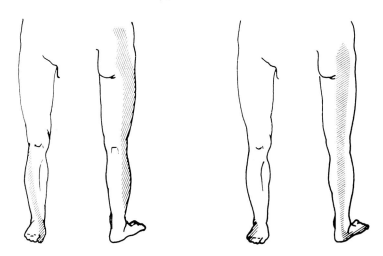

Figure 186. Travelling pain in sciatica due to the involvement of the L5 *(Left)* or S1 *(Right)*. Anterior and posterior views.

Pain is a result of two factors (de Sèze, 1951): (1) a mechanical factor, compression of the root by the disc; (2) an inflammatory factor, as a reaction to compression. There are, therefore, treatments which aim at each of these two factors:

1. Mechanical treatments such as manipulation, traction, and surgery.

2. Anti-inflammatory treatment, either drugs, general or local; or physical agents (radiotherapy).

Rest in bed is essential, in some cases with a corset or plaster so that there is complete immobilization of the involved segment. Analgesics, particularly aspirin, should be used in large quantities. One should not hesitate to use stronger analgesics or hypnotics in cases of hyperalgic sciaticas. As for the mechanical treatments, manipulation occupies a privileged position. If it is applied correctly and at the right time, it is the treatment of choice in many cases of sciatica. However, it is sometimes contraindicated. One should not forget that the method of application changes from case to case and that the maneuvers must be precise in order to insure their effectiveness and innocuousness. A standard maneuver, which is ritually applied in all cases or a manipulation carried out under poor conditions, e.g., in bed or over a table too high or too low, are dangerous to the patient. The patient's condition may suddenly worsen as a result of such procedures and the patient may then retain an unpleasant memory of a treatment that could have relieved him of his pain.

Sciatica of moderate intensity is the best indication for manipulation. However, manipulation may also be helpful in certain painful sciaticas when technical conditions necessary for application are all present. It is obvious that manipulations do not preclude medication and bed rest. Unfortunately, the excellent effect of manipulation which gives immediate relief to the patient may have undesirable results. All too often the patient, being improved, does not follow the prescription for bed rest which is essential for continued improvement.

THE COURSE OF TREATMENTS BY MANIPULATION

Sciatica is associated by antalgic scoliosis which locks the lumbosacral segment in certain movements. One distinguishes two types of antalgic postures:

1. Crossed scoliosis which is convex on the painful side.
2. Direct scoliosis which is concave on the painful side.

The rule of no pain and free movement guides the physician in his choice of the maneuver to apply in these cases as much as in any other one. Therefore, the antalgic postures, corresponding to the direction in which the movement is blocked, will contribute to the choice of the maneuver to use. However, it is preferable, even when the antalgic posture is characteristic, to carry out a careful segmental analysis of the free or limited and painful movements, as only painless maneuvers will be selected. (Fig. 187).

When the star diagram derived from an examination of a case of sciatica shows all three directions in which the movement is free, manipulation is definitely indicated. This is the most typical case of sciatica. If there are only two free directions, one should proceed with relaxing maneuvers and carefully evaluate the situation afterwards. In general such a patient does not offer a good indication for manipulation. If there is no free movement, manip-

ulation is contraindicated as the pain is very intense. The manipulation may become possible once the inflammatory condition
subsides and some movements become free. In cases of chronic

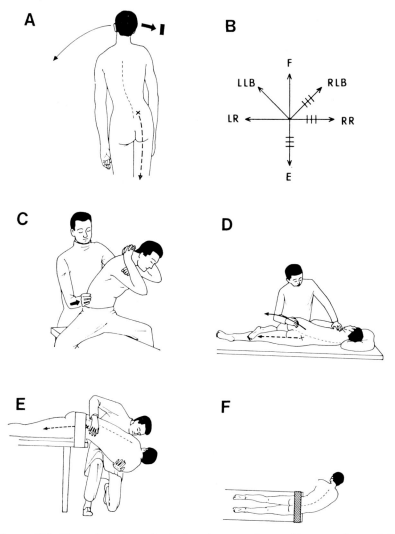

Figure 187. Example of manipulation in a patient with crossed antalgic
position. *C,* maneuver in left rotation and flexion (patient sitting); *D,*
maneuver in left rotation and flexion—patient in side-lying position; *E,*
maneuver in left lateral bending and flexion; *F,* same, upper view.

sciaticas, when the movements of the spine are not too limited and induced pain is of low intensity, the initial direction of the manipulation may be derived from other signs of the segmental examinations, for instance, the pain produced by opposed lateral pressure over the spinal processes, etc. (Fig. 188) .

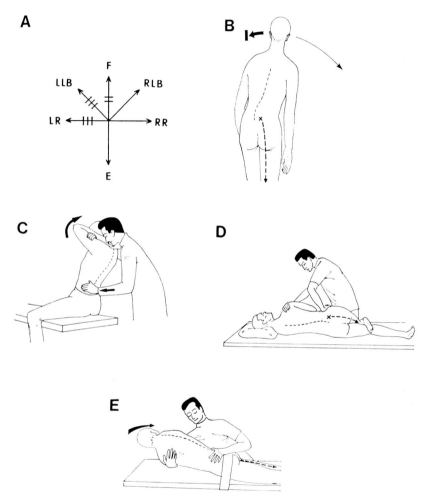

Figure 188. Example of manipulation in a case of right sciatica with direct antalgic position. *C*, maneuver in right rotation and extension (patient sitting) ; *D*, maneuver in right rotation and extension (patient side-lying) . *E*, maneuver in left lateral bending and slight extension.

At each phase of the manipulative treatment one should be guided by the following:

1. Lasegue sign, easy to elicit.
2. Forward flexion of the spine, measured by the distance separating the fingertips from the floor.
3. Subjective comments of the patient.

In no case should any additional maneuvers result in a setback. This will never occur if one correctly follows the rule of no pain and if the maneuver is carried out in a desirable position and with appropriate intensity. In general, manipulation should bring about an improvement, even a limited one. It may be ineffective in some cases, but it should never worsen the condition of the patient.

A therapeutic session should be well planned and balanced: maneuvers of relaxation first; then mobilization, then a few manipulations, no more than four; otherwise the tissues involved may become irritated. The patient should feel relieved at the end of the session and retain the improvement for at least a few hours. In 30 to 35 percent of cases one may expect that during the night following the first session the pain may be reactivated or the patient may complain of aches and stiffness for hours or even a day or two.

Once this reaction is over, the patient feels relieved again and is sometimes greatly improved for two or three days. The second manipulation should be applied four to seven days after the first one; a few days later if the initial reaction is very marked, a few days earlier if no reaction follows the first session. The third session follows the second by three to seven days. Occasionally there is no reaction following the second or third therapeutic sessions. In usual cases these three sessions are sufficient to bring about the desired improvement. In more difficult cases, additional sessions may become necessary. If there is no improvement during the initial three sessions, even a partial or temporary one, the chances of improvement during these additional sessions become questionable and a review of the case is indicated (see also Leca, 1950; Le Go, Maigne and Toumit, 1956; Levernieux, 1961; Lescure and Maigne, 1953) .

SCIATICA AND MUSCLE PAIN: A MYALGIC FORM OF THE SCIATICA

In a preceding section we mentioned the possibility of changes of consistency of certain muscle fascicles supplied by an irritated or compressed root. These muscle fascicles (the entire muscle is very rarely involved) become firm and, most significantly, are very tender to pressure. We believe that these changes play a dominant role in the genesis of persistent cases of sciatica. Yet, this observation does not seem to have attracted the attention of clinical investigators. However, the presence of such changes requires the application of different therapeutic procedures which may be contrary to those generally accepted in cases of sciatica (p. 50).

If one systematically examines each muscle within the myotome corresponding to the involved root, one may easily identify these hardened fascicles, so tender to pressure. The contrast is manifest between their consistency and that of the remaining mass of the muscles, which are often hypotonic, as it is usually the case of a muscle affected by a discogenic segmental involvement. The size of such fascicles is variable both in relation to diameter and length. At times, they may be only one or two inches long, at times they appear as long as the entire muscle. Their diameter is comparable to that of a fountain pen.

Very rarely is the entire muscle involved. Palpation gives the impression of a local contracture. Tenderness is very acute, particularly in the middle of the fascicle. If pressure is sustained, it often elicits in addition to local pain, the habitual pain of the patient which is referred to another region. Certain muscles seem to be much more involved than others: gluteus medius, medial or lower part of the gluteus maximus; tensor fascia lata, lower segment of the biceps femoris, soleus and the lateral gastrocnemius. The distribution is segmental; gluteus medius and fascia lata for the L5 segment; gluteus maximus, biceps femoris, soleus, lateral gastrocnemius for S1 neuralgias. In each of these muscles there are selected regions of tenderness; for example, the lower tendinomuscular junction for the biceps femoris, the lateral fascicles for the soleus, etc. In order to determine, particularly at the level of the buttocks, which muscle has partial hardening, one should use muscle testing along with muscle palpation. For example, one should elicit isometric abduction against resistance in the case of the gluteus medius. The muscle contraction sensitizes the involved muscle fascicles.

Such a systematic examination should permit one to discover in practically all cases of sciaticas during the acute period such areas of muscular tenderness, particularly in the gluteal muscles. However, only in about 30 per cent of cases is this partial hardening of the muscle particularly pronounced and appears to us to play a particular role. It is at this level that most patients complain of intense pain. It is quite easy, by simply pinching this fascicle or submitting them to pressure, to realize that these muscular areas are directly related to the habitual pain.

Local anesthesia, when the tender zone is large enough, immediately relieves the patient of both local pain and that referred to another region. This local hardening of the muscle, of which the patient is not aware, subsides when the discal compression is relieved. For example, following vertebral treatment, they may decrease and may completely disappear following a simple manipulation. These favorable results may last only a few hours or even minutes; in other cases, the beneficial effects are lasting. The muscle hardening generally progressively subsides during treatment, but it may survive the crisis even when the patient believes that he is completely cured. It is in such cases that the local pressure will reproduce the previous pain for the patient. Thus for example, the patient who is cured because he no longer suffers from his sciatica is unable for a prolonged time to cross his legs since the pressure over the gastrocnemius or soleus is extremely disagreeable or even painful.

There are cases where the local, painful, partial hardening of the muscles dominates the clinical picture. The spine is flexible, bed rest does not help the patient, injections or manipulations are not effective, and the patient continues to suffer. Only the treatment selectively aimed at this muscular involvement, looked for systematically, will relieve the patient of his intractable sciatica. One should realize that these cases have certain peculiarities. During the acute phase, the pain is extremely intense while the antalgic attitude is moderate. The spine is more flexible and has greater range of motion than one would expect from the intensity of the pain. The pain occurs in slow, progressively increasing waves with a sensation of crushing and prolonged acute cramps.

If one palpates the muscles during the attack, one will clearly perceive an intense contraction of its fascicles. The focus of a maximum pain is fixed: buttock or thigh or calf. There may be fasciculations and occasionally a motor deficit, usually very mild. Between the waves of pain, one may perceive painful tension at the level of the fascicles which originates the attack.

After the acute episode is over, the patient complains of persistent sciatica which does not respond to the usual treatment. The pain diminishes to moderate intensity but is influenced by the position of the legs. In certain cases, the patient will observe that when his leg is hyperflexed while he is in a sitting position the pain arises from the posterior aspect of the thigh. Examination will reveal exquisite tenderness of the lowermost fascicles of the biceps femoris; in other cases a sitting position will elicit gluteal pain which spreads to distant regions. The patient often states that exercise seems to relieve his pain and usually indicates that heat has a beneficial effect. In addition he often complains that after a fatiguing day he suffers from insomnia and consequently feels badly the next day. In such cases, one usually finds good flexibility of the spine with Lasegue sign of 45 degrees. If one slowly raises the leg, a greater angle may be obtained. Careful palpation should detect the area of muscle responsible for the pain. As soon as this area is anesthetized, Lasegue sign jumps to 90 degrees, and the patient is completely relieved.

Treatment of Myalgic Form of Sciatica

First of all, one should ascertain that the intervertebral disturbance has been reduced locally. As we stated before, the local, painful muscle hardening may often disappear after a purely vertebral treatment, and it would be poor strategy to apply local treatment without reducing a discogenic disturbance.

1. Local infiltration is sometimes an excellent treatment. We

use 0.5% of millicaine. However, this treatment is valid only in very localized forms and does not usually have complete beneficial results. With LeCorre (Maigne, 1964), we compared this treatment with injection of saline or the introduction of a dry needle into the tender fascicle. Such treatments, reminiscent of acupuncture, have been as successful as those using anesthetic.

2. For some time, we have preferred treatment by stretching. Indeed, we have noticed that the stretching of the hardened fascicles, either in transverse, or better, longitudinal direction, although eliciting temporary pain, makes the muscle more elastic and less tender. At the same time, the patient is subjectively relieved and his stiffness as well as the Lasegue sign disappear. One should keep in mind, however, that the Lasegue maneuver stretches certain muscles longitudinally such as the hamstrings and gastrocnemius, the latter by dorsoflexing the foot. One exerts progressive stretching during this maneuver which is carried out within the limit of supportable pain. The pain subsides if the progression is slow, commonly changing a Lasegue of 40 degrees to that of 80 degrees during the same maneuver. We usually perform three stretchings of two minutes each separated by one minute of rest. Simultaneous massage of the muscle fascicle under treatment may often be beneficial. It is preferable to raise both legs of the patient while he remains flat on his back, with both feet maintained in maximal dorsiflexion. In certain cases, we prefer to use more lasting maneuvers which are progressively accentuated. One often notes during these stretchings of the tender muscle fascicles that the patient perceives a burning sensation which subsides when the stretching is maintained.

Three or four sessions of this kind are usually sufficient in the majority of cases. However, if irritation of the nerve persists and particularly if the discogenic disturbance has not been reduced, it is obvious that these maneuvers cannot be tolerated. Instead of helping the patient, his pain will be awakened and exacerbated. This maneuver should therefore be carried out with a great delicacy and may serve as a test for evaluating if root irritability is present and if so, the maneuver should be discontinued.

Other physiotherapeutic procedures may also be used. For

example, one may apply pressures over the painful area exerted by the thumb, heel of the hand, or elbow. It is in the gluteal region that these maneuvers are most effective.

We have stressed for a long time the value of slow and lasting petrissage of the painful gluteus muscles at the point of maximum pain. Pressure maintained ten to fifteen seconds, with an interval of five to seven seconds and repeated ten times is often the treatment of choice while in other cases, one may sustain pressure for two to three minutes. The correct choice of one of these two methods is a result of personal experience and one should judge the situation in terms of the muscle reaction to pressure. Once more, these treatments should be very delicate and if poorly conducted, one may irritate the tissues instead of relieving the patient.

What do these localized pseudocontractures represent? The muscular localization of the pain of radicular origin may be surprising. Yet, the presence of cramps or fasciculations have been known to be a part of the clinical picture of certain sciaticas, thus expressing irritation of the ventral root. Are these partial hardenings of the muscles of the same origin and nature as a cramp? This seems to be probable because of the following observations:

1. Their coexistence is often observed.

2. Cramps often originate from these hardened muscle fascicles in certain cases of sciatica.

3. Treatment by stretching is analogous to that used in acute cramps.

The EMG tracings which we often recorded from such hardened and tender muscles did not show any particular pattern. This is why we hesitate to call these local hardenings muscle contracture. Frykholm (1951) stressed the importance of the involvement of the motor roots in the neuralgias. One may ask whether these findings lend anatomical support to this suggestion. This seems to be the case.

Are these intramuscular changes due to the response of the muscle fibers themselves or to the conjunctive tissue? One should keep in mind that these tender muscle fascicles often coexist with skin areas of cellulitis which express the trophic nature of these changes and which may be revealed by the skin-rolling technique. Whatever the case may be, lasting tenderness of certain muscle fascicles constitutes a particular aspect of certain sciaticas and therefore this myalgic sciatica should be identified as such. Etiles, 1948; Maigne, 1965, 1961, 1969; Putti, 1927; Ravault and Vignon, 1950; 1956; de Sèze, 1955; de Sèze and Ryckewaert, 1954; de Sèze and Welfling, 1957; Spurling, 1953; Troisier, 1959; Waghemacker, 1961; Walch, Nombouts, and Petit, 1949; Wilson and Ilfeld, 1952 have each discussed various aspects of sciatic pain and related subjects.

Chapter 31

Femoral Neuritis

T HE INCIDENCE of femoral neuritis is clearly not as high as that of sciatica. It is often related to irritation of L3 or L4 roots by a discal protrusion. It often starts after an effort. The pain, which is initially located in the low back, rapidly spreads to the anterior aspect of the thigh and knee. If L3 is involved, the pain will be localized at the anterior and medial aspects of the thigh and will not spread beyond the patella. If there is involvement of L4, it will spread over the anterior and lateral aspect of the thigh and then over the anterior and medial aspect of the lower leg down to the ankle (Fig. 189) . Examination will reveal (1) hyperesthesia of the L3 or L4 dermatomes; (2) absence of knee jerk (more often in the L4 involvements) ; (3) decrease of muscle strength of the quadriceps which may be hypotonic or even show local atrophy.

Lumbar examination reveals tenderness of L2-L3 or L3-L4 joints either by direct pressure over the spinal processes or still better by the examination described on p. 104. It also reveals lateral pressure over the spinal processes against resistance obtained by the pressure in the reverse sense of the adjacent spinal processes; tenderness of the supraspinous ligament; tender points at the level of the posterior joints on one side (in general, the same side as the neuritis, although not always) .

It is important, however, to keep in mind that the discal protrusion is not always responsible for femoral neuropathy. Even if one does not consider such things as tuberculosis, vertebral metastases, or neurinoma, the femoral nerve may be involved during its course by arthritis of the iliosacral joint or by appendicitis or colitis. At the level of the thigh it can be compressed by a hernia support or compressed by a node. There is also viral femoral neuritis. However, it is mostly diabetes which causes femoral neuritis.

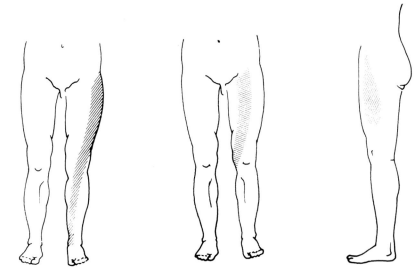

Figure 189. *Left* and *Center,* Femoral neuritis pain. Radiating pain. *Left,* L4; *Right,* Femoral meralgia. Area of pain (after de Sèze).

Manipulations carried out by the usual rules may be helpful and sometimes rapidly so when the neuralgia is due to vertebral and mechanical cause. They are affected in the same way as for sciatica and are associated with appropriate medication and bed rest. Just as in the case of sciatica, myalgic components, expressed by the presence of hardened fascicles in the quadriceps, are found. They are very localized in most cases in the lower segment of the rectus femoris which should be treated in the same way as mentioned in the preceding section.

Chapter 32

Paresthetic Meralgia

M ERALGIA IS characterized by paresthetic sensations at the anterolateral aspect of the thigh with an area having the form of a tennis racket and corresponding to the distribution of the femorocutaneous nerve (Fig. 189, right). It is nearly always unilateral. The patient complains of numbness, dead skin, crawling, pins and needles sensation. The skin is hypersensitive and even contact with clothing is very disagreeable. In most cases these sensations are elicited by prolonged ambulation or standing and are relieved by rest.

Meralgia is not as rare as it is usually considered to be. We have observed it very frequently. However, when it is mild or intermittent, the patient is affected only slightly. Inasmuch as most therapeutic attempts are ineffectual, the patient accepts his trouble and does not consult a physician any further about it.

We have often found, during systematic examination of patients who come for another painful condition, an area of hyperesthesia at the lateral aspect of the thigh. It is then that the patient usually states that he has had difficulty for five to twenty years and that it occurs in episodes separated by periods of silence when even a prolonged walk does not affect him. This is not the case in severe forms associated with a permanent disagreeable sensation which brings the patient to a physician.

Paresthetic meralgia was described by Roth (1895) who found it in German calvary men who wore tight supports which compressed the initial segment of the femoral cutaneous nerve at the level of the ilio-inguinal angle below the anterior and superior spine of the iliac bone. The cause cited for this condition, which is frequently quoted, is an irritation of the nerve by the microtraumas (carrying too heavy a load which compresses the thigh, hernia supports, etc.). In rare cases, one can see a symptomatic meralgia (corresponding to abscess or tumor). However, in most

313

cases, the examination is negative and the cause of meralgia remains unknown.

Good results may be obtained by vertebral manipulations (in about 50 percent of the cases) which suggest that at least in these cases, the etiology is vertebral. This should be suspected when a segmental examination reveals tenderness of the L1-L2 space associated with cellulitis on the same side.

Chapter 33

Coccygeal Pain

COCCYGEAL PAIN is very resistant to treatment. Massage of the muscle levetor ani and infiltrating injections are not always successful.

If the coccygeal pain occurs after a fall or following delivery, it is practically always relieved by the maneuver which is described below. Those which do not seem to follow trauma may disappear following a lumbo-sacral manipulation. However, in general "essential" coccygeal pain representing about ten per cent of cases is not relieved by this maneuver.

MANIPULATIONS

The patient is put on his knees in a genuflected position. The physician introduces his index finger into the rectum and applies the palmar aspect of the finger against the coccyx without exerting any pull. At that moment the patient is asked to lie down in a prone position. With his free hand, the physician exerts pressure over the sacrum and while he maintains this pressure for 40-50 seconds, pressing with all his weight on the sacrum, the internal finger applies pressure on the inferior tip of the sacrum simply maintaining the coccyx in hyperextension (Fig. 190B). This personal technique differs from the osteopathic technique as shown in Figure 190A.

The maneuver is then terminated. If pressure is then applied over the coccyx, one finds that it is no longer tender and the patient may sit down with ease. Sometimes it is advisable to repeat this maneuver two or three times in order to secure complete success. Renoult (1962) believes that coccygeal pain results from the sacroiliac strain.

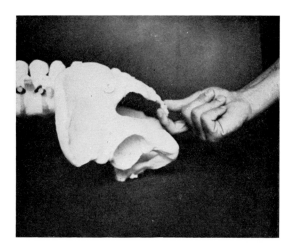

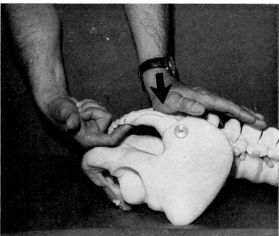

Figure 190. *Upper,* osteopathic technique; *Lower,* personal technique (see text).

PART IV

TECHNIQUES

Introduction

W E WILL DESCRIBE only the techniques which we use most frequently. There are others which are simple variants of those described, although some are quite different from them. Indeed, this book does not summarize all possible manipulative therapy, and there are certain techniques which are very difficult to describe even with the aid of photographs. In addition, as clear and precise as the description may be, it is impossible to completely explain a manipulation. Everything counts in this method and particularly what the physician himself perceives as he manipulates. An incorrect starting position of the patient or of the operator, a gesture of only limited amplitude, a poor stabilization —and the manipulation becomes impossible, ineffective, and painful (Beal and Beckwith, 1963). Thus, the physician should have a sense of movement, a sense of the precise instant when the gesture should be forced. This is a question of personal talent and particularly of long training.

Good manipulators are rare. They must spend a great deal of time before they become good. However, if a physician who is interested in these techniques is willing to follow the directives which we try to formulate, he should remember that manipulation is not a question of strength. No brutal maneuver, even if one disregards the momentary pain which is inflicted upon the patient, will ever be equal in efficacy to a delicate maneuver which is "performed by itself" because the execution is correct and the coordinates have been well chosen.

Note—In the illustrations and photographs of the techniques, direction of the movement is indicated by the arrow and the stabilized points, by a cross.

Chapter 34

Cervical Spine

MANEUVERS OF DECONTRACTION

Following are some examples of maneuvers of decontraction:

1. The patient is supine. The operator is standing at his left as in the given example (Fig. 191). With his left hand he stabilizes the right shoulder of the patient while with the tip of his right fingers he hooks the lateral mass of the neck. His left hand continues to stabilize the shoulder while he pulls the muscles of the neck toward him and then releases them by a slow, rhythmic and elastic movement.

2. The patient is supine. The operator is standing or sitting at his head (Fig. 192). With the tips of the fingers of both hands, the operator effectuates deep massage (petrissage) of the infraoccipital muscles. This maneuver is very relaxing and sedative.

3. The patient is supine. The operator, standing at his head, his hands placed at each side of the patient's neck, hooks, with the tips of his fingers, the lateral muscle groups and applies petrissage in alternation, first on one side and then on the other, pulling

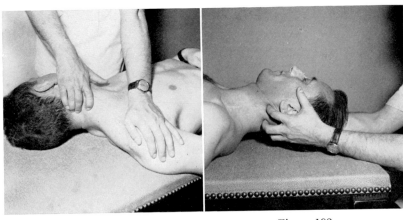

Figure 191.   Figure 192.

these muscles toward him as if he wanted to slowly separate them from the spine and then rhythmically releases them first on one side, then the other (Fig. 193).

4. The patient is seated on a stool, facing a table which supports him. His elbows are apart, forehead resting on his hands. This position permits an excellent relaxation of the infra-occipital and paravertebral muscles (Fig. 194).

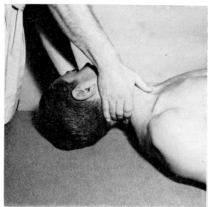 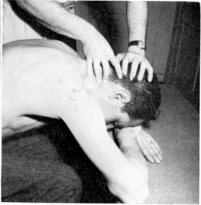

Figure 193.   Figure 194.

MOBILIZATIONS

Mobilizations can be done in traction, rotation, flexion, extension, and lateral bending.

MANUAL TRACTION

This is a very useful maneuver which is commonly employed. The head may be placed in one of two ways (Fig. 195).

In the first position (Fig. 195, left) the operator holds the head with his hands placed on each side of the base of the occiput. (It is on the basis of this maneuver that we developed an apparatus for cervical traction which does not hook the chin.) In the second position (Fig. 195, right) imitating the Sayres' apparatus, the physician immobilized the chin with one hand and places the other under the occiput. The first procedure is easier to perform for a manual traction of an extended neck. The second one is easier to perform over the neck in flexion.

The operator pulls the head slowly, steadily, progressively, and firmly toward himself, holds this traction for about ten seconds, then releases it and repeats the sequence about ten times. In order to do it well, he should use the weight of his body, and with the arms stretched, lets himself fall backwards rather than using the strength of his arms.

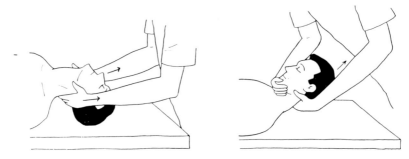

Figure 195.

In Rotation

1. *Patient in a supine position (Fig. 196).* For mobilization in left rotation, the physician holds the patient's head with his left

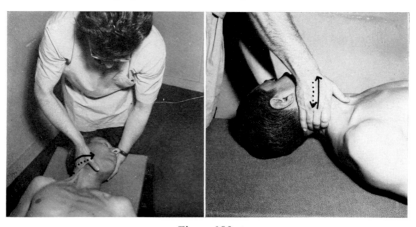

Figure 196.

hand, placing his hand at the left occipitomaxillary region. With his right fingers flat against the neck of the subject, he rotates the spine to the left, reaches the maximum of possible movement, maintains his pressure for a few seconds, then releases and repeats the sequence with a slow, rhythmic, and elastic movement.

2. *Patient in sitting position (Fig. 197).* For mobilization in left rotation, the physician passes his left forearm in front of the patient, and with his left hand grasping the right side of the patient's neck, rotates the latter to the left while his right hand, placed against the left side of the neck, applies pressure in such a way as to aid the rotation. This movement is repeated insistently, progressively, and slowly.

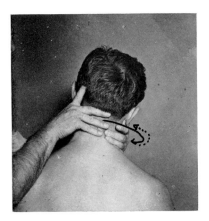

Figure 197.

In Flexion

1. *Patient in a supine position (Fig. 198).* The physician is standing at the head of the table but slightly to the side. With his left hand, he stabilizes the upper part of the anterior aspect of the thorax while his right hand, holding the occiput, pushes the head slowly forward, maintains his pressure, releases, then starts again slowly.

2. Another maneuver (Fig. 199) aims at the upper cervical spine and more particularly at the occipito-atloid joint:

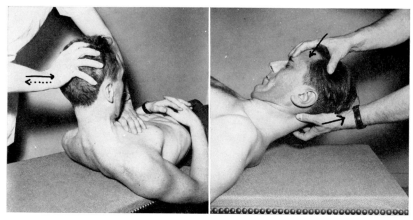

Figure 198.   Figure 199.

The patient is supine. The physician, standing at his head, grasps with his thumb on one side and the tips of the third, fourth, and fifth fingers on the other, the base of the occiput, while with the other hand, he stabilizes the forehead.

With his occipital hand, the physician pulls toward himself; with his frontal hand he pushes downwards toward the patient's feet, this bringing the head in hyperflexion. This movement, as always, is slow, rhythmic, and repeated.

3. *The patient is supine* (Fig. 200). The operator crosses his forearms behind the neck of the patient and stabilizes the sub-

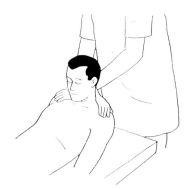

Figure 200.

ject's shoulders with his hand. With light alternating movements of flexion and extension of the wrists, using these levers, he pushes the neck in flexion and then releases it. This is a powerful maneuver to be performed very slowly and with extreme caution. It is necessary of course, to repeat it several times.

In Extension

1. *The patient is sitting on a table* with his legs hanging down. The physician standing and facing the patient places the patient's forehead against his chest. He places the balls of the fingertips on either side of the back of the neck and applies pressure. He then leans slightly backward, pulling the patient forward and upward. This maneuver induces an extension of the patient's cervical column which is well controlled by the hands of the physician. Simultaneously, the doctor accomplishes petrissage of the neck. (Fig. 201). If the left temporofrontal region rather than the forehead of the patient is against the chest of the physician, then the maneuver becomes a combined movement of extension, right lateral flexion, and right rotation. (Fig. 202).

2. *The patient is in a supine position.* The physician, standing at the side of the patient at the level of his shoulder, places his forearm (left in the picture) under the neck of the patient with his hand flat on the table. With his right hand he pushes down

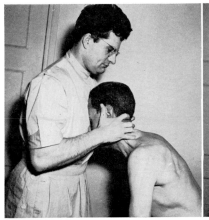 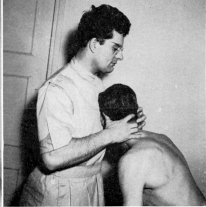

Figure 201.   Figure 202.

on the forehead; this hand remains immobile in order to exercise counterpressure (Fig. 203).

The physician then cups his left hand against the table and slowly lifts his elbow, and to a lesser degree his wrist. This moves the cervical column of the patient in extension, which is maintained for a moment, then released. This maneuver is repeated several times.

If during the preceding maneuver, the patient's head is bent to one side and the doctor's counterpressure is applied to the temporal region, the resulting mobilization will become a combined extension and lateral flexion.

In Lateroflexion

The patient is in a supine position. The physician is standing at the side toward which a lateroflexion is to be directed (left side in the picture) (Fig. 204). He exercises counterpressure with

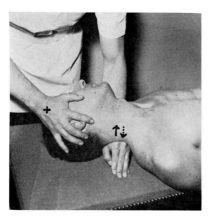

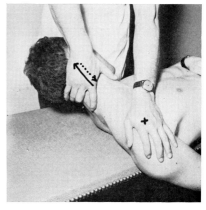

Figure 203.   Figure 204.

his left hand against the patient's left shoulder while his right hand grasps the right occipitomastoid region. It is the pulling of the neck toward him that accomplishes left lateroflexion of the cervical spine.

He pulls slowly toward him, maintains the traction for a while, then releases it by a slow, elastic, firm, supple, repeated, and rhythmic movement. He may add a movement of rotation to this movement of lateroflexion by pronating his right hand while pulling the neck toward him.

MANIPULATIONS

The neck is undoubtedly the region where it is easiest to elicit a cracking sound by any forced movement. However, the only common elements between movements associated with cracking sounds performed in a haphazard manner and rational manipulation are the appearance and the sound. It is precisely the ease with which the neck may be mobilized that makes it difficult to perform a correct manipulation. Yet, most frequently, the lack of success of manipulations at the level of the cervical column is due to the fact that the operator is content to perform a rotation in any direction and being pleased with the ease with which he elicits the cracking sound, discontinues the treatment. Performed in this fashion, twenty sessions may be carried out without achieving the benefit of one well-planned correctly applied maneuver.

The head of the patient in supine position is grasped with both hands (Fig. 205), the neck being in an intermediate position between flexion and extension. If the physician then rotates the cervical spine to the left or to the right, most of the movement takes place at the midcervical region (Fig. 206). If the same

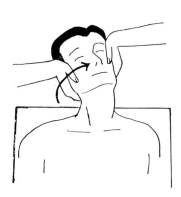

Figure 205.

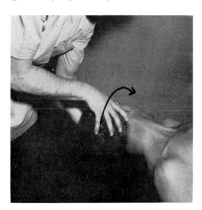

Figure 206.

maneuver is carried out with the cervical spine in flexion most of the movement will take place at a lower level (Fig. 207).

On the contrary, in a case of the neck in extension most of the movement will take place at the higher level and it is there that the cracking sound will be produced. (Fig. 208). This, therefore, permits one to localize the manipulation in rotation. However, the precision of the manipulation carried out in this fashion is only relative. This is why most of the cervical manipulations, in order to be elective and effective, should be performed according to the technique of *assisted* manipulations.

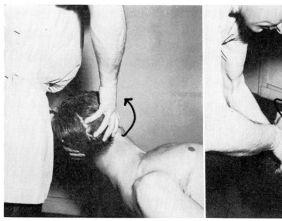
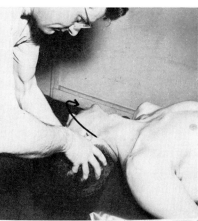

Figure 207.   Figure 208.

High Cervical Column

In Rotation: Patient Lying Down

SPINE IN EXTENSION (Figs. 209, 210, and 211). *Left rotation.* The patient is in a supine position. The physician standing at his head supports with his left hand the head of the patient placed in left rotation while pressing the lateral edge of the axis with the radial border of his right index finger. He then brings the higher level of the cervical spine to the maximum of rotation and extension, taking up the slack. This being accomplished, the physician will execute manipulation by exercising a brisk pressure with the

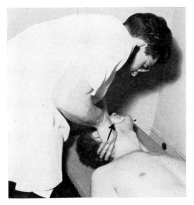

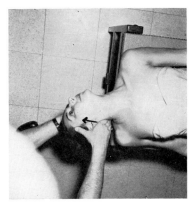

Figure 209. Left rotation in extension.

Figure 210. The same manipulation viewed at a slightly different angle.

right index finger forward and to the left in the direction of the movement. Such a maneuver will be associated of course with the habitual cracking sound. In the last phase of the maneuver, the left hand only supports the head of the patient in the proper position in an absolutely passive fashion.

SPINE IN FLEXION (Fig. 212). The same manipulation is performed here on the spine in flexion (still in a case of left rotation). Here again, the left hand supports the head placed in the correct position. The maneuver is carried out as above.

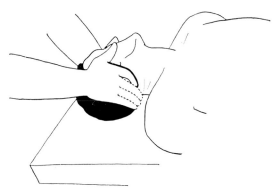

Figure 211. It is with the radial border of the index finger that the manipulation is performed.

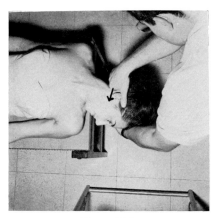

Figure 212.

Again, it is carried out with the radial border of the index finger after the slack has been taken up. The brisk and sharp movement of this finger produces the manipulation. Note in the picture the direction of the manipulating force toward the mouth of the patient.

SPINE IN LATEROFLEXION (Fig. 213). *Right rotation on a spine placed in left lateroflexion.*

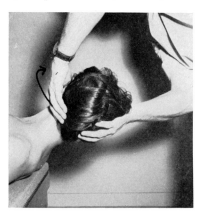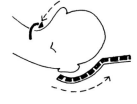

Figure 213 and Figure 214. Position of the hands. The force which they apply and maintain for the preparation and accomplishment of maneuvers is in lateral flexion. In the diagram movement of manipulation in rotation is represented by the solid line arrow.

The patient lies in a supine position with his head extending beyond the edge of the table. The right hand of the physician supports the head, while the lateral border of the left index finger presses against the lateral edge of the axis. The physician moves the spine in right rotation while he simultaneously bends the head to the left (moving his right hand upward as indicated by the broken arrow in Fig. 214) and moves his left hand (as indicated by the broken arrow in Fig. 214). By firmly maintaining this position, the physician takes up the slack in right rotation. Then by a brisk pressure of the left index finger he exaggerates the movement of rotation, thus performing the manipulation.

Right rotation on a spine in right lateroflexion (Fig. 215). The position of the head is the same as for the preceding manipulation. However, after positioning in right rotation, the physician will move the head in right lateroflexion. In order to do this, he performs a traction downward with his right hand (indicated by the corresponding arrow in Fig. 216) while he pushes upward with his left hand. The physician firmly maintains this position, then accentuates right rotation during the phase of taking up the slack and then, finally, effects the manipulation by a brisk pressure to the right with his index finger. The success of these

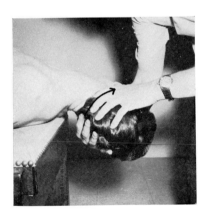 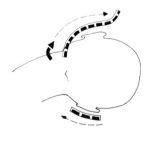

Figure 215 and Figure 216. Position of the hands. The force which they must apply and maintain for the preparation and execution of the maneuvers in lateral flexion. In the diagram, movement of manipulation in rotation is indicated by the solid line arrow.

maneuvers depends primarily upon the correct accomplishment of the positioning and of the taking up of the slack.

In Lateroflexion

EXAMPLE OF A RIGHT LATEROFLEXION. The preparation of this manipulation is done in the same way as for the one just described, but in contradistinction to the latter, the manipulation is performed in lateroflexion on the spine in rotation rather than in rotation of the spine in lateroflexion. The spine is placed in a position of complete left rotation, then is laterally flexed to the right. The thrust of the manipulative movement is directed straight downward with the pisiform of the hand of the physician. Figures (217 and 218) show the preparation. Figures 219 and 220 illustrate the maneuver, and the arrow shows the direction of the thrust. The heavy broken line in the drawing shows the position of the physician's left hand, the thin broken arrow represents the force applied by this hand in order to bring the spine into right lateral flexion. The solid arrow indicates the direction of the manipulating thrust.

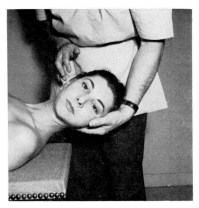
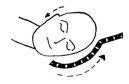

Figure 217 and Figure 218. Preparation.

In Rotation: Technique of the Immobilized Head

SPINE IN EXTENSION (Fig. 221). This technique permits one to effectuate elective and powerful maneuvers over the high

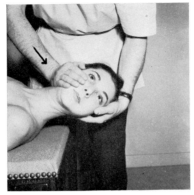 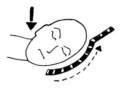

Figure 219 and Figure 220. Manipulation exaggerating the movement of lateroflexion.

cervical spine. The patient is supine. The physician immobilizes the head against his chest and grips with his left hand (in order to perform a left rotation) the chin of the patient as if he were dealing with a ball of Rugby. He turns the head in a maximal left rotation, then exercises pressure with the radial border of the first phalanx of his right index finger against the spine at the desired level. Then, still maintaining the rotation, the physician places the head in the desired degree of extension and performs the manipulation by a brief limited movement of his chest, synchronized with a sharp thrust with his right index finger to the left. One cannot overstress that the maneuver is extremely powerful and should not be attempted by an inexperienced operator.

SPINE IN FLEXION (Fig. 222). The maneuver is the same as the preceding one, but instead of placing the head in hyperextension the physician moves it in hyperflexion.

SPINE IN LATEROFLEXION (Figs. 223 and 224). Figure 223 shows the patient lying on his left side, the head being laterally flexed and directed upward, the manipulating thrust being vertical and exaggerating the lateral flexion.

In Figure 224 the patient is supine. The lateral flexion, which is poorly seen in this picture, takes place high on the cervical spine near the Atlanto-occipital Articulation. In the illustrated example, the operator directs the thrust in right rotation.

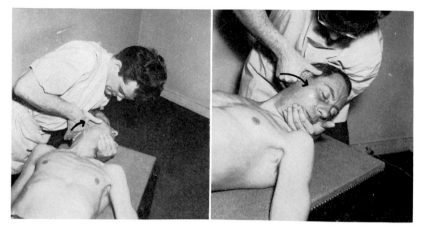

Figure 221.   Figure 222.

Note: It is well understood that other combinations are possible. For instance, the physician may, after positioning the head in extension (Figure 221), add a lateral flexion and perform the manipulation in rotation. He may, to give another example, position the head in extension and left rotation and manipulate it in right lateral flexion.

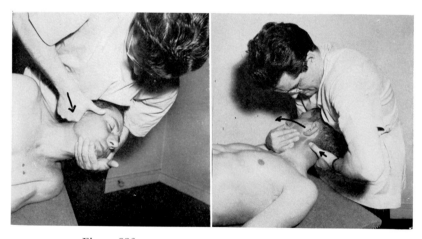

Figure 223.   Figure 224.

Rotation: Technique for a Patient in Sitting Position.

SPINE IN FLEXION (Fig. 225). The patient is in a sitting position, his legs hanging down. The physician stands behind him slightly to the side towards which he desires to rotate the head (right side in this picture). He places his right forearm in front of the neck under the chin and exerts pressure with his curved right index finger at the level of the right intervertebral point to be manipulated, while his left hand, grasping the right parietal region, applies counterpressure and places the head in the desired degree of flexion. He moves the head in right rotation. After taking up the slack and when the good positioning of the spine is secured, he applies a sharp thrust with his index finger, pulling the neck toward him, and imparts to it a slight movement of rotation. This will achieve the manipulation at the level of which the index finger is located.

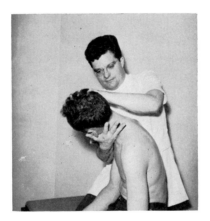

Figure 225.

SPINE IN EXTENSION (Fig. 226). The same maneuver may be carried out on a spine in extension; the preparation and the execution are the same, but the direction of the traction of the manipulating finger is changed.

Note: It is possible, obviously, to add lateroflexion to a manipulation in flexion or in extension.

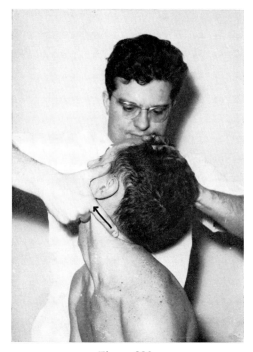

Figure 226.

Middle and Low Cervical Spine
In Rotation with the Patient Lying Down

EXAMPLE OF RIGHT ROTATION. The patient is supine, the physician standing at the head of the table. He supports the head of the patient with his left hand and exerts a counterpressure to the force which he applies with the radial border of his right index finger which is placed against the joint to be manipulated (Fig. 227). Then he positions the head, for example in extension and left rotation, before taking up the slack in left rotation. A sudden thrust with the right index finger will locally exaggerate this movement which constitutes the manipulation. This manipulation in rotation may be accomplished at any level of the cervical spine placed either in flexion or extension. The physician may also add a certain degree of lateral flexion as the manipulated joint has to occupy the summit of the curve.

Figure 228 shows this maneuver applied to the lower cervical spine in flexion. Note the position of the left hand of the physician who places and supports the head in a fashion needed for the maneuver. The taking up of the slack being effected, this hand will remain immobile while the right index finger alone achieves the manipulation. Analogous maneuvers may be effected in extension.

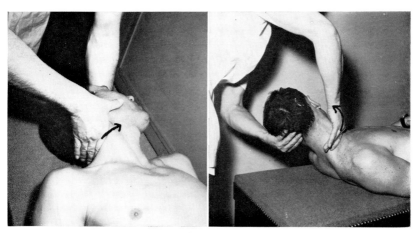

Figure 227.　　　　　　　　　Figure 228.

Rotation with Patient in a Sitting Position

Spine in Extension. The patient is in a sitting position with his legs hanging down. The physician is at the side toward which the rotation is to be effected; in this case, the right side (Fig. 229).

The physician, with his right hand in front of the neck of the patient places his right index finger against the transverse process of the vertebrae which is to be manipulated, while his left hand exerts pressure over the right frontoparietal region, and brings the head and the spine to the desired degree of extension as he moves the neck in maximum right rotation. After taking up the slack, it is with the curved index finger that the physician effects a sudden thrust to the right and forward, thus exaggerating locally the movement of right rotation. This constitutes the manipulation.

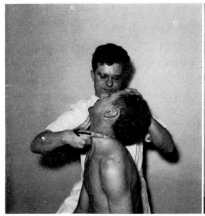

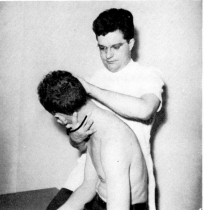

Figure 229.   Figure 230.

Figure 231 shows the same maneuver applied to the lower cervical spine.

SPINE IN FLEXION. The same type of maneuver by the operator using only his index finger for the high cervical spine. It is easier to use other fingers at other levels of the spine; for example, the third one for the middle cervical spine (Fig. 230) and the ulnar border of the little finger for the low cervical spine (Fig. 232).

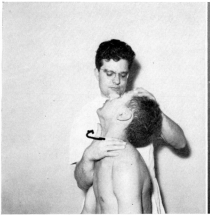

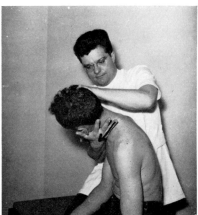

Figure 231.   Figure 232.

A VARIANT. This is a personal technique which is related to those of the preceding page. The physician places his active hand behind the neck of the patient instead of placing it in front of it, the curved active finger (index or third finger usually) being applied to the joint to be manipulated (Figure 233, the left index finger effecting right rotation).

The right hand exerts pressure on the left side of the forehead of the patient or else grips his chin. It is with this hand that the physician positions and takes up the slack in the illustrated fashion. Finally, it briskly exaggerates the movement of rotation assisted by a synchronized pressure with the left index finger (Fig. 234).

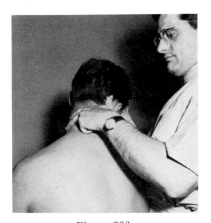

Figure 233.

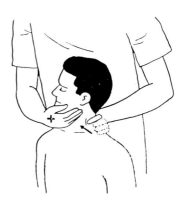

Figure 234.

OPPOSED MANIPULATION. The physician stands behind the patient (Fig. 235) in order to achieve a manipulation in right rotation. For example, he exerts pressure with his right thumb against the spinal process of the vertebrae located just below the segment to be manipulated, while with his left hand he grasps the top of the patient's head. He rotates the head and the cervical spine to the right. The right thumb exerts a counterpressure below the joint to be manipulated while the physician, after taking up the slack, briskly exaggerates the movement of rotation of the head with his left hand. This is an "opposed manipulation."

Low Cervical Spine

The patient is in a sitting position with the physician standing behind him. The example is a manipulation in right lateroflexion (Fig. 236).

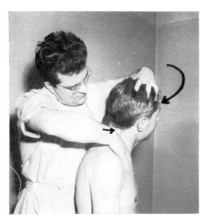

Figure 235.

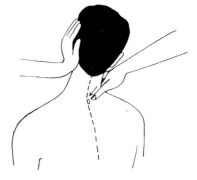

Figure 236.

The physician with his left hand exerts pressure against the left parietal region of the patient, moving his neck in right lateroflexion. He pinches, with his right thumb and index finger, the right part of the vertebrae located just below the joint to be manipulated. The operator takes up the slack and with a brisk thrust of his right hand effects the manipulation, the left hand remaining strictly immobile.

This useful technique may be applied from C5 to D3. It is very useful in treating cervicobrachial pain and the scapulohumeral periarthritis.

Chapter 35

Cervicodorsal Junction

CERVICODORSAL junction, i.e. the junction between the two last cervical and the higher dorsal vertebrae, constitutes a region which is considered a difficult one by those who practice manipulation because "it is more difficult to elicit cracking sounds in this area." In fact, as we have said previously, a precise manipulation is more delicate in the regions where the cracking sounds are easy to elicit. We believe that the cervico dorsal region is the easiest one for the average operator.

MANEUVERS OF DECONTRACTIONS
Patient in Sitting Position (Fig. 237)

The patient is sitting on a stool with his head resting on his crossed forearms placed on the edge of a table. This is an excellent position for a decontraction maneuver which is so useful in this region. This maneuver is effected with the thumbs by performing a deep petrissage of the muscles, effecting simultaneously a kind of traction directed from the midline upward and sideways.

The same maneuver may be effected with the patient in a prone position.

Patient in a Supine Position (Fig. 238)

The physician stands on the opposite side of the side to be treated. With the hand nearest the head of the patient, he grips the lower part of the mass of the lateral muscles of the neck, pulls it towards him, then releases it by a slow, repeated, rhythmic, elastic movement, while the other hand exerts a counterpressure over the shoulder.

MOBILIZATIONS
In Flexion

The patient is resting on his elbows in a prone position (Fig. 239) . The physician exerts pressure with one hand over the upper dorsal region and with the other over the occiput. He performs a slowly alternating movement of slight pressure and release over the occiput, then does just the opposite: he maintains a constant pressure over the occiput and exerts the alternating movement of intermittent pressure over the high dorsal spine, thus mobilizing flexion of the cervico dorsal junction.

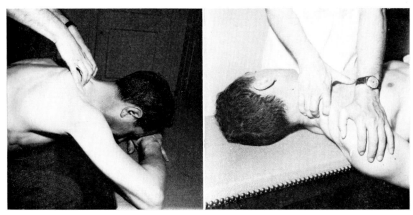

Figure 237.   Figure 238.

In Rotation, Extension and Lateroflexion

The patient lies on his right side and the operator stands facing him (Fig. 240). With his left hand the physician supports

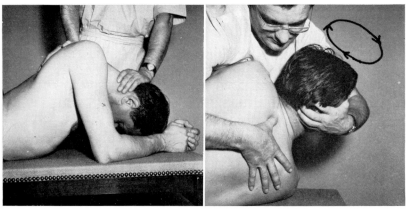

Figure 239.   Figure 240.

the head while he holds the patient's left shoulder under his arm. He then imparts to the cervicodorsal spine, mobilization in circumduction, with lateroflexion or with extension, or with flexion. With his right thumb he controls and thus localizes the movement. Obviously, the mobilization is slow, supple, continuous and gentle. This technique may be used for a maneuver of manipulation (see below).

MANIPULATION

In Lateroflexion

The patient is in a sitting position with the physician standing behind him (Fig. 241) (personal technique). The figure depicts the maneuver in left lateral flexion. The physician immobilizes the head of the patient by his hand and forearm (see Figs. 241 and 242). The left thumb exerts pressure over the lateral part of the spine at the level of the neck-shoulder angle. With his right hand the operator slowly bends the neck forward and to the left to a point where he feels that the movement is performed at the level of the cervicodorsal junction. After being sure of the correct position of the thumb, the physician makes a brisk thrust with his thumb along the line which bisects the neck-shoulder angle and thus performs the manipulation.

This manipulation is very powerful; it has to be performed

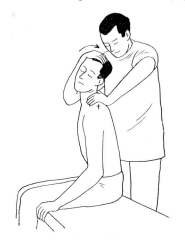

Figure 241.

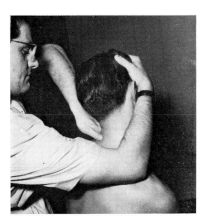

Figure 242.

with a great deal of restraint. It must be perfect in order not to cause pain. Its success obviously depends upon the precise localization of the pressure.

This technique permits one to act upon the levels C5-D3.

In Lateroflexion and Rotation

PATIENT IN A PRONE POSITION (Fig. 243). The physician is standing at the head of the patient. With his right thumb (left lateroflexion) he exerts pressure on the transverse process of the first or second vertebrae, while with his left hand applied to the right temporomaxillar region, he moves the head and the neck in left lateroflexion. The right thumb exerts counterpressure. With his left hand, the physician pulls the neck toward him, bent to the left and placed in slight right rotation. After taking up the slack, he exaggerates the pressure either in rotation or in lateroflexion, the chin serving as a pivot. This completes the manipulation.

First Variant. In contradistinction to the above, the left hand of the operator is immobilized until the slack has been taken up. It is a brisk thrust of the thumb downward and forward (in relation to the operator) which performs the manipulation.

Second Variant. The head of the patient extends beyond the table. The left hand of the operator grasps the chin and the right side of the maxilla while the right hand localizes and assists the manipulation which is performed by a brisk exaggeration of the pressure exerted by the left hand (Fig. 244).

PATIENT IN A SIDE-LYING POSITION. The technique about to be described permits one to manipulate in all possible combinations of flexion, extension, rotation, and right or left lateroflexion. It is particularly useful for the cases of cervicobrachial neuritis:

1. *Combined lateroflexion and rotation in the same direction exerted upon the spine in flexion.* (Fig. 246). We will give an example of left lateral flexion. The patient is lying on his right side. The physician is standing facing the patient. With his left hand the physician maintains the head of the patient at the level of the temporomaxillar region, while he firmly holds the left shoulder of the patient under his right arm and exerts pressure

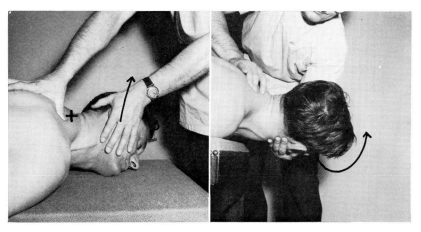

Figure 243.   Figure 244.

with his right thumb upon the left edge of the spinal process of
D2, D1, or C7, whatever the case may be. The left hand, which
supports the head, moves the neck in left lateral flexion, then
rotates it to the left. The physician changes slightly the degree of
bending to the point where he feels the angulation to be made
just at the level of the manipulated joint which becomes in this
position the point of least resistance. He takes up the slack with
the left hand and gives an additional brisk thrust while he exerts

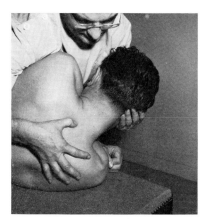

Figure 245. Initial Position: Left lateroflexion upon spine in flexion.

pressure over the spinal process downward, thus exaggerating the left rotation of the vertebrae.

2. *Lateroflexion and rotation in the opposite direction with the spine in flexion.* (Fig. 247). The patient is in the same position as for the preceding maneuver. The physician moves the head

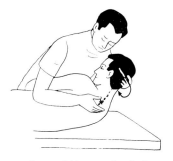

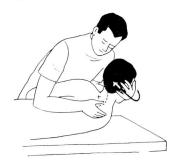

Figure 246. Manipulation of left rotation. The thumb assists the movement.

Figure 247. Manipulation of right rotation. The thumb opposes the movement.

of the neck in left lateroflexion, then he adds the movement in right rotation. The right thumb, then, does not have to assist the movement, but on the contrary, should maintain a firm pressure directed downward. It is by brisk exaggeration of both lateroflexion and rotation that the left hand performs the manipulation upon the joint located just below the point of counterpressure.

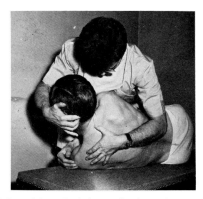

Figure 248. Initial position: Left lateroflexion of the spine in extension.

3. *Lateroflexion and rotation in opposite direction upon the spine in extension* (Fig. 249). Positions of the patient and physician are the same as above.

The physician, with his left hand moves the cervical spine in maximal extension, then he moves it in left lateroflexion and right rotation which produces a kind of screwing motion of the cervical spine, which is immobilized by this maneuver. A brisk exaggeration of the movement in lateroflexion and rotation effected by the left hand mobilizes the joint located just below the vertebra pressed by the thumb.

4. *Lateroflexion and rotation in the same direction upon the spine in extension* (Fig. 250). After placing the cervical spine in complete extension, the physician rotates it and moves it in left lateral flexion. He exaggerates the rotation of the vertebra upon which he exerts the pressure when he feels that the latter becomes the point of least resistance, thus completing the manipulation. The physician assists the movement with his right thumb pressing downward.

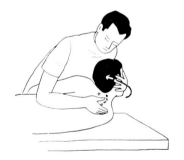 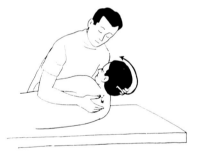

Figure 249. Manipulation in right rotation. Thumb opposes the movement.

Figure 250. Manipulation in left rotation. Thumb assists the movement.

Chapter 36

Dorsal Spine

MANEUVERS OF DECONTRACTION

1. The patient is in a prone position with his head turned to the side opposite the one to be treated.

The physician stands on the opposite side of the side to be treated, applying his hands to the paravertebral region, the fingers being well separated and thumbs touching each other, being placed along a parallel line to that of the spinal processes (Fig. 251).

With a "rod" made of both thenar eminences and the thumbs, the operator produces a slow traction of the mass of paravertebral muscles as if he wanted to separate it from the spinal processes as well as from the deeper structures. When the traction is at a maximum, the physician ceases the movement for a while and slightly exaggerates the pressure, then releases it. This maneuver must be quite rhythmic and continuous without losing contact even during periods of relaxation. Under such conditions, this movement is very sedative and quite helpful in both acute and chronic back pain.

2. The patient is in a side-lying position, the upper arm against his side. The physician stands facing him with his hand near the head of the patient gripping the mass of the paravertebral muscles at the root of the spinal processes, while, with the other hand introduced under the arm of the patient, he performs the same gripping maneuver below the area held by the right hand. The physician should pull the muscles toward him, separating his hands slightly, then release this traction. This movement should be performed slowly, rhythmically, continually, regularly, and elastically (Fig. 252).

3. The patient and the physician remain in the same position. The physician hooks the medial border of the scapula with the tips of his fingers and moves both scapula and shoulder in a slow

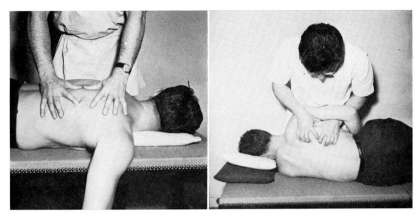

Figure 251.   Figure 252.

circumduction pulling them at times toward the head (Figs. 253 and 254), at times toward the legs while exercising a deep petrisage of the muscles. During these maneuvers, the upper arm of the patient rests at times upon one arm of the physician and at other times over the other arm (Fig. 255).

MOBILIZATIONS
Extension

The mobilizations in extension at the level of the dorsal spine, just as those in rotation, are particularly helpful. There are many

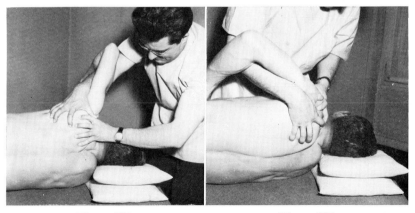

Figure 253.   Figure 254.

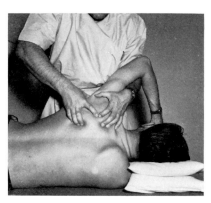

Figure 255.

techniques for these movements. Here are a few which we have used frequently:

1. *The upper dorsal spine* (Fig. 256). The patient is sitting on the table with his forearms crossed in front of his forehead. The physician, standing, faces him and introduces his arms under the forearms of the patient, placing his hands over the regions to be mobilized. With his hands he pulls toward him by slightly elevating his elbows and takes a short step backward. Thus a lever is formed, acting upon the upper dorsal spine which is mobilized in extension. Then the physician releases his pull by advancing a short step and lowering his elbows, only to repeat the movement several times slowly and elastically (Fig. 257). (The physician

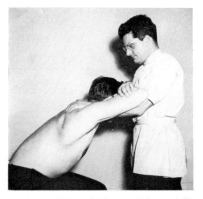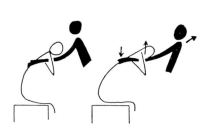

Figure 256 and Figure 257. Mobilization in extension high dorsal spine.

may, pulling to the right or left, mobilize the patient in a combined extension and lateral flexion.)

2. *Middle and lower regions of the dorsal spine* (Fig. 258). The following technique is excellent: The patient is sitting on a table with his feet resting on the bar of a stool and his arms projected forward. The physician is at his side with one foot on the stool, his forearm sustaining the outstretched arms of the patient. The physician rests his forearm on his knee and with the other hand exerts pressure on the dorsal region to be mobilized. While he accentuates this pressure, he moves his knee laterally, thus effecting a traction of the dorsal spine in extension. Then he releases it and thus effects a series of slow, alternating, rhythmic, elastic movements (Fig. 259).

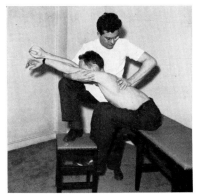

Figure 258.

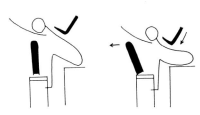

Figure 259.

3. *Other techniques.* Here are other techniques equally useful and effective:

a) The patient straddling the table bends slightly forward and holds the edges of the table with his stretched hands. The physician, behind him, with his extended arm, applies his hand on the region to be mobilized, imparting an alternating pressure by a slow and elastic repeated movements (Fig. 260).

b) This is a maneuver which resembles the one represented on the preceding page but which concerns particularly the mid-dorsal region. This time, it is the patient, who with his forearm crossed in front of his forehead, rests on the chest of the physician who stands facing him. The physician places his hands at either side of the region to be mobilized. In order to mobilize in extension, he pulls toward him, taking a short step backwards, then releases his pull by taking a short step forward; then repeats the movement smoothly (Fig. 261).

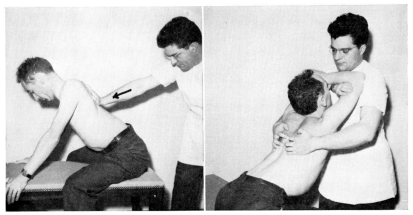

Figure 260.   Figure 261.

c) The patient sits on a stool facing a table on which he rests his elbows. The physician, behind him, exerts pressure combined with the lateral push. This is an excellent maneuver for scoliotic patients (Fig. 262).

d) The patient is in a prone position with his elbows resting on the table, supporting his chin in his hands. The physician exerts pressure over the dorsal region to be mobilized with one hand, while the other hand applies a counterpressure by gripping the belt of the patient. The movement is again slow and rhythmic (Fig. 263).

e) The patient is in a sitting position with his forearm crossed on his chest. The physician, behind him, immobilizes his chest by grasping his right arm (Fig. 264). He places his right elbow on his right thigh which permits him to exert a pressure with his right hand on the region to be mobilized in extension. By moving his thigh forward, the physician increases the pressure of his hand over the spine while he exerts counterpressure with his left forearm backwards, pulling the upper part of the chest.

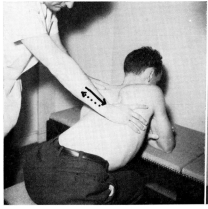

Figure 262.

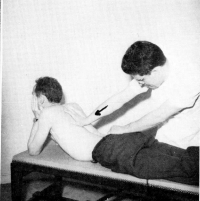

Figure 263.

In Rotation (Fig. 265)

The patient, with his hands clasped behind his neck, straddles the end of the table. The physician stands behind him slightly to the side toward which the rotation is directed (left side on the example illustrated in Fig. 265). With his left arm he grasps the right arm of the patient and pulls toward him, moving the chest

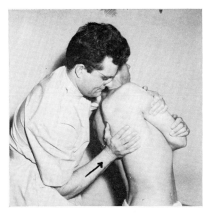

Figure 264.

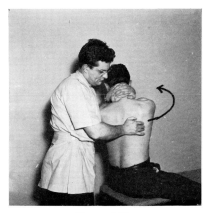

Figure 265.

in left rotation. With his right hand he helps this movement by exerting pressure on the area to be mobilized in the direction of rotation. This movement is, as always, slow, elastic, and repeated, the right forearm of the physician being perpendicular to the patient's back.

In Flexion (Fig. 266)

The patient, in a prone position, rests on his crossed arms with his head bent downward. One hand of the physician secures the anterior flexion of the head while the other exerts pressure according to a tangential direction toward the patient's feet.

In Lateroflexion (Fig. 267)

In right lateroflexion, the patient, with his arms crossed over his chest, straddles the end of the table. The physician, standing at his left, places his left arm under the left arm of the patient and grasps with his left hand the right shoulder of the patient. Using his left forearm as a lever, he lifts the left axilla of the patient while his left hand depresses his right shoulder. This produces lateroflexion of the dorsal spine at a level which varies according to the degree of the depression of the shoulder. With his right hand the physician controls or assists the movement.

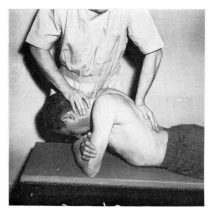

Figure 266.

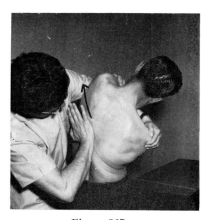

Figure 267.

MANIPULATIONS

The technique which we are going to describe below is certainly the one most commonly used by those who practice vertebral maneuvers. However, in the majority of cases it is incorrectly used as a standard maneuver which is able to easily elicit cracking sounds in the middle of the spine. In fact, this maneuver permits one, by changing the points of application, to effectuate helpful manipulations of the upper, middle and lower dorsal spine either in flexion or in extension. In addition, one may add a certain degree of lateral flexion and rotation during this maneuver, if necessary.

The patient is sitting on the table with his legs hanging and his hands clasped behind his neck. The physician, standing behind him, introduces his forearms under the arms of the patient and grasps his wrists (Fig. 268). He exerts pressure with his sternum against the region to be manipulated. This constitutes the positioning. Taking up the slack is achieved by lifting the patient as the physician pushes his inflated chest forward. The important point is *not to* exert any pressure on the wrists of the patient which otherwise would cause a painful hyperflexion of the neck. The manipulation is performed by lifting the axillae of the patient with an additional thrust while the physician simultaneously increases the pressure exerted by his sternum (Fig. 269). How-

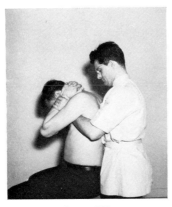

Figure 268.

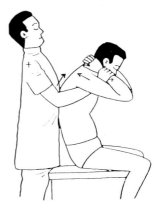

Figure 269.

ever, if this maneuver is applied without careful localization, it
will not be effective.

In Flexion: Patient in Sitting Position

The area to be manipulated corresponds to the top of the
dorsal curvature when the patient is placed in a position for
manipulation. In order to produce the necessary angulation for
this curvature at a high dorsal level, the patient has to be pulled
backwards way beyond the edge of the table (Fig. 272). On the
other hand, in order to produce a curvature at the lower segment,
the patient must bend forward (Fig. 270).

Low Dorsal Region (Figs. 270 and 271). The physician must
elicit a significant forward flexion of the spine (see the picture).
This is achieved by the maneuver described above.

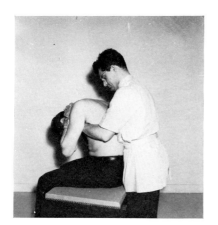

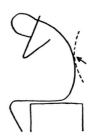

Figure 270.   Figure 271.

Upper Dorsal Region (Figs. 272 and 273). The patient must
be pulled way back beyond the table so that the physician elicits a
kyphosis at a high level. As above, the physician should not force
a flexion of the cervical spine at the terminal phase of the manipulation. Once the slack has been taken up the pressure over the
neck should remain constant.

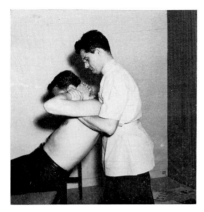

Figure 272.

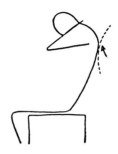

Figure 273.

In Extension

Patient in sitting position. It is by changing the position of his hands that the physician pulls the patient backwards and places the back in extension (Figs. 274 and 275). For the rest, the maneuver is performed as above.

A VARIANT OF THE POSITION OF THE HANDS (Fig. 276). This technique is very helpful in a patient with a frozen or painful shoulder. The patient is in a sitting position, his hands hanging. The physician introduces his forearms under the arms of the patient, one hand is applied behind the neck (the left in the

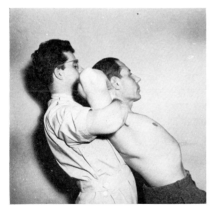

Figure 274.

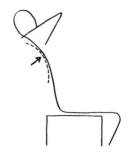

Figure. 275.

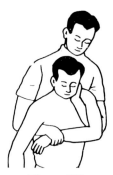

Figure 276.

picture): it is this hand which will permit the physician to achieve a desired degree of flexion. The other hand grasps the contralateral wrist of the patient. The flexion is therefore elicited by the left hand of the physician. The latter should be immobile once the slack has been taken up. The right hand serves to support the left wrist pushed against the thorax but should not exert any traction on the wrist. This technique was divised essentially for manipulations of the back in flexion to which rotation and lateral bending may be added.

In Flexion: Patient in a Supine Position *(Fig. 277)*

The patient is supine, his hands clasped behind his neck and his elbows projected forward. The physician, standing to the right of the patient, grasps the patient's elbows with his left hand. He places the thenar eminence of the other hand (the right one in

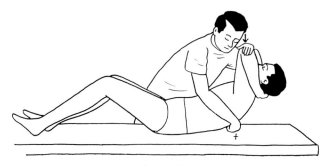

Figure 277.

the picture) at the level of the region to be manipulated, while his left hand moves the spine to the degree of flexion necessary to take up the slack in the joint under treatment (Fig. 278). After this phase has thus been accomplished, a brisk and brief thrust with the left hand directed toward the right hand effects the manipulation (Fig. 279).

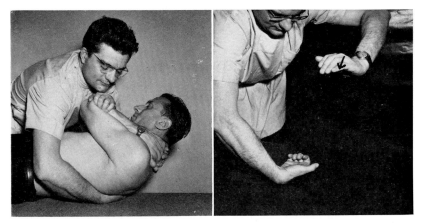

Figure 278.   Figure 279.

Diagrams 280 and 281 illustrate how the manipulation may be obtained on either upper or lower dorsal spine in flexion.

One may also change the effect of manipulation by moving the point of pressure exerted by the hand which supports the back of the patient. This pressure may be on the midline or else exerted laterally (at the level of the transverse apophysis). In the latter case, the manipulating thrust adds a movement, of left or right rotation to the vertebra under treatment, according to the locus of the application of pressure.

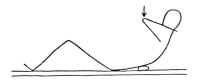

Figure 280.

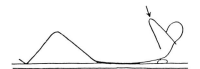

Figure 281.

A Variant of the Preceding Manipulation (Figs. 282, 283, and 284). The preceding maneuver may be modified if it is desirable to avoid stretching the neck of the patient. The patient crosses his arms over his chest. With his own thorax, the physician applies pressure (through an interposed small pillow) while his forearm and hand (left on figure 282) support the dorsal spine in the degree of necessary flexion and the counterpressure is effected as previously by the physician's right hand cupped lengthwise.

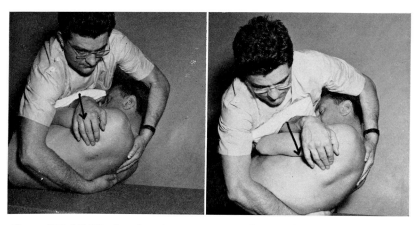

Figure 282. Middle dorsal region.   Figure 283. Low dorsal region.

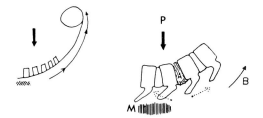

Figure 284.

P, Vertical force exerted by the chest of the operator.

B, Force in hyperflexion exerted by the arm of the operator.

M, The hand of the operator applying a counterpressure.

The result of this maneuver is hyperflexion of the joint located just above the point of counterpressure.

Knee Technique: Patient in Sitting Position

This technique permits one to effect extremely precise manipulations of the dorsal spine (Fig. 285). The patient is sitting on a stool with his hands behind his neck. The physician, standing behind him, places his knee against the region to be manipulated, then grasps the wrists of the patient by introducing his forearms under the arms of the patient.

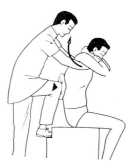

Figure 285.

In FLEXION. According to the level of manipulation, high middle or low, the operator effects the backward traction of the trunk of the patient either placed in a normal position or bent forward in such a way that the top of the resulting curvature corresponds to the manipulated point (Figs. 286 and 287). The knee of the physician exerts pressure, through a small pillow either over the spinal process or over the transverse process (in the latter case a slight rotation will be performed) of the vertebra located just below that to be manipulated. The knee *remaining immobile,* the physician takes up the slack in the region to be treated by lifting the axillas of the patient upward and toward him without using the wrists of the patient as a leverage. The manipulation consists of a simple exaggeration of this traction without exerting too much effort.

Note: The region just below the point of application of the knee may be flexed to the right or to the left as well as rotated in either direction at the time of taking up the slack. This will significantly change the effect of the maneuver.

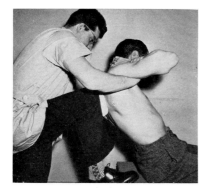

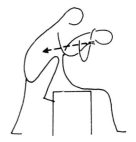

Figure 286. In Flexion: upper dorsal region.

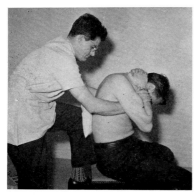

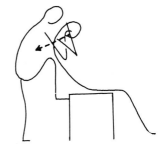

Figure 287. In Flexion: lower dorsal region.

IN EXTENSION. The same maneuver by the physician brings the back of the patient into hyperextension (Figs. 288 and 289). In order to do so, he must be very close to the patient and therefore stands bent forward on his supporting leg. In this case, the point of application should be above the point to be manipulated.

Note: In contradistinction to what one might expect or what might occur with poor execution, these remarkably precise manipulations are absolutely painless.

In Rotation: Patient in Sitting Position

The patient straddles the end of the table. The physician stands behind him. The patient clasps his hands behind his neck. The physician introducing his left arm (in the case of manipulation in left rotation) under the patient's left arm, grasps the

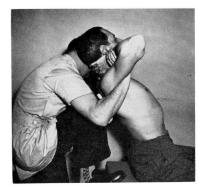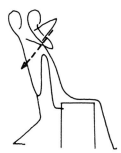

Figure 288. In extension.

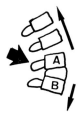

Figure 289. In extension.

right arms or right shoulder of the patient whom he rotates to the left. At the same time, he places his right thumb at the level of the transverse process of the vertebra to be manipulated. (Fig. 290).

It is known that when the spine is in an intermediate position between flexion and extension, the movement takes place essentially at the level of the lower dorsal spine. Pressure, exerted by the thumb precisely at the time of the rotation elicited by the left arm of the operator, permits one to localize very precisely the level of the manipulation directed to this region.

For the other levels of the dorsal spine, the precise localization will be favored by an additional lateral bending with the top of the curvature at the level of the point to be manipulated. In the present example, the lateroflexion will be elicited by the operator by lifting the right shoulder of the patient and depressing his *left arm* (with a continuous counterpressure with the right arm against the chest of the patient) . In order to do this, it is better that the operator introduce his arm, not under the left arm of the patient but between his arm and his forearm in the case of a mid-dorsal manipulation. In the case of the dorsal lumbar manipulation, the physician's arm should be introduced under the arm of the patient.

The movement of rotation by the shoulder of the patient has a small radius in the case of the high thoracic region (Fig. 291).

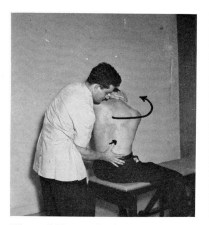 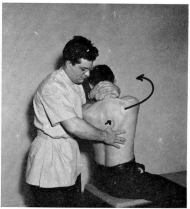

Figure 290. Manipulation in dorsal lumbar rotation.

Figure 291. Manipulation in rotation at a middorsal level.

When this radius increases, the movement attaining greater amplitude, the localization of the manipulation involves lower levels of the spine (Fig. 292).

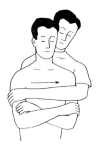 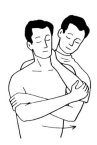 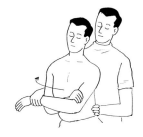

Figure 292. These diagrams show three other positions of the hands during this maneuver.

Direct Pressures

These are chiropractors' techniques:

1. Single point of pressure (Fig. 293). The point of pressure is either on the spinal process or over the region of the transverse processes. This produces a manipulation *in extension* with a slight rotation, if the pressure is lateral).

2. Bilateral points of pressure. The right hand is applied at the level of the transverse process of a vertebra on one side and the left hand against the transverse process of the other side corresponding to a vertebra located just below the preceding one (Fig. 294). One hand exerts a counterpressure while the other elicits the manipulating thrust producing rotation and extension of the corresponding intervertebral point.

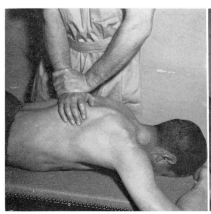
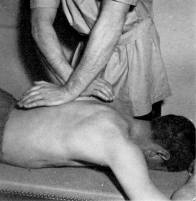

Figure 293.   Figure 294.

These techniques are well liked by the beginners or those who are not thoroughly experienced, inasmuch as they permit one to easily obtain the cracking sounds. However, they achieve mediocre results, are painful, and may be followed by complications. They cannot be evaluated in the same way as the maneuvers with long leverage which we prefer, inasmuch as the *facility* of these maneuvers using direct pressure is only apparent.

Chapter 37

Articulations of the Ribs

I<small>T MAY SEEM</small> strange that one should consider manipulations of the joints of the ribs. However, there may be blocking of the ribs which we described under the name of costal sprain, either in the costal joints or chondrocostal joints which may be responsible for acute and chronic pain (see p. 275). This may happen particularly in the dorsolumbar region with the involvement of the false ribs. The maneuvers described in a previous section may permit one to relieve this pain simply, immediately, and definitely. In addition, this kind of pain, which is often intractable without such treatment, may lead to diagnostic or therapeutic errors.

The maneuver which is illustrated in Fig. 295 permits one to correct the global costo-vertebral block, helpful in patients with respiratory insufficiency, and preliminary to all respiratory exercises.

The patient is in a supine position with hands clasped behind his neck. The physician, at his head, introduces his forearms between the arms and the forearms of the patient and grasps with

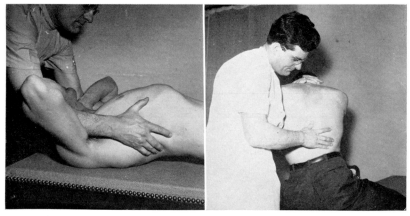

Figure 295. Maneuver of "costo-vertebral deblocking." *Left,* Posterior "costo-vertebral deblocking"; *Right,* Global "costo-vertebral deblocking."

366

each of his hands the side of the patient's chest. He asks the patient to breathe deeply and during each inspiration exerts a leverage with his forearms. This amplifies the movement of the ribs.

In another maneuver, the patient straddles a stool as in the case of manipulation of the back (see p. 353). The physician exerts pressure by applying his hand flat against the chest, at 10 cm from the midline. When he rotates the trunk of the patient, the thoracic hand increases its pressure in order to mobilize the ribs. (This maneuver repeated on each side may increase, instantaneously, the thoracic parameter by 5 to 10 cm.)

The maneuvers described below are not directed toward the rib cage as a whole but involve a single rib, the one that is blocked in poor position and which is painful; in other words exhibits a costal subluxation. These maneuvers are of both diagnostic and therapeutic value. The operator, with his thumb, index finger, or with the tips of the other fingers, hooks the lower border of the rib and pulls it upward. This maneuver is then repeated, this time by hooking the upper border and pulling it downward. One of these maneuvers will increase pain while the other is either

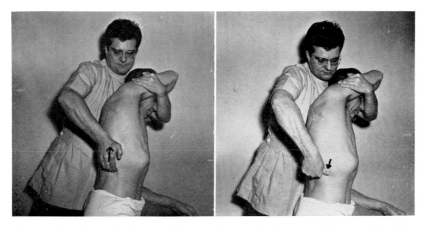

Figure 296. *First Technique:* The patient is sitting astraddle a table. The physician is behind him. The patient is in lateral bending to the side opposite to pain. The physician hooks the last rib with his finger tips and pulls upward during the end of expiration.

painless or pain relieving. It is the painless maneuver which should constitute manipulation. We call it rib maneuver.

Figure 296 shows one technique for the maneuver for the false ribs. The patient is sitting astraddle a table. The physician is behind him. The patient bends to the side opposite the painful one. The physician hooks the tips of his fingers under the lowest rib and pulls it upward when the patient is at the end of the expiratory phase (Fig. 296, left). Figure 296, right, is the same maneuver but the physician applies a downward pressure to the rib. Figure 297 shows another technique for the same maneuver.

Another maneuver designed for the same purpose is as follows:

The patient straddles the end of the table with his hands clasped behind his neck. The physician grasps the right arm of the

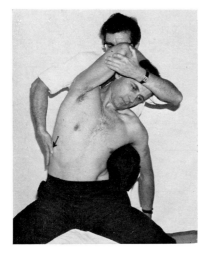
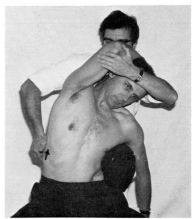

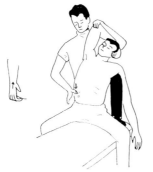

Figure 297. *Second Technique:* The patient is sitting astraddle a table or a stool. The physician places his knee (at the side of the manipulation) under the arm of the patient and pulls in maximal lateral bending. The maneuver is also exerted at the end of the expiration. (Note position of the arms.)

patient with his left hand introduced under the left arm of the patient and moves the trunk of the latter in flexion and rotation, so that the intercostal space to be acted upon becomes fully accessible. The maneuver (Fig. 298) permits one to apply upward pressure (left) or downward pressure (right) to the rib.

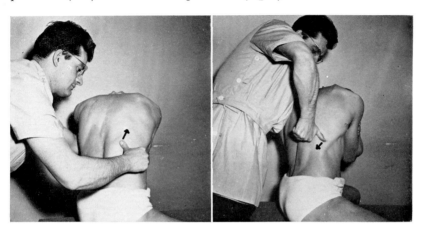

Figure 298. Maneuver with associated rotation. This maneuver is applied to lower ribs, but is also valid for midthoracic region. The patient sits astraddle a table, his hands crossed behind the neck. The physician imparts a movement of left rotation and lateral bending with his left hand if manipulation is exerted on the right side. The movement of his right hand is associated with the movement of rotation, imparting to the rib an upward pressure, either by the radial border of the right index or by the right thumb, in the same time as rotation takes place. The maneuver may be exerted in the opposite direction (pushing the rib downwards, the contact with the upper border of the rib being made by the ulnar border of the index or by the radial border of the thumb which are applied along the manipulated rib). While the left hand of the physician imparts to the trunk a global movement of left rotation, the right hand simultaneously opposes this movement and "holds" the rib, by pressing it downwards.

There are also chondrocostal "subluxations" following direct trauma or an awkward movement. These subluxations are often erroneously taken for the Tietze syndrome. They usually respond well to manipulations. The technique of the manipulation is as follows:

The patient is in a supine position. The physician, with the tips of his thumbs butted together, applies pressure on the upper or lower rib to be manipulated according to the respiratory movement present at that time (upward pressure in inspiration, downward pressure in expiration) (Figs. 299 and 300).

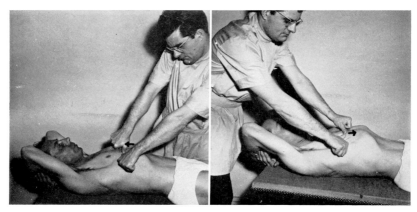

Figure 299.

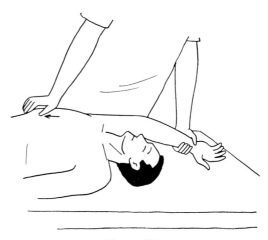

Figure 300.

Figure 301 is a variant for the manipulations of the false ribs. In certain difficult cases, this technique with the patient standing is very useful. A better precision is obtained and the lateroflexion is more complete.

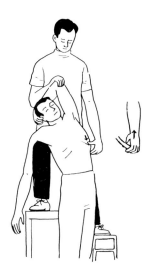

Figure 301. A variation in position for manipulation of false ribs.

Chapter 38

Lumbar Spine

MANEUVERS OF DECONTRACTION

Patient in Prone Position (Fig. 302)

WITH HIS LEFT hand the physician exerts a deep pressure downward and laterally on the lumbar muscles while the right hand applies a counterpressure on the iliac crest. This maneuver consists of alternating deep pressure and relaxation, applied slowly, rhythmically, and continuously.

Patient in Side-lying Position with Flexed Hips and Knees (Fig. 303)

In this figure the patient is in side-lying position with his hips and knees flexed. The physician stands facing him. He applies pressure with his right forearm on the iliac crest and with his left forearm on the shoulder of the patient. With his hands close together and his fingers hooked, he grasps the mass of the left paravertebral muscles. This maneuver is applied as follows: while the physician pulls the muscular mass toward him and upwards,

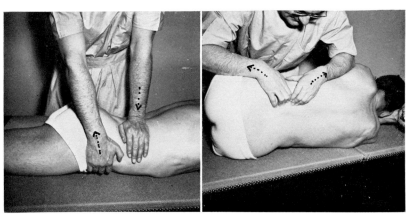

Figure 302.   Figure 303.

he spreads his elbows in a fanlike fashion, pushing both the shoulder and the iliac crest.

Patient in Supine Position (Fig. 304)

The physician sitting at the side of the patient introduces both hands under the lumbar region. He exerts traction on the mass of the lumbar muscles on that side with the tips of his fingers applied against the spinal processes. While using the leverage formed by his wrists, he also applies pressure upward with his fingers. This combined pressure-traction is maintained for some time, then released, to be renewed again. This maneuver is very sedative for acute lumbago.

Patient Supine with Hips and Knees Flexed (Fig. 305)

The physician stands at the side of the patient (to the right in this figure). He grasps both knees with his right hand, while his left hand holds the mass of the left lumbar muscles. He then pushes the knees away from him while pulling the muscles toward him. This is a slow and very rhythmic movement.

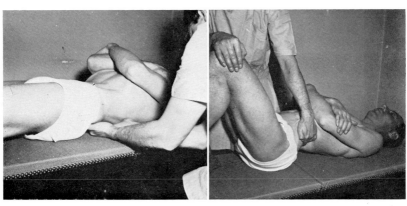

Figure 304.   Figure 305.

Patient In a Prone Position (Fig. 306)

Petrissage of the muscles of the external iliac fossa, particularly of the gluteus medius, constitutes an important phase in the treatment of low back pain and sciatica.

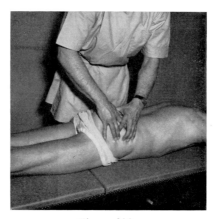

Figure 306.

MOBILIZATIONS

In Flexion

1. *The patient is in a supine position* with both hips and knees flexed (Fig. 307). The physician, exercising pressure on both knees, exaggerates this pressure in the direction of the head of the patient, thus causing lumbar hyperflexion. This maneuver is repeated slowly with increased pressure each succeeding time.

2. This again is a maneuver in flexion but here the *subject is in a side-lying position* (Fig. 308, right) his hips and knees flexed.

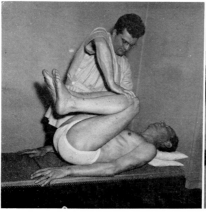
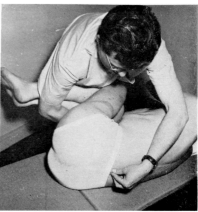

Figure 307.   Figure 308.

The physician, facing the patient, supports the legs with his right forearm while he exerts a counterpressure on the left shoulder with his left elbow. He imparts a movement toward the thorax to the knees of the patient, thus placing the lumbar spine in flexion. He controls this movement by simultaneously palpating the lumbar region with his left hand.

3. *The physician stands at the side of the patient* (right side in this example) facing the head. His left hand exerts pressure on the right shoulder of the patient while his right hand grasps the left bent knee, and pushes it toward the ipsilateral shoulder (Fig. 309). He makes alternating movements of pressure and release. This is pure mobilization in flexion. However, if the physician pushes the knee of the patient toward the contralateral shoulder, he produces a flexion-traction in rotation. The same movement is repeated with progressively increased pressure (Fig. 310). The physician may also, by exaggerating the rotation, push the knees toward himself. It is preferable in this maneuver to apply the counterpressure on the arm of the patient crossed over the chest.

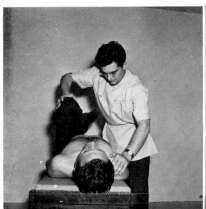 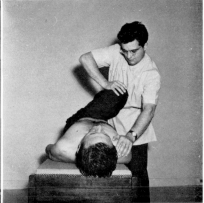

Figure 309.   Figure 310.

In Rotation (Fig. 311)

1. *The patient straddles the table* with his arms crossed over his chest. The physician, standing behind him, grasps the right arm with his left hand while his right hand applies pressure on

the lumbar paravertebral region and thus exaggerates locally the movement of rotation which is imparted to the lumbar spine by the left hand of the physician. This maneuver may be more effective if the operator braces his right elbow against his thigh. It is in this way, by rotating his pelvis to the left and forward, that he imparts to his right hand the necessary strength for mobilization. Simultaneously, he uses his left shoulder to rotate the trunk of the patient to the left.

2. *The patient is sitting on the table* with hands clasped behind his neck and elbows projected forward (Fig. 312). This figure exemplifies right rotation. The physician stands behind the patient. He introduces his right hand under the right arm of the patient and grasps the left arm. His left hand grasps the edge of the table firmly between the legs of the patient while his left forearm immobilizes the left thigh. Pulling to the right with his right hand, he rotates the lumbar region of the patient in lateroflexion and causes a movement of continuous circumduction: flexion, right rotation, etc. The degree of these different movements may be diversely applied. This is an excellent technique for the mobilization of the high lumbar region. (It may be simply transformed in a manipulative technique by taking up the slack in rotation and by briskly exaggerating the movement. However, a manipulation applied in this way lacks precision).

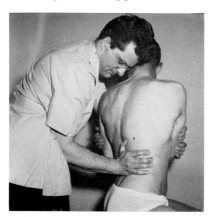

Figure 311.

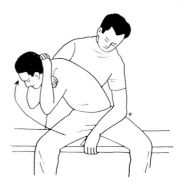

Figure 312.

In Lateroflexion

Figures 313 and 314 exemplify left lateroflexion. *The patient is in right side-lying position* with hips and knees flexed, each at 90 degrees. The physician stands to the right of the patient. With his left elbow he immobilizes the left shoulder of the patient; with his right hand he grasps the ankles of the patient and exerts pressure with the knees of the patient against his abdomen. The physician himself has his hips and knees slightly flexed. He then produces simultaneously the following: he lifts and pulls the ankles toward him while he exerts a counterpressure with his pelvis. This produces left lumbar lateroflexion. This is an excellent maneuver, but because of the power exerted, it has to be prudently executed, being repeated slowly and with progressively increased strength.

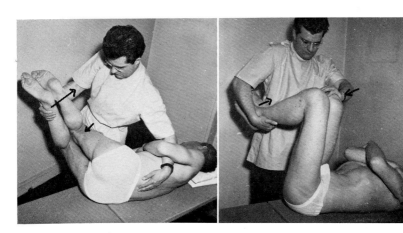

Figure 313. Figure 314.

In Extension

The patient is in a prone position (Fig. 315) with the physician standing at his side. The physician grasps the contralateral thigh near the knee and while exerting pressure over the lumbar region with his other hand, he applies sychronous movements of the elevation of the thigh and pressure over the lumbar region.

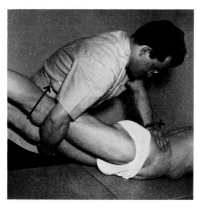

Figure 315.

MANIPULATIONS

First Group of Techniques

The patient is in the side-lying position with the physician standing at one side facing him. The physician applies pressure with one hand against the shoulder and pressure against the buttock with the other. The hand holding the shoulder remains immobile while the other hand imparts a movement of rotation to the lumbar spine. When the slack has been taken up, he briskly exaggerates the pressure which constitutes the manipulation. This is essentially the typical maneuver. In reality this way of practicing manipulation offers no precision but we will show all the possibilities offered by this basic technique.

It is evident that the effect of the maneuver will change with the position of the plane of the shoulders as related to the plane of the table, with a different degree of hip flexion, and with the posture in either kyphosis or lordosis imparted to the lumbar spine at the time of the application of the manipulating thrust. The following diagrams (Fig. 316) show how this movement varies from that in *almost pure flexion-traction* to a movement of *rotation in extension,* with possibly an *almost pure rotation* (without flexion or extension) with the possibility of having all other intermediate positions. It is certain that the maneuver which is represented in A can be used in almost every one of low back

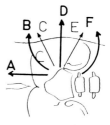

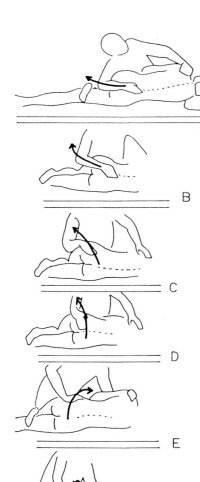

Figure 316. These diagrams show how it is possible to obtain a *different direction* of the manipulation starting with the same position (patient in a side-lying position with the upper leg flexed at the hip and at the knee). *A,* The forearm exerts pressure on the sacrum, being in the direction of the spine. This movement produces, essentially, traction in kyphosis. There is practically no rotation. There is always a slight lateral flexion upward. *B,* The pressure is exerted with the distal end of the forearm against the ischial tuberosity. This is still manipulation in *kyphosis* with a certain degree of rotation. This is the *"helicoidal traction"* of de Sèze and Thierry-Mieg (1955). *C,* Pressure is exerted in the mid-region of the buttock. There is a *significant rotation* of the lumbar spine in *slight kyphosis. D,* The same localization of the pressure but with the direction of the manipulative thrust perpendicular to the axis of the spine. There is a *very pronounced rotation* of the lumbosacral juncture in the *intermediary position* between kyphosis and lordosis. *E,* Pressure is applied against the iliac crest. This is a movement of *rotation* but with the spine in *lordosis.* The manipulation is in extension. *F,* The same localization of the pressure but the direction of the manipulating thrust is perpendicular to the axis of the spine producing a pronounced *rotation* in extension or marked lordosis.

pain or sciatica. However, this maneuver alone is not sufficient to completely correct a discogenic disturbance. The others may be adapted to particular cases according to the rules formulated previously and thus become more specific and more effective.

Among all the possibilities which we have just reviewed concerning lumbar manipulation with the technique involving the patient in a side-lying position, three are the most common. We are going to describe each of these techniques in detail. In each of these maneuvers there is always a slight lateroflexion of the spine above.

Rotation of the Spine in Flexion (in kyphosis) (Fig. 317)

This is the technique illustrated in Figure 316B and Figures 318 and 319. The patient is in right side-lying position, his head resting on a small pillow and the upper leg (left one in figure) flexed at both hip and knee. The movement is in left rotation. The physician, facing the patient, pulls the right arm toward him so that the plane of the shoulders is at a 45-degree angle to the plane of the table. He then places his left hand on the left

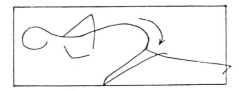

Figure 317.

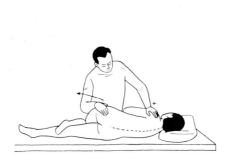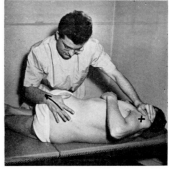

Figure 318 and Figure 319. The left hand holds the shoulder immobile.

shoulder of the patient, the hand exerting no other movement. With the distal portion of his right forearm the physician exerts pressure on the ischial tuberosity. He then exaggerates this pressure by pulling the left half of the pelvis toward him and to the right, thus producing traction in kyphosis with a slight left rotation. When the slack has been taken up, the physician stops a moment and then exaggerates the pelvic rotation by a sudden limited movement of his forearm.

Rotation of the Spine in a Position Intermediate Between Flexion and Extension (Fig. 320)

This maneuver may be performed the same as the maneuver in Figure 316 which is also represented in Figure 329. However, it may achieve the same result as the following technique (Fig. 321):

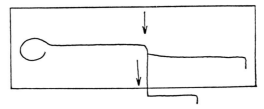

Figure 320.

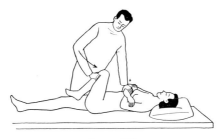

Figure 321.

The patient, supine, with his arms crossed on his abdomen, has his left leg flexed in the hip and knee. The physician, standing facing him firmly grasps the left wrist with his left hand while he holds the left leg below the knee with his hand and brings the thigh to 90 degrees flexion over the pelvis, then pulls it along a line directed *downward* (see also Fig. 322).

Rotation of Spine in Extension (lordosis) (Fig. 323)

The position of the patient very much resembles that of the maneuver for rotation in flexion. He is in a side-lying position with his lower leg extended and his upper leg flexed in both hip

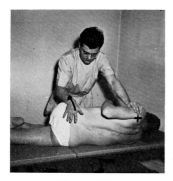

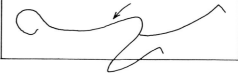

Figure 322.   Figure 323.

and knee, his head resting on a small pillow. The following maneuver, however, differs from the above maneuver. The physician still exerts pressure against the shoulder of the patient with his hand. In this technique the shoulders are perpendicular to the plane of the table; it is even possible to have the anterior aspects of the upper shoulder almost facing the plane of the table, making a sharp angle with this plane. Neither the hand which manipulates nor the forearm of the operator any longer exerts pressure against the ischial tuberosity but rather against the superior and anterior portion of the *iliac crest*. This is the essential point of this manipulation, during which the lumbar spine is no longer in kyphosis as was the case in Figure 317 but rather in *lordosis*. In other words, when the operator has positioned the patient he will make certain that the leg that is below is pulled backwards, which results in a large arc of the circle with the posterior concavity (Fig. 323), while Figure 317 illustrates the presence of a larger arc of the circle with a posterior convexity. The hand which exerts pressure against the shoulder remains immobile while the active hand exerts pressure toward the operator and downward, tangentially to the iliac crest.

Lumbar Manipulation in Rotation With the Spine Slightly Flexed

The maneuver illustrated in Figures 324 to 326 is very much like the maneuver described previously in rotation and kyphosis.

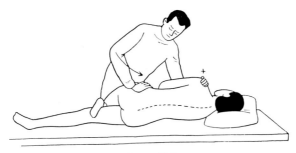

Figure 324.

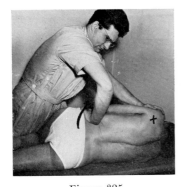

Figure 325.

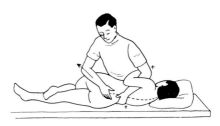

Figure 326.

But in the last Figure, the doctor no longer exerts counterpressure against the shoulder with his hand, but rather introduces his forearm under the arm of the patient.

This maneuver permits the doctor to have better control of the exact area at the level of which the rotation is effected by both hands which are able to perceive the precise point where the movement takes place when the operator takes up the slack. By changing the direction of the plane of the shoulders, the flexion of the upper thigh, and the direction of the manipulating thrust, the physician may perform this maneuver with extreme precision and efficacy.

Other Techniques

Maneuver with a Belt

The patient is in a prone position. (Fig. 327) A strong belt immobilizes his sacrum against the table. The physician is standing at the side toward which the rotation and lateroflexion are performed. (left in figure). He kneels on one knee and introduces his arm (the one closest to the head of the patient; left in the figure) under the upper part of the patient's chest in order to grasp the countralateral shoulder (right). Then with this hand he pulls the patient toward him while he asks him to place his other arm (left) on his left shoulder. The physician now supports the patient with his left arm while he applies his left shoulder against the left axilla of the patient. With his right hand he controls the lumbar movement. The physician then lateroflexes the patient by pulling him upwards. When the satisfactory degree of lateral bending is achieved, while still supporting the patient solidly with his left hand, the physician progressively increases the pressure with his left shoulder forward, thus eliciting a trunk rotation of the patient localized mostly in the lumbar sacral region. After slack has been taken up, a slight additional push with his left shoulder will complete the manipulation.

Warning. Never force the patient in lordosis. This very powerful movement may be dangerous. This type of manipulation should not be practiced by beginners. The slightest fault makes the manipulation extremely dangerous in view of the powerful leverage involved in this maneuver.

A very interesting variant of this technique, which allows one to minimize the lordosis, consists in applying the belt to the end of the table with the lower extremities extending beyond the table (P. Piedallu, 1947). The patient then has a much less pronounced lordosis.

Manipulation with the Knees

IN EXTENSION. The patient is sitting on a stool with his hands clasped behind his neck. The physician sits behind him on a slightly higher stool. He grasps the wrists of the patient with his forearms under the arms of the patient. He then presses both knees against the sacrum or slightly above, according to the area he intends to manipulate. He pulls the trunk of the patient in extension toward him, then lifts his forearms while continuing to pull the trunk which takes up the slack of the lumbar spine. A brisk, though slight exaggeration of this movement, with the knees exerting a counterpressure, accomplishes the manipulation (Fig. 328).

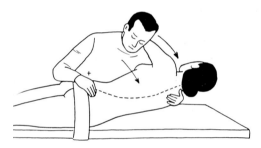

Figure 327.

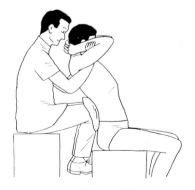

Figure 328.

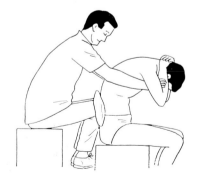

Figure 329.

IN FLEXION. Instead of pulling the shoulders of the patient toward him, the physician bends his trunk with a resulting kyphosis of the lumbar spine; it is necessary that the patient bends far enough forward to create a rounded back (Fig. 329). The knees apply counterpressure just below the joint to be manipulated. The physician takes up the slack by lifting the shoulders of the patient while maintaining them at a distance. The manipulation consists of a brief exaggeration of this movement by pulling the forearms upward and toward the physician.

Manipulation in Extension

The patient is in a prone position (Fig. 330), the physician standing against the middle of the table at the side of the patient toward which the rotation and lateroflexion are to be performed. With one hand the physician holds the thigh above the knee while the thumb of the other hand exerts pressure at the level of the transverse process of the vertebra under consideration. The physician pulls the thigh toward him in order to obtain lateroflexion which spreads the intervertebral spaces on the opposite side. He also exerts traction upward to extend the spine. The manipulation may be performed either by a direct pressure of the thumb following a correct positioning and taking up the slack of the spine, or with the thumb remaining immobile but briskly exaggerating the extension (resisted manipulation).

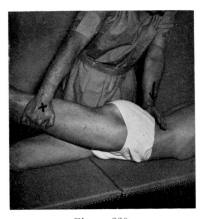

Figure 330.

In Rotation

The patient is astraddle the table. This technique permits one to realize all possible movements: flexion, extension, rotation, and lateroflexion in a precise manner. Its only drawback is the inability to achieve sufficient segmental traction. It may be used for both mobilization and manipulation. It permits one to manipulate either globally or precisely by either assisted or resisted maneuvers. It is moreover, as we saw, an excellent position for the examination and evaluation of lumbar movements, offering the possibility of detecting the slightest limitation of the range of motion and revealing tender points. The patient straddles the end of the table with his hands clasped behind his neck, or as in Figure 331, one hand behind the neck and the other grasping the

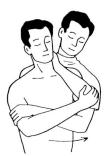

Figure 331.

elbow. The operator introduces his forearm under the arm of the patient and grasps the countralateral arm, while the other hand is placed against the lumbar spine at the level of the area to be manipulated (Fig. 335). The physician is then free to place the patient either in extension or flexion. He may bend him to the right or to the left or rotate him to the left if it is the left arm of the physician which is in front of the patient, or to the right if it is his right arm. The figures show examples of these different possibilities. Here, just as before, the combinations of different movements must place the point to be manipulated on top of the curvature produced by the maneuver (Figs. 332, 333, and 334). The best application of this technique is the case of assisted

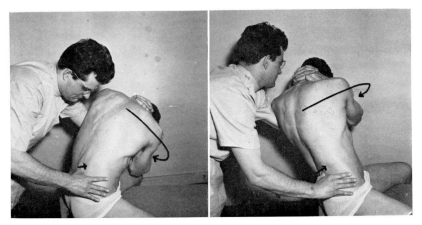

Figure 332.   Figure 333.

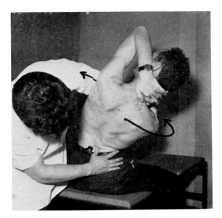

Figure 334.

manipulations. The general direction and the gross localization of the manipulation are determined by the hand of the patient which holds the shoulder. It is therefore by this arm that the positioning and taking up the slack are achieved. Finally a slight and brisk exaggeration of this movement will be responsible for the manipulation which will be assisted and localized very precisely by the thumb or the hyperthenar eminence of the lumbar hand of the physician.

Resisted Manipulation

In the case of the high lumbar spine, the following maneuver permits one to perform resisted manipulations: the lumbar hand now exerts counterpressure. For example, the forward hand of the physician produces the right rotation of the patient's trunk while with his left hand he applies counter pressure against the right transverse process of the vertebra just below the joint to be manipulated in right rotation (Fig. 335).

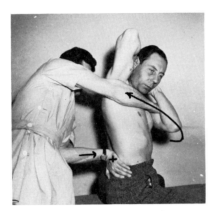

Figure 335.

Chapter 39

Sacro-iliac Manipulation Maneuvers

I T IS IMPOSSIBLE to speak of manipulations without saying a word about "sacro-iliac subluxations." The osteopaths first, followed by specialists in physical medicine and orthopedic surgery in England, discussed the sacroiliac subluxations (strain) responsible for low-back pain, acute lumbagos, and even sciaticas. It was mostly Mennell (1949) who focused attention on this sacro-iliac strain and described several signs of this condition.

In France, it was Pascal Piédallu (1947, 1952) who emphasized this condition. Let us sum up the essential arguments:

1. The sacro-iliac is a mobile articulation. This is true more or less according to different morphological types (Delmas, 1950); however, it is very mobile in pregnant women.

2. This joint may be blocked on one side in "nutation" or in contranutation (Mennell, 1949) (see p. 109) (for Piedallu, 1952, only the pinching in nutation may persist).

3. This block in one of the extreme positions may be responsible for (a) lumbosacral pains and (b) sciatica due to the play of muscular contractions. Piedallu does not believe that these "direct" sciaticas exist. According to this author the sacro-iliac block, in most cases is the origin of the dysfunction of the lumbosacral system which generates discal fatigue and discogenic diseases, thus facilitating the genesis of sciaticas and low-back pain.

Mennell specifically describes the following signs of the sacro-iliac strain:

1. The patient is in a sitting position; posterior and superior iliac spine is below the one on the opposite side if the iliac bone is blocked in posterior rotation over the sacrum. This situation is corrected following successful manipulation. This sign was described by the osteopaths.

2. Mennell describes an antalgic attitude in what he calls an acute sacro-iliac strain which is a direct antalgic attitude.

3. In the presence of sciatica the Lasègue is intensified by dorsiflexion of the foot if sciatica is of a discogenic nature. However, it is not the case in sacro-iliac strain.

4. For Mennell (1949) the contralateral Lasègue is in favor of a sacro-iliac strain. According to him, straight leg raising on the normal side produces, at the end, the movement of the sacrum and then increases the sacro-iliac strain on the other side.

5. Finally lateroflexion is not painful in either direction (with the exception of very acute strain) while this maneuver is not tolerated by the patient in discal protrusion.

6. In the case of sciatica, obviously the trunk of the nerve is affected.

For Piédallu the principal signs of the sacro-iliac block are as follows:

1. Superior and posterior iliac spine is lowered in a patient sitting on a hard surface. This is also true in a patient standing but this may be due to a true shortening of the leg on that side.

2. However, if one asks the patient to bend his trunk forward in either sitting or standing position, the superior and posterior iliac spine ascends more on the involved side than on the normal side so that the spine on the noninvolved side may be lower than the other at the end of the forward bending. This may be explained by the block and by the contractions which maintain the sacrum rigidly attached to the iliac bone on the involved side, a condition which does not exist on the normal side where there is a certain degree of free play.

3. A frequent incidence of a false shortening of the leg on the same side. Radiologically the legs are of equal length but clinically one appears to be shorter than the other. A successful manipulation instantaneously suppresses all these signs.

These are the principal signs described by the proponents of the "sacro-iliac block." We are not going to discuss these important but unsolved problems in detail.

What are we to conclude from all this?

1. The discovery of the above described signs suggest the usefulness of the *specific maneuvers* which we are going to describe.

2. A successful maneuver suppresses the above described signs and symptoms which are not reduced by other maneuvers.

3. These signs appear in a certain distorted fashion in some low-back pain or sciatica of pregnant women near term in whom the sacro-iliac points are particularly mobile. This appears to us as the best argument in favor of the existence of the sacro-iliac strain although even this argument is not a definitive one.

The above signs, when present, suggest certain maneuvers which may suppress them, together with the associated symptoms. Does it mean then that the sacro-iliac strain exists? It is quite plausible but there is no absolute proof, since these maneuvers are the same as those which when conducted according to our rule of no pain, may reduce certain sciaticas of true radicular and discal origin.

SO-CALLED SACRO-ILIAC MANIPULATION

Some of these manipulations were described by us among the manipulations of lumbosacral juncture. They are aimed at rotating the iliac bone either forward (most frequently) or backward (very seldom).

1. *A technique for two operators.*

a) Patient is in side-lying position (Fig. 336). Operator number one places his hand against the anterior portion of the iliac crest and the other against the ischial tuberosity. Both hands exert a pressure aimed at rotating the iliac bone forward (most frequently). Operator number two pulls the leg briskly in a

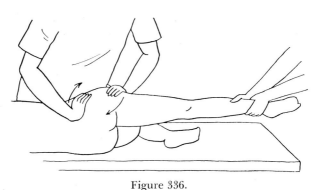

Figure 336.

slightly elevated position while operator number one firmly maintains his pressure.

b) The same maneuver but operator number one rotates the iliac bone backwards (Fig. 337) .

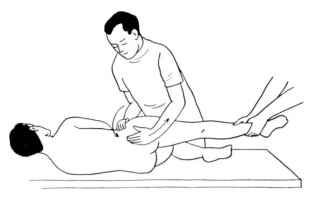

Figure 337.

2. The maneuver which we described as a lumbar manipulation in extension (p. 383) may be considered as a maneuver of the sacro-iliac joint having for its goal the forward rotation of the iliac bone (Fig. 338) .

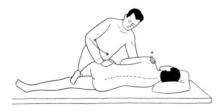

Figure 338.

3. *Patient in Sims Position* (Fig. 339) . The operator exerts pressure against the iliac crest aiming at rotating it forward while with the other hand he supports the knee of the upper leg by pulling it upward and backward.

4. *Patient in prone position* (on a very low table) (Fig. 340). The physician is standing at the side of the patient (contralateral

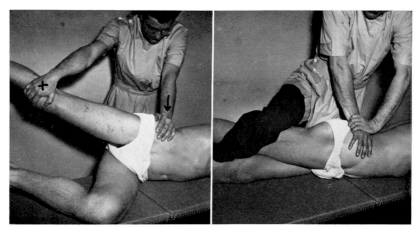

Figure 339.   Figure 340.

to the manipulating one, left in this figure). He is supported by
his left leg while the right leg maintains the right leg of the patient above the table while both hands apply pressure over the
iliac bone in order to rotate it forward.

Bibliography

Alajouanine, T. *La douleur et les douleurs.* Masson, Paris, 1957.

Alajouanine, T., and Nick, J. L'algie occipitale d'origine psychique ou syndrome d'Atlas. *Sem Hop Paris, 25:*852, 1949.

Alajouanine, T., Castaigne, P., Cambier, J., and Liantonokis, E. Le role des positions anormales et prolongées de la tete et du cou dans le determinisme de certains accidents vasculaires du tronc cerebral. *Bull Soc Med Hop Paris, 74:*1, 1958.

Alajouanine, T., and Petit-Dutallis, D. Compression de la queue de cheval pa une tumeur du disque intervertebral; operation, guerison; presentation du malade. *Bull Soc Int Chir, 54:*1452, 1928.

Alajouanine, T., and Petit-Dutaillis, D. Le nodule fibrocartilagineux de la face posterieure des disques intervertebraux. Etude clinique et therapeutique d'une variete nouvelle de compression radiculo-medullraie extradurale. *Presse Med, 38:*1749, 1930.

Arlet J., LaPorte, C., and Toussaint, J. Les dorsalgies benignes de l'adulte. *Rhumatologie, 4:*139, 1952.

Arlet, J. Les dorsalgies benignes de l'adulte. *Rev Rhum, 21:*303, 1954.

Aubry, M. Les troubles labyrinthiques dans les traumatismes craniens et cranio-cervicaux. *Concours Med, 12:*7109, 1964.

Baastrup, C. L. Proc. Spin. Vert. Lumb. und einige zwischen diesen liegende Gelenkbildungen mit pathologischen Prozessen in dieser Region. *Fortschr Roentgenstr, 48:*430, 1933.

Balland, Grozelier. La gymnastique corrective. Amedee Legrand, Paris, 1952.

Barbizet, J. *Comment traiter les nevralgies.* Flammarion, Paris, 1957.

Barbizet, J. Les accidents nerveux des manipulations du rachis cervical. *Rev Prat Paris, 19:*2235, 1958.

Barbor, R. A treatment for chronic low back pain. In *Comptes rendus du 4th Congress International de Med. Phys.* Excerpta Medica, Ansterdam. 1966, pp. 661-664.

Barcelo, P., and Vilaseca, J. M. Clinica y radiologia de las afecciones degenerativas de las pequenas articulationes vertebrales. In *Contemporary Rheumatology* Elsevier, Amsterdam, 1956, p. 218.

Barre, J. and Lieou. Syndrome sympathique cervical posterieur. *Paris Med, 15:*266, 1925.

Barre, J. Sur un syndrome sympathique cervical posterieur et sa cause frequente: l'arthrite cervicale. *Rev Neurol, 1:*1246, 1926.

Bartelink, D. L. The role of abnormal pressure in relieving the pressure on the lumbar intervertebral discs. *J Bone Joint Surg, 38-B:*718-725, 1957.

Bartschi-Rochaix, W. Troubles encephaliques apres des lesions meconnues de la colonne cervicale: "la migraine cervicale." *Paris Med, 37*:178, 1947.

Bartschi-Rochaix, W. La migraine cervicale traumatique et ses rapports avec le S.S.C.P. *Rev Otoneuroophtal, 19*:16, 1947.

Beal, M. C. A review of short leg problem. *J Amer Osteopath Ass, 49* (Oct), 1950.

Beal, M. C., and Beckwith, G. C. Studies of vertebral motion. *J Amer Osteopath Ass, 63*:319, 1963.

Belin du Coteau, M. Les coudes du tennis. *Rev Path Comparee Hygiene Generale,* (Nov.) N. 470, 1935.

Benassy, J., and Wolinetz, E. Quadriplegie apres manoeuvre de chiropraxie. *Rev Rhum, 24*:555, 1957.

Blanc, C. Electroencephalographie et syndrome subjectif des traumatises cervico-craniens. *Concours Med, 12*:7117, 1964.

Bloch, J., and Fischer, F. K. L'enraidissement de l'epaule. Documenta Geigy, No. 15, J. R. Geigy, Basle, 1958.

Bonduelle, M. Les acroparesthesies. *Gaz Med France, 55*:233, 1948.

Boudin, G., *et al.* Syndrome grave du tronc cerebral apres manipulations cervicales. *Bull Soc Med Hop Paris, 73*:562, 1957.

Braaf, M. M., and Rosner, S. Meniere-like syndrome following whiplash injury of the neck. *J Trauma, 2*:494, 1962.

Bradford, F. K., and Spurling, R. G. *The Intervertebral Disc.* Thomas, Springfield, 1945.

Brain, W. R., Northfield, D., and Wilkinson, M. The neurological manifestations of cervical spondylosis. *Brain, 75*:187, 1952.

Bret, A. J., and Bardiau, M. Les algies de la colonne dorsale au niveau de D4 et D7 au cours des syndromes gynecologiques attribues a l'hyperfolliculinie. *Gynec Obstet, 50*:85, 1951.

Brocher, J. E. W. Maladie de Scheuermann. *Rev Rhum, 15*:181, 1948.

Broscol, M., and Claessens, M. Les lesions tramatiques des parties molles de l'epaule. *Acta Orthop Belg, 2*:97, 1957.

Brugger, A. Les syndromes vertebraux radiculaires et pseudoradiculaires. Documenta Geigy, Basle, 1961.

Buck, C. A., Dameron, F. B., Dow, M. J., and Skowlund, H. V. Study on normal range of motion in the neck utilizing a bubble goniometer. *Arch Phys Med, 40*:390, 1959.

Burke, G. L. *Backache from Occiput to Coccyx.* W.E.G. MacDonald, Vancouver, 1964.

Cailliet, R. *Neck and Arm Pain.* Blackwell, Oxford, 1964.

Camprell, A. M. C., and Phillips, D. G. Cervical disc lesion with neurological disorder. *Brit Med J, 5197*:481, 1960.

Carp, L. Tennis elbow (epicondylitis) caused by radiohumeral bursitis; anatomic, clinical, roentgenologic and pathologic aspects with suggestions as to treatment. *Arch Surg, 24*:905, 1932.

Cecile, J. P., Laine, E., Riff, G., and Waghemacker, R. L'angiographie vertebrale. (3ᵉ Journees d'Etudes et de Perfectionnement des Manipulations Vertebrales) . In *Ann Med Phys, 9, 3:*250, 1966.

Chapuis-Phankim, M. L'arthrographie dans la periarthrite scapulohumerale.
Thesis, Paris, 1957.

Chrisman, O. D., Mittnacht, A., and Snook, G. A. A study of the results
following rotating manipulation in the lumbar intervertebral disc syndrome. *J Bone Joint Surg, 4A:*517, 1964.

Claessens, H., and Anciaux-Ruysen, A. L'arthrographie de l'epaule. *Acta
Orthop Belg,* 3-4, 289, 1956.

Cloward, R. B. The clinical significance of the sinu-vertebral nerve of the
cervical spine in relation to the cervical disc syndrome. *J Neurol Neurosurg Psychiat, 23:*321, 1960.

Codman, E. A. *The Shoulder.* Todd, Boston, 1934.

Colachis, S. C., Worden, R. E., Bechtol, C. O., and Strohm, B. R. Movement of the sacroiliac joint in the adult male: a preliminary report.
Arch Phys Med Rehab, 44, 9, 490, 1963.

Copeman. *Textbook of the Rheumatic Diseases.* Livingstone, Edinburgh,
1953, pp. 14-38.

Coste, F., Cayla, J., Verspyck, R., and Vallee, G. L'arthrographie de l'epaule
en rhumatologie. In *Compte-rendu du IXeme Congres International de
Rhumatologie.* Toronto, 1957, p. 312.

Cyriax, J. Rheumatism and soft tissue injuries. Hamish Hamilton, London,
1960.

Cyriax, J. Lumbago mechanism of dural pain. *Lancet, 1:*427, 1945.

Cyriax, J. Pros and cons of manipulation. *Lancet, 1:*571, 1964.

Debeyre, J., de Sèze, S., and Patte, D. Une nouvelle technique chirurgicale
de reparation des ruptures de la coiffe musculotendineuse de l'epaule.
*Rev Rhum, 29:*303, 1962.

Dechaume, J., Antonietti, C., Bouvier, A., and Duroux, P. Sympathique et
arthroses cervicales. Documents anatomiques. *J Med Lyon,* 493, 1961.

Dechaume, J., Duroux, P., and Antonietti, C. Alterations topographiques
de la chaine sympathique dite "latero-vertebrale" dans les arthroses et
discopathies de la colonne lombosacree. *J Med Lyon,* 769, 1959.

Decroix, G., Waghemacker, R., Nicolas, G., Massol, P., and Grailles, M. A.
L'electronystagmographie et la cupulometrie, moyen objectif d'evaluation semeiologique et de controle d'efficacite des manipulations vertebrales dans le syndrome de l'artere vertebrale. *Ann Med Phys, 8:*3, 1965.

Degenring, F. W. Die Bedeuturg der Muskerlketten fur das zervikobrachiale
Syndrom und seine Analyse. *Med Welt, 17:*1915, 1966.

Delmas, A. Fonction sacro-iliaque et statique du corps. *Rev Rhum, 17:*475,
1950.

Denis, A. Contribution a l'etude du role du tendon du long biceps dans
le syndrome douloureux de l'epaule. Thesis, Paris, 1952.

De Palma, A. F. *Degenerative Changes in the Sternoclavicular and Acromioclavicular Joints in Various Decades.* Thomas, Springfield, 1957.

Depoorter, A. E. Indications et contraindications des manipulations vertebrales. In *Comptes-rendus du 4ᵉ Congres International de Medecine Physique. Excerpta Medica.* Amsterdam, 1966, pp. 150-155.

De Sèze, S. *Algies vertebrales d'origine statique.* Expansion Scientifique, Paris, 1951.

De Sèze, S. La sciatique dite banale, essentielle ou rhumatismale et le disque lombo-sacre. *Rev Rhum, 6:*986, 1939.

De Sèze, S. Reflexions sur le probleme pathogenique de la sciatique dite "essentielle" (a propos de 3 cas chirurgicalement verifies de sciatique par hernie discale posterieure lombaire). *Presse Med, 49:*222, 1941.

De Sèze, S. *Huit entretiens sur le role du disque intervertebral dans les syndromes douloureux de la charniere lombo-sacre.* Expansion Scientifique, Paris, 1953.

De Sèze, S. Les attitudes antalgiques dans la sciatique discoradiculaire commune. *Sem Hop Paris, 39:*2291, 1955.

De Sèze, S. Les manipulations vertebrales. *Sem Hop Paris, 39:*2313, 1955.

De Sèze, S. Le syndrome douloureux vertebral tropho-statique de la postmenopause. *Ann Med Phys 2, 1:*1, 1959.

De Sèze, S. *Breviaire de rhumatologie a l'usage du praticien,* 2nd ed. Expansion Scientifique, Paris, 1961.

De Sèze, S. *et al. Aux confins de la rhumatologie.* Expansion Scientifique, Paris, 1962.

De Sèze, S., Debeyre, A., and Godlewski, S. Recherches anatomiques sur les rapports osteoarticulaires des racines cervicales inferieures dans le canal rachidien et dans les canaux de conjugaison. *Rev Rhum, 16:*89, 1949.

De Sèze, S. Djian, A., and Abdelmoula, M. Etude radiologique de la dynamique cervicale dans le plan sagittal; une contribution radio-physiologique à l'etude pathogenique des arthroses cervicales. *Rev Rhum, 18:*111, 1951.

De Sèze, S., Godlewski, S., and Barbizet. Le probleme des cephalees d'origine cervicale. *Rev Prat (Paris), 2:*20, 1952.

De Sèze, S., Kahn, M. F., Thierry-Mieg, J., and Renoult, C. Les accidents des manipulations vertebrales. In *L'actualite rhumatologique.* Expansion Scientifique, Paris, 1966.

De Sèze, S., and Ryckewert, A. *Maladie des os et des articulations.* Flammarion. Paris, 1954.

De Sèze, S., Ryckewaert, A., and Welfling, J. Les lesions anatomiques de l'epaule senile. Rapport au Congres Europeen des Maladies Rhumatismales. Istanbul, Sept., 1959.

De Sèze, S., Robin, J., and Levernieux, J. Vertebrotherapie par manipulation et vertebrotherapie par traction. *Rev Rhum, 15:*337, 1948.

De Sèze, S., and Thierry-Mieg, J. Les manipulations vertebrales, *Rev Rhum, 22:*9, 1955.

De Sèze, S., and Welfing, J. Interpretation et interet du signe de Lasegue dans les sciatiques avec attitude antalgique laterale. *Sem Hop Paris, 33:* 1013, 1957.

Dittrich, R. J. Radiohumeral bursitis (tennis elbow). Report of two cases. *Amer J Surg, 7:*411, 1929.

Dreyfus, P., and Phankim-Koupernik, M. Les acroparesthesies nocturnes *Rev Prat (Paris), 14:*3247-3254, 1964.

Dreyfus, P., and Levernieux, J. Les hernies discales dorsales. In *L"actualite rhumatologique.* Expansion Scientifique, Paris, 1966.

Eshougues, R. J., Ferrand, J., Barsotti, J., and Smadja, A. Lombalgies pures et hernie discale à la lumiere de la radiculographie lombo-sacree. *Algerie Med, 64:*353, 1960.

Etiles, E. C. Backache and sciatica in the army. *J Roy Army Med Corps, 3:*151, 1948.

Falconer, M. A., McGeorge, M., and Begg, A. G. Observations on the cause and mechanism of symptom-production in sciatica and low back pain. *J Neurol Neurosurg Psychiat, 11:*13, 1948.

Feld, M. Subluxations et entorses sous-occipitales, leur syndrome fonctionnel consecutif aux traumatismes craniens. *Sem Hop Paris, 31:*1952, 1954.

Ferrand, J., d'Eshougues, R., and Barsotti, J. *La radiculographie lombo-sacree par substance iodee hydrosoluble et resorbale.* Expansion Scientifique Paris, 1961.

Fielding, W. Normal and selected abnormal motion of the cervical spine from the second to the seventh cervical vertebra based on cineroentgenography. *J Bone Joint Surg, 46A:*1779, 1964.

Fischer, E. D. Report of a case of ruptured intervertebral disc following chiropractic manipulation. *Kentucky Med J, 41:*14, 1943.

Florent, J., and Gillot, C. Elements d'anatomie fonctionnelle du rachis cervical. 3e Journees d'Etude et de Perfectionnement des Manipulations Vertebrales. In *Ann Med Phys, 9:*206, 1966.

Ford, R. F., and Clark, D. Thrombosis of the basilar artery with softenings in the cerebellum and brain stem due to manipulation of the neck. *Johns Hopkins Hosp Bull, 98:*37, 1956.

Freudenberg, G. H. Contribution a l'etude du blocage des apophyses articulaires de la charniere lombo-sacree. Thesis, Paris, 1956.

Froment, R., Gonin, A., and Bruel, P. Les angors intriques. *J Med Lyon, 32:*1017, 1951.

Frykholm, R. Deformities of dural pouches and strictures of dural sheaths in the cervical region producing nerve-root compression. *J Neurosurg, 4:*403, 1947.

Frykholm, R. J. Cervical nerve root compression resulting from disc degeneration and root sleeve fibrosis. *Acta Chir Scand,* Suppl. 160, 1951.

Galmiche, P., and Lenormand, C. Les cephalees d'origine cervicale poster-ieure. *Vie Med*, 80-83, 1951.

Godlewski, S. Les anomalies congenitales de la jonction craniorachidienne. 3e Journees d'Etude et de Perfectionnement des Manipulations Verte-brales. In *Ann Med Phys*, 9:224, 1966.

Godlewski, S., and Dry, J. *Les anomalies congenitales de la charniere cervico-occipitale*. Expansion Scientifique, Paris, 1964.

Goldthwait, J. E. The lombosacral articulation. An explanation of many cases of lumbagos, sciaticas, and paraplegias. *Boston Med Surg J, 174:* 365, 1911.

Goldthwait, J. E., and Osgood, R. B. Considerations of the pelvic articula-tions from an anatomical, pathological and clinical standpoint. *Boston Med Surg J,* May 25 and June 2, 1905.

Good, M. G. Die primare rolle der muskulatur in der pathogenese der rheu-matischen kraukheit und die therapeutische losung des rheumaproblems. *Med Klin, 13:*450, 1957.

Granit, R., Leksell, L., and Skoglund, C. R. Fibre interaction in injured or compressed region of nerve. *Brain, 67:*125, 1944.

Grossiord, A. Les accidents neurologiques des manipulations. 3e Journees d'Etude et de Perfectionnement des Manipulations Vertebrales. In *Ann Med Phys*, 9:283, 1966.

Guilleminet, M., and Stagnara, P. Role de l'entorse vertebrale dans les rachialgies. *Presse Med*, 60:274, 1952.

Hackett, G. S. *Ligament and Tendon Relaxation Treated by Prololo-therapy*. Thomas, Springfield, 1956.

Harris, R. I., and MacNab, J. Structural changes in lumbar intervertebral discs. *J Bone Joint Surg, 368:*304, 1954.

Held, J. P. Les atteintes de l'axe cerebro-spinal au cours des traumatismes cervicaux mineurs. *Ann Med Phys*, 8:13, 1965.

Held, J. P. Pieges et dangers des manipulations cervicales en neurologie. 3e Journees d'Etude et de Perfectionnement des Manipulations Verte-brales. In *Ann Med Phys*, 9:251, 1966.

Herbert, J. J. Lombalgies, etude mecanique: traitements orthopediques et chirurgicaux. *Rhumatologie*, 5:295, 1953.

Herbert, J. J., and Fenies, M. T. Syndrome de la queue de chaeval et trac-tions vertebrales. *Rev Rhum*, 26:299, 1959.

Holt, E. P. Fallacy of cervical discography. *JAMA, 188:*799, 1964.

Hovelacque, A. *Anatomie des nerfs rachidiens et du systeme grand sympa-thique*. Doin, Paris, 1927.

Hubault, A. Les manifestations neurologiques des cervicarthroses. *Vie Med, 43:*187-200, 1962.

Ingelrans, P., and Oberthur, H. Les arthrites sacroiliaques non tuberculeuses. *Paris Med, 40:*1, 1950.

Inman, V. T., Saunders, M., and Abbot, L. C. Observation on the function of the shoulder joint. *J Bone Joint Surg, 26:1,* 1944.

Isemein, L., and Perdrix, L. Les cephalees d'origine cervicale. Leur traitement physique. *Ann Med Phys, 3:13,* 1960.

Isemein, L., and Ramis, J. Le Syndrome sympathique cervical posterieur en rhumatologie. *Rev Rhum, 24:183,* 1957.

Jacquemart, M., and Piedallu, P. Le torticolis "congenital" est il simplement un torticolis obstetrical? *Concours Med, 86:4867,* 1964.

Jung, A., and Brunschwig, A. Recherche histologique sur l'innervation des articulations des corps vertebraux. *Press Med, 40:316,* 1932.

Junghanns, H. Pathologie der Wirbelsaule. In *Henke-Lubarsch: Handbuch der speziellen pathologischen Anatomie und Histologie.* Berlin, 1939, Tome IX, vol. 4, pp. 280-284.

Junghanns, H. Erkennung und Behandlung vertebragener Krankheiten. *Med Klin,* 208-213, 252-256, 1958.

Junghanns, H. Die insufficientia intervertebralis und ihre Behandlungsmoglichkeiten. In *Beitrage zur manuellen Therapie.* Hippocrates Verlag, Stuttgart, 1959.

Junghanns, H. Die patho-physiologischen Grundlagen fur die manuelle Wirbelsaulentherapie. In *Comptes-rendus du 4eme Congres International de Medecine Physique.* Excerpta Medica, Amsterdam, 1966, pp. 141-144.

Keegan, J. J. Diagnosis of herniation of lumbar intervertebral discs by neurological signs. *JAMA, 126:868,* 1944.

Keegan, J. J. Dermatome hypalgesia with posterolateral herniation of lower cervical intervertebral disc. *J Neurosurg, 4:115,* 1947.

Kellgren, J. H. On the distribution of pain arising from deep somatic structures with charts of segmental pain areas. *Clin Sci,* 35-46, 1939.

Kessel, A. W. Arthrography of the shoulder joint. *Proc Roy Soc Med, 17:* 418, 1950.

Keyes, D. C. and Compere, E. L. The normal and pathological physiology of the nucleus pulposus of the intervertebral disc; anatomical, clinical and experimental study. *J Bone Joint Surg, 14:897,* 1932.

Klapp, B. *Das klappische kriechverfahren.* G. Thieme, Stuttgart, 1955.

Kleyn, A de, and Nieuwenhuyse, P. Schwindelanfalb und nystagmus bei einer bestimmten. Stellung des Koptes. *Acta Otolaryng (Stockholm), 11:* 155, 1927.

Kohlrausch, W. *Massage des zones reflexes dans la musculature et dans le tissu conjonctif.* Masson, Paris, 1961.

Kottke, F. J., and Mundale, M. O. Range of mobility of the cervical spine. *Arch Phys Med, 40:379,* 1959.

Koupernik, C. Colloque sur le syndrome subjectif des traumatismes cervicocraniens. Introduction. *Concours Med, 12:7097,* 1964.

Krayenbuhl, H., and Klingler, M. Zur diagnose und differential diagnose der lumbalen diskushernien. *Verh. Deutsch Ges Inn Med, 55:137,* 1949.

Kuhlendahl, H. Uber die beziehungen zwischen anatomischer und funktioneller lasion der lumbalen zwischenwirbelscheiben und den klinischen erscheinungsbilden der kreuzschmerzen und ischialgien. *Artzl Wschr, 5:* 281, 1950.

Lacapere, J. Rhumatismes et syndromes radiculaires douloureux. *Rev Rhum, 20:*1, 1933.

Lacapere, J. Nevralgie cervico-brachiale. *Sem Hop Paris, 26:*2685, 1950.

Lacapere, J. Rhumatisme vertebral et degenerescence discale. *Rhumatologie, 6:*99, 1954.

Lacapere, J., and Maigne, R. Presentation d'un serre-tete pour tractions cervicales. *Rev. Rhum, 25:*299, 1957.

Lacapere, J., and Souplet, P. Les dorsalgies fonctionnelles. *Readaptation, 64:*17, 1959.

Lapresle, J. Nevralgies dorsales et lombaires. *Sem Hop Paris, 55:*1690, 1950.

Lazorthes, G. *Le systeme neuro-musculaire.* Masson, Paris, 1941.

Lazorthes, G. *Le systeme nerveux peripherique.* Masson, Paris, 1955.

Lazorthes, G. La vascularisation de la moelle epiniere. *Rev Neurol, 106:*535, 1962.

Lazorthes, G. Le rachis cervical. Donnees anatomiques et physiologiques recentes. 3e Journees d'Etude et de Perfectionnement des manipulations vertebrales. In *Ann Med Phys,* 9, *3:*193, 1966.

Lazorthes, G., Despeyrou, L., and Juskiewenski, S. Les branches posterieures des nerfs rachidiens et la medecine physique. *Ann Med Phys,* 8, *1:*67, 1965.

Lazorthes, G., and Poulhes. Etudes sur les nerfs sinu vertebraux lombaires. *C. R. Assoc. Anatomistes,* 317, 1947.

Leca, A. Le traitement des lombalgies et des lombo-sciatiques par les manipulations vertebrales. Thesis, Paris, 1950.

Le Corre, F., and Maigne, R. L'entorse des dernieres cotes. Son traitement par manipulation. In Comptes-rendus du 4eme Congres International de Medecine Physique. Excerpta Medica, Amsterdam, 1966, pp. 173-174.

Le Go, P., Maigne, R., and Toumit, R. Le traitement des lombalgies et des sciatiques aigues en medecine physique. *Informations Med. S.N.C.F.,* 60, 47, 1956.

Le Goaer, M. Interet du traitement sclerosant de Hackett dans les hyperlaxites ligamentaires vertebrales et sacro-iliaques post-traumatiques. *Ann Med Phys, 3:*162, 1960.

Leriche, R. Effets de l'anesthesie à la novocaine des ligaments et des insertions tendineuses periarticulaires dans certaines maladies articulaires. *Gaz Hop, 103:*1294, 1930.

Lescure, R. Etude critique d'un traitement par manipulation dans les algies d'origine rachidienne. Thesis, Paris, 1951.

Lescure, R. Incidents, accidents, contre-indications des manipulations de la colonne vertebrale. *Med Hyg Geneve, 12:*456, 1954.

Lescure, R. Le pseudo-asthme infantile par insuffisance respiratoire mecanique. Ses caracteristiques et sa reeducation. *Ann Med Phys, 1:*57, 1959.

Lescure, R. Physiologie vertebrale du cou. *Rhumatologie, 4:*167, 1959.

Lecure, R. Reponses a quelques questions concernant les tractions et manipulations des syndromes cervicaux. *Med Hyg, Geneve, 17:*761, 1959.

Lescure, R., and Maigne, R. Commentaires sur les effects d'un traitement par manipulations dans une premiere serie de lombalgies. *Rhumatologie, 6:*398, 1953.

Lescure, R., and Renoult, C. Manipulations articulaires à longue echeance en reeducation. In *Comptes-rendus du 4ᵉ Congres International de Medecine Physilgue. Excerpta* Medica, Amsterdam, 1966, p. 166.

Lescure, R., and Thierry-Mieg, J. Manipulations des arthroses vertebrales et leurs effets therapeutiques; tentative d'explication basee sur certaines deformations nucleaires et la distribution harmonieuse des mouvements segmentaires. In *Contemporary Rheumatology.* Elsevier, New York, 1956, p. 323.

Lescure, R., Trepsat, P., and Waghemacker, R. Sur les possibilites des traitements par manipulations dans la therapeutique des rhumatismes. *Rhumatologie, 2:*71, 1953.

Levernieux, J. *Les tractions vertebrales.* Expansion scientifique, Paris, 1961.

Lewis, T., and Kellgren, J. H. Observations relating to referred pain, viscero-motor reflexes and other associated phenomena. *Clin Sci, 4:*47, 1939.

Lewis, T. *Pain.* MacMillan, New York, 1942.

Licht, S. *Massage, Manipulation and Traction,* Elizabeth Licht, New Haven, Conn., 1960.

Lieou, Yong Choen. Syndrome sympathique cervical posterieur et arthrite chronique de la colonne cervicale: etude clinique et radiologique. Thesis, Strasbourg, 1928.

Lievre, J. A. Paraplegie due aux manoeuvres d'un chiropractor. *Rev Rhum, 20:*708, 1953.

Lievre, J. A. Paraplegie due aux manoeuvres d'un osteopathe. *Rev Rhum, 20:*707, 1953.

Lindblom, K., and Palmer, L. Arthrography and Roentgenography on ruptures of the tendons of the shoulder joint. *Acta Radiol, 20:*548, 1939.

Lovett. *Lateral Curvature of the Spine and Round Shoulders.* Bilkeston Beard and Co., Philadelphia, 1907.

Luschka, H. Die nerven des menschlichen wirbelkanals. H. Laupp, Tubingen, 1850.

MacConnail, M. A. Mechanical anatomy of motion and posture. In *Therapeutic Exercise.* Elizabeth Licht, New Haven, Conn., 1958.

Maigne, R. Manipulations vertebrales et manipulateurs. *Sem Hop Paris, 29:*1944, 1953.

Maigne, R. Les manipulations vertebrales: indications, contreindications, techniques et resultats. *J Med Paris, 11:*405, 1955.

Maigne, R. Les entorses costales. *Rhumatologie, 9:*35, 1957.

Maigne, R. Le traitement des epicondylites. *Rhumatologie, 9:*293, 1957.

Maigne, R. Epicondylalgies, rachis cervical et articulation radiohumerale. *Ann Med Phys, 3:*299, 1960.

Maigne, R. Dorsalgies, sequelles des traumatismes cervicaux mineurs. Communication au 3e Congres de Therapie Manuelle, Nice, 1962.

Maigne, R. *Les Manipulations Vertebrales.* Expansion Scientifique. Paris, 1960.

Maigne, R. Le massage dans les sciatiques. Comm. Congres Nat. de Medecine Physique, Nice, 1961.

Maigne, R. La dorsalgie benigne interscapulaire. Son origine cervicale frequente. *Rhumatologie, 14:*457, 1964.

Maigne, R. The concept of painlessness and opposite motion in spinal manipulations. *Amer J Phys Med, 44:*55, 1965.

Maigne, R. Sur l'origine cervicale de certaines dorsalgies benignes et rebelles de l'adulte. *Rev Rhum, 31:*497, 1964.

Maigne, R. L'application rationnelle des manipulations vertebrales. In *Proc. of the IVth International Congress of Physical Medicine.* Exerpta Medica, Amsterdam, 1966, pp. 145-159.

Maigne, R. Le choix des manipulations dans le traitement des sciatiques. *Rev Rhum, 32:*366, 1965.

Maigne, R. La mobilisation passive de la region lombaire. In *Journees de Reeducation.* Expansion Scientifique, Paris, 1965.

Maigne, R. Une doctrine pour les traitements par manipulations: la regle de la non-douleur et la regle du mouvement contraire. *Ann Med Phys, 8:*37, 1965.

Maigne, R. Une forme frequente de dorsalgie commune de l'adulte; l'algie interscapulovertebrale. Son origine cervicale. Diagnostic et traitement. *Maroc Med, 47:*73, 1967.

Maigne, R. A propos du mecanisme de la douleur dans les dorsalgies dites des "couturieres". Le point interscapulo-vertebral. *Rev Rhum, 34:*636, 1967.

Maigne, R. La douleur musculaire dans les sciatiques. *Ann Med Phys, 1:*45, 1969.

Maigne, R., and LeCorre, F. L'algie interscapulo-vertebrale. Forme frequente de dorsalgie benigne. Son origine cervicale. *Ann Med Phys, 7:*1, 1964.

Maigne, R., Lescure, R., Renoult, C., and Waghemacker, R. Une fiche d'identite pratique des manipulations vertebrales. *Ann Med Phys, 4:*47, 1965.

Maitland, G. D. Lumbar manipulation: does it do harm? A five year follow-up survey. *Med J Austr, 11:*546, 1961.

Maitland, G. D. *Vertebral Manipulation.* Butterworths, London, 1964.

Maitrepierre, M. J. Les manipulations vertebrales. *Rev Lyon Med,* 1959, pp. 1111-1118.

Mennell, J. B. *The Science and Art of Joint Manipulation.* Vol. 1: *The Extremities.* Vol 2: *The Spinal Column.* J. A. Churchill, London, 1949.

Mennell, J. M. *Joint Pain.* J. A. Churchill, London, 1964.

Mennell, J. M. Assessment of residual symptoms from a "whiplash" injury. In *Comptes-rendus du 4e Congres International de Medecine Physique.* Excerpta Media, Amsterdam, 1966, pp. 528-529.

Michelsen, J. J., and Mixter, W. J. Pain and disability of shoulder and arms due to herniation of the nucleus pulposus of cervical intervertebral disks. *New Eng J Med, 231,* 1944.

Mills, G. P. Treatment of tennis elbow. *Brit Med J, 2:212,* 1937.

Mitchell, P. E., Hendry, N. G., and Billewica, W. Z. Chemical background of intervertebral disc prolapse. *J Bone Joint Surg, 41B:237,* 1961.

Morris, J. M., Lucas, D. B., and Bresler, B. The role of the trunk in the stability of the spine. *J Bone Joint Surg, 43A:327,* 1961.

Mostini, G. Les manipulations vertebrales en rhumatologie. *Ann Med Phys, 3:219,* 1960.

Moure, M. Jr. Radiohumeral synovitis. *Arch Surg, 64:501,* 1952.

Nachlas, L. W. Pseudo-angina pectoris originating in the cervical spine. *JAMA, 323,* 1934.

Oger, J. Les accidents des manipulations vertebrales. *J Belge Med Phys Rhum, 19:2,* 1964.

Olivier, G., and Olivier, C. *Mecanique articulaire.* Vigot, Paris, 1963.

Osgood, R. B. Radiohumeral bursitis, epicondylitis, epicondylalgie (tennis elbow). *Arch Surg, 4:420,* 1922.

Peillon, M. Traitement des maladies de la charniere lombo-sacree par le mouvement. *Ann Med Phys, 1:18,* 1958.

Peillon, M. Cinesitherapie de la region cervicale. *Ann Med Phys, 2:213,* 1959.

Piedallu, P. *L'osteopathie, ses rapports avec la gymnastique analytique.* Biere, Bordeaux, 1947.

Piedallu, P. *Problemes sacro-iliaques.* Homme sain. No. 2, Biere, Bordeaux, 1952.

Putti, W. New conception in the pathogenesis of sciatic pain. *Lancet, 53:* 213, 1927.

Rageot, E. Les accidents et incidents des manipulations vertebrales. In *C. R. du IX Congres Int. de Med. Phys.* Exerpta Medica, Amsterdam, 1966, pp. 170-172.

Rageot, E., Maigne, R., and Nataf. Les troubles dits sympathiques du membre superieur: Maladie de Raynaud et algo-neurodystrophie reflexe et leurs rapports avec le syndrome du canal carpien. *Angeiologie, 6:5,* 1968.

Raney, A. A. Post-traumatic headache. *Bull Los Angeles Neurol Soc, 16:209,* 1951.

Raney, A. A., and Raney, R. B. Headache: a common symptom of cervical disk lesions. *Arch Neurol Psychiat (Chicago), 59:603,* 1948.

Raney, A. A., Raney, R. B., and Hunter, C. R. Chronic post-traumatic headache and the syndrome of cervical disc lesion following head trauma. *J Neurosurg, 6:*458, 1949.

Raou, R. J. P. *Recherches sur la mobilite vertebrale en fonction des types rachidiens.* Thesis, Paris, 1952.

Ravault, P. P., and Vignon, G. Les manipulations vertebrales dans le traitement des lombalgies, des sciatiques et des nevralgies cervico-brachiales. *Lyon Med, 39:*193, 1950.

Ravault, P. P., and Vignon, G. *Rhumatologie Clinique.* Masson, Paris, 1956.

Reich, N. E., and Fremont, R. E. *Chest Pain. Systematic Differentiation and Treatment.* MacMillan, New York, 1961.

Renoult, C. Epicondylalgie, epicondylite, epicondylose ou coude du tennis. Thesis, Paris, 1951.

Renoult, C. Le tennis elbow. *Rev Rhum, 21:*593, 1954.

Renoult, C. Les manipulations: Acte medical de reeducation. In *Journees de Reeducation.* Expansion Scientifique, Paris, 1965.

Renoult, M. *La coccygodynie, algie statique.* Thesis, Paris, 1962.

Ricard, A., Girard, P. F., and Dupasquier, P. *Les discopathies cervicales.* Dugas, Lyon, 1948.

Riederer, J., and Rettig, H. Beobachtungen eines akuten Basedow nach chiropraktischer Behandung der Habswirbelsaule. *Med Klin, 50:*1911, 1955.

Rieunau, G. Indications et pieges de la Medecine physique. *Ann Med Phys, 4:*201, 1961.

Rieunau, G. Pieges et dangers des manipulations vertebrales en orthopedie. 3e Journees d'Etude et de Perfectionnement des Manipulations Vertebrales. In *Ann Med Phys, 9:*260, 1966.

Rissanen, P. M. Comparison of pathologic changes in intervertebral discs and intervertebral ligaments of the lumbar spine in the light of autopsy. *Acta Orthop Scand, 34:*54, 1964.

Roge, R. Donnees pratiques concernant les cephalees d'origine neuro-chirurgicale. *Vie Med,* 749-761, 1964.

Roofe, P. G. Innervation of annulus fibrosus and posterior longitudinal ligament. *Arch Neurol Psychiat (Chicago), 44:*100, 1940.

Rotes-Querol, J. Anatomie, physiologie et radiologie des articulations sacro-iliaques. *Rhumatologie, 6:*284, 1954.

Roth, W. K. *Meralgia paraesthetica.* S. Karger, Berlin, 1895.

Roud. *Mecanismes des articulations et des muscles de l'Homme.* Lausanne, 1913.

Rouviere, H. *Anatomie humaine.* (3 vol.). Masson, Paris, 1943.

Rubens-Duval, A. Activites et mefaits des chiropractors. *Rev Rhum, 25:*438, 1958.

Saidman, *Les maladies de la colonne vertebrale.* (2 vol.). Doin, Paris, 1950.

Sardina, J. A propos du syndrome d'insuffisance dorsale douloureuse; sur la valeur d'un facteur constitutionnel. Thesis, Paris, 1959.

Schmincke, A., and Santo, E. Zur normalen pathologischen anatomie der jalswirbelsaule. *Zbl Allg Path Anat, 55:*369, 1932.

Schmorl, G., and Junghanns, H. *Clinique et radiologie de la colonne vertebrale normale et pathologique.* Doin, Paris, 1965.

Schwartz, G. A., Geiger, J. K., and Sapno, A. V. Posterior inferior cerebellar artery Sd. of Wallenberg after chiropractic manipulation. *Arch Intern Med, 3:*352, 1956.

Seligmann, F. Les sequelles affectives des traumatismes craniens et leurs eventuels rapports avec des alterations electroencephalographiques. *Rev Neuropsychiat Infant, 13:*517, 1965.

Serre, H., and Simon, L. Les limites de l'arthrose de la charniere cervico-occipitale. *Ann Med Phys, 7:*19, 1964.

Serre, H., Simon, L., Claustre, J., and Serre, J. C. Le syndrome du canal carpien: ses incidences dans la pathologie du membre superieur. *Ann Med Phys, 8, 4:*347-365, 1965.

Simon, L. Pieges et dangers des manipulations cervicales en rhumatologie. 3e Journees d'Etude. et de Perfectionnement des Manipulations Vertebrales. In *Ann Med Phys, 9, 3:*272, 1966.

Soum, P. Un test pathogenique dans les syndromes cervicarthrosiques. *Vie Med, 43:*232, 1962.

Souplet, P., and Boulet-Gercourt, J. Dorsalgies organiques et dorsalgies fonctionnelles. *Gaz Med Franc, 69:*2517, 1962.

Spurling, R. G. *Lesions of Lumbar Intervertebral Discs.* Thomas, Springfield, 1953.

Stack, J. K. and Hunt, W. S. Radiohumeral synovitis. *Quart Bull Northwestern Univ. Med School, 20:*394, 1946.

Still, A. T. *Philosophy of Osteopathy.* A. T. Still, Kirksville, Mo., 1899.

Sureau, C. Notions nouvelles sur l'anatomie et la physiologie de l'articulation sacro-iliaque. *Presse Med, 67:*947, 1959.

Taillard, W. *Les spondylolisthesis.* Masson, Paris, 1957.

Taptas, J. N. *Maux de tete et nevralgies, douleurs cranio-faciales.* Masson, Paris, 1953.

Tatlow, W. F. T., and Bammer, H. G. Syndrome of vertebral artery compression. *Neurology, 7:*331, 1957.

Tavernier. Algies rachidiennes par apophysite epineuse. *Lyon Chir,* 1949.

Terrier, J. C. *Manipulation, Massage.* Hippocrates Verlag, Stuttgart, 1958.

Terrier, J. C. Les bases de la therapeutique manipulative de la colonne vertebrale. *Med et Hyg, 17:*390, 1959.

Testut, L. *Traite d'anatomie humaine.* (5 vol.) Doin, Paris, 1929.

Testut, L., and Latarjet, A. *Traite d'anatomie humaine.* (1 vol.) Doin, Paris, 1931.

Thierry-Mieg, J. Interet de la physiotherapie manipulative dans les algies faciales. *Ann Med Phys, 2:*52, 1959.

Thierry-Mieg, J. Indications, mode d'action et resultats des manipulations dans le traitement des nevralgies cervicobrachiales. In *Entretiens de Bichat.* (vol. Therapeutique). Expansion Scientifique, Paris, 1963.

Thierry-Mieg, J. Resultats des manipulations vertebrales dans le traitement de la periarthrite scapulo-humerale. In *Comptes Rendus du 4e Congres International de Med. Physique.* Excerpta Medica, Amsterdam, 1966, p. 665.

Thierry-Mieg, J. Technique des manipulations vertebrales utilisees dans le traitement des cruralgies discales. Indications, contreindications et accidents. *Sem Hop Paris, 43:*401, 1967.

Timbrell-Fischer, A. G. *Treatment by manipulation.* H. K. Lewis, London, 1944.

Tiry, A. Etude radio-anatomique sur les articulations posterieures du rachis cervical dans leur rapport avec l'artere et les nerfs vertebraux. Thesis, Lille, 1957.

Tomlinson, K. M. Purpura following manipulation of the spine. *Brit Med J,* no. 4224, 1260, 1955.

Töndury, G. Uber den ramus meningiecus nervi spinalis. *Priaxis, 26:*3, 1937.

Töndury, G. Le developpement de la colonne vertebrale. *Rev Chir Orthop, 39:*553, 1953.

Toole, J. F. The influence of head position upon flow through the vertebral and internal carotid artery, a post-mortem study. *Arch Neurol, 3:*3, 1960.

Toussaint. Les dorsalgies benignes de l'adulte. Thesis, Toulouse, 1951.

Travell, J. Referred pain from skeletal muscles; the pectoralis major syndrome of breast pain and soreness and the sternomastoid syndrome of headache and dizziness. *NY State J Med, 55:*331, 1955.

Troisier, O. Les paresses musculaires des membres inferieurs dans les compressions radiculaire discales. *Ann Med Phys, 2:*21, 1959.

Troisier, O. Remarques sur la physiologie du sus-epineux. *Ann Med Phys, 3:*37, 1960.

Troisier, O. *Traitement non chirurgical des lesions des disques intervertebraux.* Masson, Paris, 1962.

Troisier, O. Douleurs rachidiennes d'origine ligamentaire. In *Comptes-rendus du 4e Congres International de Med. Physique. Exerpta Medica,* Amsterdam, 1966, pp. 659-669.

Waghemacker, R. La methode de Klapp dans les scolioses. In *Journees de Reeducation 1959.* Expansion Scientifique, Paris, 1959.

Waghemacker, R. "Sciatiques Paralysantes." Etude pathogenique. *Ann Chir, 4:*1573, 1961.

Waghemacker, R. Les bases physiologiques des manipulations vertebrales. Reunion Internationale de Medecine Physique et Rehabilitation. Turin, 1961. *Minerva Fisioterapica, 7:* (Suppl. 4) 21-24, 1962.

Waghemacker, R. Controle de l'efficacite des manipulations vertebrales dans le syndrome de l'artere vertebrale par l'electronystagmographie et la cupulometrie. *Ann Med Phys, 8:3,* 1965.

Waghemacker, R. Applications nouvelles de la cinesitherapie grace aux progres de la cinesiologie. *Ann Med Phys, 8:51,* 1965.

Waghemacker, R., Cecile, J. P., Bonte, G., and Decoulx, P. Arthrographie de l'epaule. Indications, technique et resultats. *J Radiologie Electrol, 44:* 337, 1963.

Waghemacker, R., Cecile, J. P., and Buise, A. Dissociation du syndrome periarthrite de l'epaule grace aux renseignements fournis par l'arthrographie: les consequences au point de vue reeducation. *Ann Med Phys, 6:1,* 1963.

Waghemacker, R. Lasselin, and Bertin, J. Douleurs vertebrales, syndrome radiculaires associes et medecine psychosomatique. *Rev Rhum, 9:*693, 1955.

Waghemacker, R., Lasselin, and Bertin, J. "PSH" rebelles et Medecine Psycho-somatique. *Rhumatologie, 5:*184, 1955.

Walsh, A., Nombouts, R. and Petit, Y. L. Funicalgies rachidiennes dépendant des lésions discales. *Acta Orthop Belg, 4:*105-180, 1949.

Wattebled, R. Les acroparesthesies des membres superieurs. *Vie Med, 45:* 1549, 1964.

Weiser, H. I. Early manipulative treatment of acute back pain following accidents in hospital personnel. In *Comptes-rendus du 4° Congres International de Med. Physique,* Excerpta Medica, Amsterdam, 1966, p. 163.

Weisl, H. Les mouvements de l'articulation sacroiliaque. *Acta Anatomica, 2-3* (No.1) 80-91, 1954.

Welfling, J., de Sèze, S., and Tellier, M. L'epaule bloquee et sa reeducation. *Ann Med Phys, 6:*114, 1963.

Wiberg, G. Back pain in relation to the nerve supply of the intervertebral disc. *Acta Orthop Scand, 19:*211, 1949.

Wilson, J. N. ,and Ilfeld, F. W. Manipulation dans la hernie du disque intervertebral. *Amer J Surg, 83:*173, 1952.

Wolinetz, E. Sur six cas de thrombose du tronc basilaire. *Sem Hop Paris, 27:*1305, 1963.

Name Index

411

Subject Index

415